The Hands-on Guide to Clinical Reasoning in Medicine

The Hands-on Guide to Clinical Reasoning in Medicine

Mujammil Irfan

MBBS, MRCP(UK), MSc Medical Education
SCE Respiratory Medicine
Consultant Respiratory Physician
Copenhagen, Denmark

WILEY Blackwell

Registered Office(s)
John Wiley & Sons, Inc., 111 River Street, Hoboken, NJ 07030, USA
John Wiley & Sons Ltd, The Atrium, Southern Gate, Chichester, West Sussex, PO19 8SQ, UK

Editorial Office
9600 Garsington Road, Oxford, OX4 2DQ, UK

For details of our global editorial offices, customer services, and more information about Wiley products visit us at www.wiley.com.

Wiley also publishes its books in a variety of electronic formats and by print-on-demand. Some content that appears in standard print versions of this book may not be available in other formats.

Library of Congress Cataloging-in-Publication Data

Names: Irfan, Mujammil, author.
Title: The hands-on guide to clinical reasoning in medicine / Mujammil Irfan.
Other titles: Clinical reasoning in medicine
Description: Hoboken, NJ : John Wiley & Sons, 2019. | Includes bibliographical references and index. |
Identifiers: LCCN 2018027395 (print) | LCCN 2018027969 (ebook) | ISBN 9781119244073 (Adobe PDF) | ISBN 9781119244004 (ePub) | ISBN 9781119244035 (pbk.)
Subjects: | MESH: Physical Examination–methods | Medical History Taking–methods | Clinical Decision-Making | Clinical Competence
Classification: LCC RC76 (ebook) | LCC RC76 (print) | NLM WB 200 | DDC 616.07/51–dc23
LC record available at https://lccn.loc.gov/2018027395

Cover Design: Wiley
Cover Images: © jhorrocks/Getty Images; © Andrew Brookes/Getty Images;
© Thomas Northcut/Getty Images; © Hero Images/Getty Images; © fStop/Getty Images

Set in 8.5/10.5pt TimesNewRoman by SPi Global, Pondicherry, India

Printed in Singapore by C.O.S. Printers Pte Ltd

10 9 8 7 6 5 4 3 2 1

Dedicated to my grand-parents
Syed Maqboolullah Sha Khadri
Zahedunnisa
Noorunnisa Begum

Contents

Foreword

Teaching Clinical Medicine is both an art and a science. In its simplest form it has several components: history taking or gathering information relevant to the patient's problem, clinical methods, or how to examine the patient, differential diagnosis, or what is the most likely condition affecting the patient, and, a management plan or what investigations one should undertake and what treatment to start. Arguably, history taking and clinical examination are two of the easiest to teach. One could even use tick-boxes for history and examination to teach and assess the students. The most difficult component of clinical medicine is teaching the art and science of arriving at a diagnosis and formulating an appropriate action plan, in other words, Clinical Reasoning.

Clinical experience and analytical thinking are both extremely important in making an accurate diagnosis but not yet available or developed in a medical student. Furthermore, uncertainties and complexities of clinical medicine make reliance on experience wholly inadequate. A more structured approach is required both by the teacher and by the student to employ clinical reasoning at every step of the process of making a diagnosis.

This book explores, with practical examples, the process of learning through reasoning. It enables the student (and his teacher) to approach the patient with an open mind. It helps him to collect relevant information, both positive and negative, whilst at the same time critically evaluating its relevance to clinical diagnosis.

Dr. Irfan has long had an interest in teaching and this book is, but one example of his commitment to teaching medical students. He should be commended for approaching this difficult aspect of clinical teaching in a unique and conversational way, using medical students, and, with complex medical scenarios that get resolved through critical analysis and reasoning. I would have carried this book and the accompanying booklet with me both as a final MB student and as a house officer. These new and exciting methods in clinical teaching enable one's mind to think so the eyes can see.

Dr B S Dwarak Sastry OBE
DL FRCPI FRCP

Preface

All through medical school we are taught to find one diagnosis that fits the clinical picture. We are taught to decipher clinical information in black and white, and investigate and initiate treatments evidenced by randomised controlled trials. We are trained to move in a linear fashion from data collection (history taking, clinical examination, investigations) to diagnosis, treatment, and prognosis. Armed with this knowledge and practice we start as doctors in the real world and quickly feel insecure in the face of uncertainty.

The real world as we know it is a bit more unforgiving! Clinicians are faced with incomplete data, uncertain circumstances; and difficult diagnostic, investigational, and therapeutic decisions on a daily basis. A pure subjective stance favouring astute clinicians who rely heavily on their past experience in solving the present diagnostic problem can be fatally flawed. Enter evidence based medicine (EBM) which aims to take away all that subjectivity and usher in the era of objective science based on statistical analyses and clinical practice rooted in guidelines and protocols. There is however a glitch: several clinical problems have no evidence, and when there is some it can be insufficient or even conflicting. Hence, rigid adherence to guidelines in these settings can lead to uncomfortable outcomes as at the end of the day we are dealing with people, not numbers (Sniderman et al. 2013).

Through the course of this book I shall aim to sow the seeds of a 'thinking doctor.' One who not only heeds best practice evidence and follows evidence based guidelines, but also remains attuned to human communication. One who knows where each of these attributes is to be used. For, you will soon be exposed to vague symptoms, complex histories and complex disease presentations. Circumstances where protocols and guidelines do not venture, where there are no randomised controlled trials that show you that 'a' is better than 'b.' Yet you are expected to give this person sitting in front of you an answer as to what is wrong with him or her and suggest a solution, all with an ever dwindling commodity in modern medicine, called time. Medicine is an inexact science. We have to learn to be comfortable with uncertainty.

Clinical reasoning is not only tested in all your exams including objective structured clinical examinations (OSCEs) but will be constantly tested throughout your careers as clinicians. You will eventually develop into a unique practicing clinician who will have their own world view, with all its accompanying fallacies and quirks. So long as you remember to consciously develop yourself every step of the way you are unlikely to go wrong and heaven forbid help someone who is ill!

I have used a unique conversational style in this book utilizing two imaginary students and addressing the reader directly. My humble attempt at teaching clinical reasoning is not the only way to learn this art. There will be many who will not agree with everything that I say and that is the beauty of clinical reasoning in medicine where dissent with dogma is the key to progress. The thrill of solving a clinical dilemma is unmatched. I would like you to enjoy every moment of it and thrive in those grey areas where few dare to tread!

Sniderman, A.D., LaChapelle, K.J., Rachon, N.A. et al. 2013. The necessity for clinical reasoning in the era of evidence-based medicine. *Mayo Clinic Proceedings* 88(10), pp. 1108–1114.

Acknowledgements

I would like to thank John Wiley & Sons Limited and their editorial team for publishing this book and for their patience and forbearing. I am grateful for the help of Jonathan Ayling-Smith, Foundation Year Doctor, Glan Clwyd Hospital and Emily Murphy, Medical Student at Cardiff University for providing invaluable insight into what the students would want to see in such a book. I thank the countless patients that I have encountered in my clinical practice who have provided me with the experience to write this book and all the reviewers for their valuable input in reviewing the accuracy of the content. Last but not the least I would like to thank my wife Leila for having endured the vagaries of book writing and assisting in revising the book.

Reviewers

Cardiology
Dr Andy Wai Tze Jong BMedSci, MBChB, MRCP (UK)
Cardiology Specialty Registrar
West of Scotland Deanery

Nephrology
Dr Aled G. Lewis, MD FRCP
Consultant Nephrologist
Glan Clwyd Hospital, BCULHB

Endocrinology
Dr Stephen Wong
Consultant Endocrinologist
Diabetes & Renal Centre
Glan Clwyd Hospital, BCUHB

Neurology
Dr Tom Hughes FRCP MD
Consultant Neurologist
Clinical Director (Medical Neurosciences)
University Hospital of Wales
Heath Park, Cardiff

Geriatric Medicine
Dr Hamsaraj Shetty BSc, MBBS, FRCP
(London & Edinburgh)
Consultant Physician with an interest in Stroke Medicine
University Hospital of Wales, Cardiff

Gastroenterology
Dr Laith AlRubaiy MRCP(UK), PhD
Clinical Lecturer
Swansea University School of Medicine
Dr. Lavanya Shenbagaraj MBBS MRCP (UK)
Specialty Registrar in Gastroenterology
University Hospital of Wales, Cardiff

Rheumatology
Dr Anurag Negi MBBS, MD, FRCP (London), CCT
(rheumatology)
Consultant Rheumatologist
University Hospital of Wales, Cardiff

Dr Julian Nash BSc, MB Bch, PhD, FRCP
Consultant Rheumatologist
Morriston Hospital, Swansea

Abbreviations

A&E	Accident and emergency unit	DIP	Distal interphalangeal joint
A-a	Alveolar-arterial gradient	DKA	Diabetic ketoacidosis
ABG	Arterial blood gas	DM	Diabetes mellitus
ACEi	Angiotensin converting enzyme inhibitor	DNAR	Do not attempt resuscitation
ACPA	Anti-citrullinated protein antigen	DVT	Deep vein thrombosis
ACR	Albumin-creatinine ratio	EBM	Evidence based medicine
ACS	Acute coronary syndrome	EBV	Epstein Barr virus
ACTH	Adreno-corticotropin hormone	ECF	Extracellular fluid
ADH	Anti-diuretic hormone	ECG	Electrocardiogram
ADL	Activities of daily living	EF	Ejection fraction
AF	Atrial fibrillation	eGFR	Estimated glomerular filtration rate
AG	Anion gap	EMG	Electromyogram
AIN	Acute interstitial nephritis	ESR	Erythrocyte sedimentation rate
AKI	Acute kidney injury	ESRD	End-stage renal disease
ALP	Alkaline phosphatase	ET	Exercise tolerance
ALS	Advanced life support	GBS	Guillain Barre syndrome
ALT	Alanine transferase	GCA	Giant cell arteritis
AMT	Abbreviated mental test	GCS	Glasgow coma scale
ANA	Antinuclear antibody	GERD	Gastro-esophageal reflux
ANCA	Anti-nuclear cytoplasmic antibody	GGT	Gamma glutamyl transpeptidase
APKD	Adult onset polycystic kidney disease	GIB	Gastrointestinal bleed
APTT	Anti-prothrombin clotting time	GI	Gastrointestinal
ARB	Angiotensin receptor blocker	GN	Glomerulonephritis
ARDS	Acute respiratory distress syndrome	GORD	Gastro-oesophageal reflux
ARR	Absolute risk reduction	GP	General practitioner
ATN	Acute tubular necrosis	GTCS	Generalised tonic clonic seizures
AV	Atrioventricular	GTN	Nitroglycerine
AVM	Arteriovenous malformation	H/O	History of
AXR	Abdominal X-ray	HAP	Hospital acquired pneumonia
BE	Base excess	Hb	Haemoglobin
BMI	Body mass index	HBV	Hepatitis B
BMs	Blood sugars	HCM	Hypertrophic cardiomyopathy
BP	Blood pressure	HHS	Hyperosmolar hyperglycaemic state
BPH	Benign prostatic hyperplasia	HIV	Human immunodeficiency virus
bpm	Beats per minute	HPA	Hypothalamo-pituitary-adrenal axis
BTS	British Thoracic Society	HPOA	Hypertrophic pulmonary osteoarthropathy
CABG	Coronary artery bypass graft	HR	Heart rate
CAM	Confusion assessment method	HRCT	High resolution computerised tomography
CAP	Community acquired pneumonia	HSV	Herpes simplex virus
CCF	Congestive cardiac failure	HT	Hypertension
CDT	Clock drawing test	IBD	Inflammatory bowel disease
CGA	Comprehensive geriatric assessment	IBS	Irritable bowel syndrome
CK	Creatinine kinase	ICD	Implantable cardioverter defibrillator
CKD	Chronic kidney disease	ICH	Intracranial haemorrhage
CMV	Cytomegalovirus	ICP	Intracranial pressure
CNS	Central nervous system	ICS	Intercostal space
COPD	Chronic obstructive pulmonary disease	IGRA	Interferon gamma release assay
CRP	c-reactive protein	IHD	Ischaemic heart disease
CSF	Cerebrospinal fluid	IIH	Intracranial hypertension
CT	Computerised tomography	ILD	Interstitial lung disease
CTD	Connective tissue disease	INR	International normalised ratio
CTPA	Computerised tomography pulmonary angiogram	IPF	idiopathic pulmonary fibrosis
CVA	Cerebrovascular accident	ITU	Intensive care unit
CVS	Cardiovascular system	IV	Intravenous
CXR	Chest x-ray	JVP	Jugular venous pressure
DI	Diabetes insipidus	LBBB	Left bundle branch block

LDH	Lactate dehydrogenase		PPM	Permanent pacemaker
LFT	Liver function test		PR	Per rectal
LGIB	Lower gastrointestinal bleed		prn	As required
LHF	Left heart failure		PSC	Primary sclerosing cholangitis
LIF	Left iliac fossa		PT	Prothrombin time
LMN	Lower motor neurone		PTH	Parathyroid hormone
LMWH	Low molecular weight heparin		PUD	Peptic ulcer disease
LP	Lumbar puncture		PVD	Peripheral vascular disease
LR	Likelihood ratio		py	Pack year
LV	Left ventricle		RAAS	Renin-angiotensin-aldosterone system
LVF	Left ventricular failure		RF	Rheumatoid factor
LVH	Left ventricular hypertrophy		RHF	Right heart failure
MAP	Mean arterial pressure		RR	Respiratory rate
MC&S	Microscopy, culture and sensitivity		RS	Respiratory system
MCI	Mild cognitive impairement		RVH	Right ventricular hypertrophy
MCV	Mean corpuscular volume		SAAG	Serum ascities albumin gradient
MI	Myocardial infarction		SAH	Subarachnoid haemorrhage
MMSE	Mini mental state examination		SARD	Systemic autoimmune rheumatic disease
MODS	Multi-organ dysfunction syndrome		sats	Oxygen saturations
MRI	magnetic resonance imaging		SDH	Subdural haemorrhage
MRA	Magnetic resonance angiogram		SHO	Senior house officer
NASH	Non-alcoholic steatohepatitis		SIADH	Syndrome of inappropriate ADH secretion
NCS	Nerve conduction studies		SIRS	Systemic inflammatory response syndrome
NIV	Non-invasive ventilation		SLE	Systemic lupus erythematosis
NMJ	Neuromuscular junction		SOB	Shortness of breath
NNT	Number needed to treat		SOBOE	Shortness of breath on exertion
NOAC	Newer oral anticoagulants		SOL	Space occupying lesion
NPH	Normal pressure hydrocephalus		SpA	Spondylarthropathy
NSAIDs	Non-steroidal anti-inflammatory drugs		SBP	spontaneous bacterial peritonitis
NSTEMI	Non-ST elevation MI		SQs	Semantic qualifiers
O/E	On examination		STEMI	ST elevation MI
OA	Osteoarthritis		SVCO	Superior vena cava obstruction
OCP	Oral contraceptive pill		TB	Tuberculosis
OGD	Oesophagogastroduodenoscopy		TFTs	Thyroid function tests
OSCE	Objective structured clinical examination		TIA	Transient ischaemic attack
PA	Per abdomen		TLOC	Transient loss of consciousness
P-A	Postero-anterior		TSH	Thyroid stimulating hormone
PCKD	Polycystic kidney disease		U&E	Urea and electrolytes
PCP	Pneumocystis carinii pneumonia		UACS	Upper airway cough syndrome
PCR	Polymerase chain reaction		UGIB	Upper gastrointestinal bleed
PE	Pulmonary embolism		UMN	Upper motor neurone
PESI	Pulmonary embolism severity index		UOP	Urinary output
PFT	Pulmonary function test		URTI	Upper respiratory tract infection
PMH	Previous medical history		USG	Ultrasonography
PMN	Polymorphonuclear cell count		UTI	Urinary tract infection
PMR	Polymyalgia rheumatica		V/Q	Ventilation/perfusion
PND	Paroxysmal nocturnal dyspnoea		VSD	Ventricular septal defect
PNS	Peripheral nervous system		VTE	Venous thrombo-embolism
PPI	Proton pump inhibitor		WCC	White cell count

Normal Reference Ranges

Biochemistry

Renal function

Urea and electrolytes (U&Es)

Sodium (Na$^+$)	135–145 mmol l^{-1}
Potassium (K$^+$)	3.5–4.5 mmol l^{-1}
Urea	2.5–6.7 mmol l^{-1}
Creatinine	53–106 µmol l^{-1}
Chloride (Cl$^-$)	95–105 mmol l^{-1}
Bicarbonate (HCO$_3^-$)	24–30 mmol l^{-1}

Liver function tests

Bilirubin	3–17 µmol l^{-1}
Alanine aminotransferase (ALT)	5–35 IU l^{-1}
Aspartate aminotransferase (AST)	5–35 IU l^{-1}
Alkaline phosphatase (ALP)	30–150 IU l^{-1}
Albumin	35–50 g l^{-1}
Total protein	60–78 g l^{-1}
Globulin	18–36 g l^{-1}
Gamma-glutamyl transpeptidase (GGT)	
Male	11–58 IU l^{-1}
Female	7–33 IU l^{-1}
Alpha fetoprotein (AFP)	0–40 mcg l^{-1}

Bone profile

Corrected calcium (Ca^{2+})	2.1–2.65 mmol l^{-1}
Phosphate (PO$_4^{3-}$)	0.8–1.45 mmol l^{-1}
Alkaline phosphatase (ALP)	30–150 IU l^{-1}
Albumin	35–50 g l^{-1}

Miscellaneous

Amylase	25–125 U l^{-1}
C-reactive protein	<10 mg l^{-1}
Creatine kinase (CK)	
Male	25–195 IU l^{-1}
Females	25–170 IU l^{-1}
Lactate dehydrogenase (LDH)	70–250 IU l^{-1}
Plasma osmolality	280–300 mosmol kg^{-1}
Troponin I	<0.1 µg l^{-1}
Troponin T	<0.03 µg l^{-1}
Urate	0.15–0.5 mmol l^{-1}

Drug levels

Digoxin (6 h post dose)	0.8–2 nmol l^{-1}
Lithium	0.5–1.5 mmol l^{-1}

Endocrinology

Free thyroxine (free T$_4$)	7.6–19.7 pmol l^{-1}
Total thyroxine (T$_4$)	70–140 nmol l^{-1}
Thyroid-stimulating hormone (TSH)	0.4–4.5 mU l^{-1}

Hematology

Full blood count (FBC)

Hemoglobin (Hb)	
Males	135–180 g l^{-1}
Females	115–160 g l^{-1}
Mean cell volume (MCV)	76–96 fl
Red cell distribution width	12–15%

Packed cell volume (PCV) or hematocrit (Hct)

Males	0.4–0.54
Females	0.36–0.46
Red cell count (RCC)	
Males	4.5–6.5 × 10^{12} l^{-1}
Females	3.8–5.8 × 10^{12} l^{-1}
White cell count (WCC)	4–11 × 10^9 l^{-1}
Differential cell count	
Neutrophils	2–7.5 × 10^9 l^{-1}
Lymphocytes	1.5–4 × 10^9 l^{-1}
Eosinophils	0.04–0.4 × 10^9 l^{-1}
Monocytes	0.2–0.8 × 10^9 l^{-1}
Basophils	0.0–0.1 × 10^9 l^{-1}
Platelets	150–400 × 10^9 l^{-1}
Reticulocytes	05–2.5% of red blood cells

Clotting profile

Prothrombin time (PT)	12–16 s
Activated partial thromboplastin time (APTT)	35–45 s
Fibrinogen	2–4 g l^{-1}
D-dimer	<0.5 mg l^{-1}

Haematinics

Iron studies	
Iron	11–32 mol l^{-1}
Total iron-binding capacity (TIBC)	42–80 mol l^{-1}
Ferritin	12–200 µg l^{-1}
Folate	>2 µg l^{-1}
Vitamin B$_{12}$	>150 ng l^{-1}

Miscellaneous

Cerebrospinal fluid (CSF)

Total protein	<0.45 g l^{-1}
Glucose (2/3 of plasma glucose)	2.5–4.4 mmol l^{-1}
White cell count (WCC)	<5/mm^3
Red cell count (RCC)	0/mm^3

Urine

Creatinine clearance (Ccr)	
Male	85–125 ml min^{-1}
Female	75–115 ml min^{-1}
Osmolality	250–1250 mosmol kg^{-1}
Protein	<0.2 g day^{-1}

Ascitic fluid

Total protein	<0.45 g l^{-1}
Glucose (2/3 of plasma glucose)	2.5–4.4 mmol l^{-1}
White cell count (WCC)	<5/mm^3
Red cell count (RCC)	0/mm^3

ABG on air

pH	7.35–7.45
PaCO$_2$	4.7–6 kpa
PaO$_2$	11–13 kpa
HCO$_3^-$	7.35–7.45
Base excess (BE)	−2 to +2
Saturations	>94%

Icons Explained

 Activity requiring written answers

 Answer key

 Activity requiring 'thinking'

 Remember me!

 Summary

About the Companion Website

This book is accompanied by a companion website:

www.wiley.com/go/irfan/clinicalreasoning

The website includes a reflective action guide.

1 Introduction: The Skeleton Laid Bare

▼

This chapter discusses the basic layout of this book

▲

1.1 THE BONES OF THE BOOK

Clinical reasoning is an enigma that has been the subject of research over the last few decades. It pertains to how physicians not only arrive at a diagnosis, but then use their clinical judgement to decide the next best course of action. This could be ordering another test, initiating treatment or the most curious course of just observing and not acting at all.

Current thinking revolves around the dual processing theory, which is an amalgamation of all the research thus far. It incorporates analytic and non-analytic strategies of clinical reasoning, which interact at different phases of the patient encounter and are called into play when needed. Non-analytic strategies (unconscious/reflexive) include pattern recognition, heuristics, illness scripts, and semantic qualifiers. Analytic strategies (conscious) include causal reasoning and probabilistic reasoning, where logic and critical thinking are given importance. Meta-cognition, an awareness of one's own thinking, overarches the analytic and non-analytic processes of cognition directing the clinician to the diagnosis.

An example in action:

An 82 year old lady presents with acute confusion. The doctor, using pattern recognition and heuristics (mental shortcuts) thinks this is likely to be a urinary tract infection (UTI), because he has seen this all too often. He notes the lady was on warfarin, so wonders if he is missing something (meta-cognition). He telephones her carers querying any recent falls with head injuries (analytic strategies). It turns out she had a head injury a week ago, following which she became increasingly confused and drowsy. This leads him to a working diagnosis of subdural haematoma, which gets confirmed on a CT scan.

If he had not been consciously aware of his own thinking (meta-cognition) he would have settled on the diagnosis of a UTI and ascribed a raised white cell count and low-grade temperature as confirmatory – thereby missing a significant diagnosis that carried a greater burden on the patient concerned.

You could argue that an experienced clinician would have got this diagnosis right first time. However, there are several contextual factors at play, which can easily mitigate in-depth analysis. Patient factors, such as an acutely confused person unable to give a clear story; environmental factors such as a busy A&E department and physician factors such as fatigue and sleep deprivation can all impact the decision-making process, leading to an unpleasant outcome for all concerned. Remember that experience does not equate with expertise.

Norman (2005) has suggested that clinical reasoning can only be imbibed by 'deliberate practice' wherein the learner encounters a plethora of examples, rather than just learning the strategies of clinical reasoning. In other words, practice, practice, and more practice will develop you into a skilful clinician. You can read this book to master the strategies of clinical reasoning, but unless you put them into practice, it will continue to remain an enigma.

The Hands-on Guide to Clinical Reasoning in Medicine, First Edition. Mujammil Irfan.
© 2019 John Wiley & Sons Ltd. Published 2019 by John Wiley & Sons Ltd.
Companion website: www.wiley.com/go/irfan/clinicalreasoning

This book has been divided into sections relating to the clinical placements you may find yourselves in. This allows you to work with the book whilst on your placements, transferring knowledge into practice. The topics include those often felt to be poorly covered, and are a treasure trove of common conditions that you will encounter.

The book does not claim to be an exhaustive resource on clinical medicine, but rather a route map, showing the intricacies of clinical reasoning. I shall start with a personal perspective of some rules-of-thumb for diagnostic reasoning, followed by rules-of-thumb for decision making to guide investigations and treatments. This will be followed by a unique way of approaching patients that should make your life a lot easier.

If there is one thing I would like you to take from this book, it is to always be open to diagnostic possibilities, ensuring that the thinking process never stops.

Rules of Thumb for Diagnostic Reasoning – A Personal Perspective:

1. **Commit to a diagnosis**
   'Collapse query(?) cause' is a common colloquial term in UK practice amongst junior doctors and is touted as the diagnosis for someone presenting with collapse. This is not a diagnosis. All you are doing is elaborating the fact you do not know the cause of their collapse. The first step in learning to diagnose is to commit to a diagnosis. We all make mistakes along the way, but not committing to a diagnosis is cognitively far more dangerous than making one and learning from it – as long as it does not put a patient at risk. If in doubt, ask a senior clinician for help in making those mental connections, but make sure you at least have a working diagnosis. Occasionally, a diagnosis maybe elusive, in which case a plan of action still needs to be formulated whilst acknowledging uncertainty and ensuring follow-up. Often, diagnoses emerge in the fullness of time, hence adequate follow-up is essential.

2. **Link to the past medical history**
   When trying to make a diagnosis, remember that any presentation in medicine is usually linked to the past medical history or medication list. When that train of thought does not yield a diagnosis, a new diagnosis should be entertained. If someone is known to have ischemic heart disease, they are likely to be breathless because of that than due to say, 'Churg-Strauss syndrome.'

3. **Common things are common**
   Use disease prevalence as a yardstick to know what is common. Epidemiologically speaking, a middle-aged male smoker in the developed world is likely to have vascular risk factors such as hypertension, hypercholesterolemia, and diabetes mellitus, predisposing him to ischemic heart disease and strokes.

4. **Explain the symptoms**
   Patients seek help because they are having symptoms not because they have an abnormal electrocardiogram, test result, or radiograph. Hence always try to explain the symptom/-s, and you'll hit the diagnosis.

5. **Explain all the findings**
   Can you explain all the findings (history, clinical examination, and investigations) with the diagnosis you have made (Kassirer and Kopelman 1991)? If there are any unexplained findings, re-visit the diagnosis.

6. **Think of all the alternatives**
   Always pause just before you make the final diagnosis and think of all the alternatives that can present in a similar fashion. Rule them out consciously before accepting the favoured one.

7. **ABC buys you time**
   All treatment, from intravenous fluids and antibiotics, to intensive care, is a temporary holding measure to buy time and allow the body to recover. The way you do it is by stabilising the physiological parameters, thus buying time to make a diagnosis. The ABC (airway, breathing, circulation) of emergency medicine is just this.

Rules of Thumb for Management Plans – A Personal Perspective

1. **Risk vs. benefit ratio**
   This should form the basis for decisions regarding patient management, including investigations.

2. **Mortality and morbidity**
   Most interventions in medicine are designed to prolong life (improve mortality) or reduce suffering (morbidity). Hence, the best treatment (anchored on evidence-based medicine) should improve mortality, and the second best should reduce morbidity. Of course, quality-of-life issues and patient choice trump all of this, but again, symptom control (alleviating morbidity) plays a big role even here.

3. **Will it alter my management?**
   Before ordering any test, be it a blood test or an MRI scan, ask yourself 'Will it alter my management?' This will ensure you do not do unnecessary tests.

4. **Masterly inactivity**
   Not intervening can also be a part of your management, e.g. observing a patient to see how their disease evolves before invasive tests are ordered or treatments initiated. This skill requires expertise – hence the phrase 'masterly' inactivity.

5. **Patient autonomy**
   Patients' informed decisions of not having further tests or treatments are to be respected at all times – despite how bizarre they may sound.

1.2 HEURISTICS

Some of the points elaborated above are called mental shortcuts or heuristics. Physicians use these to develop hypotheses – especially when confronted with incomplete information. They form part of the non-analytic strategies at the discretion of a clinician. Knowing when to use them and when to avoid them is a skill we must develop. When heuristics lead you down the wrong diagnostic pathway, we label them cognitive errors or biases (Croskerry 2002, p. 1201). With experience you will develop your own heuristics, but make sure they are based on accurate clinical knowledge (e.g. use disease prevalence to know what is common) and not faulty reasoning. This will ensure they do not turn into cognitive biases.

1.3 CLINICAL REASONING IN ACTION

When a junior doctor is presenting someone with acute central chest pain to the Consultant Physician, the latter is paraphrasing the information into digestible chunks, and listening intently to elicit whether the pain is pleuritic, positional, or exertional. The junior doctor may well have got lost in the sea of information ascertained from the patient, but the Consultant just picks what is relevant. You too can learn to do this. The starting point is to paraphrase the presentation using precise medical terms. The chunks of relevant information that you paraphrase from the data are called semantic qualifiers (SQs).

Allow me to illustrate:

A 56 year old man presents with a one hour history of right-sided weakness. This developed suddenly whilst sitting in a chair. He is a 30 pack year smoker and drinks 40 units of alcohol per week. He has a history of hypertension, diabetes mellitus, and hypercholesterolemia. He takes ramipril 2.5 mg od, gliclazide 80 mg od, and simvastatin 40 mg od.

Semantic Qualifiers
Middle aged man + acute neurological deficit + vascular risk factors

A *middle aged* man presents with an *acute* onset right sided weakness on a background of *smoking* and *alcohol excess*. He has *vascular risk factors* including hypertension, diabetes mellitus, and hypercholesterolemia.

A middle aged man with vascular risk factors presenting with an acute (sudden onset) focal neurological deficit is very likely to have had a vascular event. I'm thinking he has had a stroke. This is one of several possibilities, but we have made a start (Figure 1.1).

Presenting complaint + vital signs + end-of-the bed appearance = Provisional diagnosis + severity of illness
Past medical history (if unavailable, medication list)

Figure 1.1

You see what I did there? Paraphrasing the data into chunks lets you pick the relevant details and thread them into a coherent line of thinking.

We use these chunks to create a working space or 'context' which in this case is 'a neurological problem.' This is then refined in light of further history, examination, and so on.

We shall be using this technique throughout this book and hopefully you will learn to incorporate it into your daily practice.

1.4 ARRIVING AT THE PROVISIONAL DIAGNOSIS

Having paraphrased the clinical problem into meaningful chunks I then use a combination of vital signs and end-of-the-bed appearance (a 'bed-o-gram' in common parlance) to give me a measure of physiological derangement and the rapidity with which I need to formulate a working diagnosis (Figure 1.1).

Using the example above, his vital signs read: HR 110 bpm, BP 180/90, Temperature 38 °C, RR 28 per minute and Saturations of 92% on air. To this I normally add blood sugars (BMs), which read 'low.' He has marked physiological derangement with a strikingly low blood sugar. I combine this marked physiological derangement with his end-of-the-bed appearance – he appears drowsy and confused, and conclude that he is 'very ill.' I need to act *quickly* (translation: 'rule out life-threatening diagnoses first'). Life-threatening diagnoses in this case would include a stroke, low blood sugars causing neurological symptoms (neuroglycopaenia) (McAulay et al. 2001) and subdural hematoma due to history of alcohol excess (although the acute onset makes this unlikely). Life-threatening conditions need timely treatment and a delay in diagnosis will put your patient on the slope of deterioration that can be fatal.

The astute amongst you may have noticed our initial suspicion of stroke is now being called into question with more data (Figure 1.2). This is a reflection of the real world. We must keep an open mind to all possibilities before we accept any particular diagnosis. Premature closure is something we should be wary of.

Provisional diagnosis refined by history + examination + investigations = Working diagnosis

Figure 1.2

Obviously, correcting the hypoglycaemia would be the first step but I would not rule out a stroke just yet. If the symptoms resolve with a normal blood sugar then you have confirmed your diagnosis, if not you request a CT scan of his head to rule out a stroke. Remember to constantly re-visit your diagnosis and be prepared to change it if new data demands (Figure 1.3).

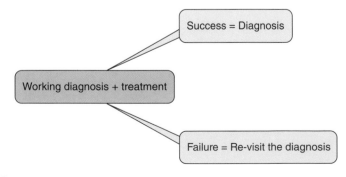

Figure 1.3

Our next task is to explain all the findings. I wonder why he has a low blood sugar. Why are his vital signs so deranged? Are we missing something? To recap: HR 110 bpm, BP 180/90, Temperature 38 °C, RR 28 per minute, Saturations 92% on air and BMs 'low.'

This can be overwhelming, but is truly very easy. I want you to now look at the beautiful orchestra of physiology, which is trying to tell you the diagnosis. His RR is high – there is something wrong physiologically; his saturations are low – there must be something wrong with his 'gas-exchange area' (the alveolar – capillary interface of the lung). I must ask if he has had any chest symptoms (breathlessness, chest pain, cough, etc.) and examine his heart and lungs. His blood pressure is raised at 180/90, with a pulse of 110 bpm indicating sympathetic activation. He must be sweaty and clammy too (the inner Sherlock speaking). This could just be a response to the hypoglycaemia, or to the neurological deficit. But, why is his temperature raised? Has he had any infective symptoms? Or is it secondary to the neurological problem?

It turns out he has had a cough with discoloured phlegm for the last four days with increasing breathlessness, lethargy, and poor oral intake. I seem to be localising a problem to his lungs. I listen to his chest – he has signs compatible with consolidation. A CXR confirms my suspicions. An ABG reveals hypoxia and metabolic acidosis – the latter secondary to sepsis and acute renal impairment detected on the bloods.

The sequence of events seems to be:
Pneumonia → acute kidney injury and sepsis → ↓BMs (secondary to poor oral intake + accumulation of gliclazide due to renal impairment) → new focal neurological deficit.

He improves with intravenous glucose and antibiotics and is discharged five days later.

Thus far we have discussed the six basic principles of clinical reasoning. To recap:

1. Frame a 'context' upon first contact with the data. Use semantic qualifiers to paraphrase the data and come up with a provisional diagnosis/-es.
2. Use vital signs and end-of-the-bed appearance to establish the severity of illness and elicit inconsistencies between the data and your provisional diagnosis.
3. Refine this with further data from history and clinical examination to arrive at a working diagnosis.
4. Outline further investigations and/or treatment based on this working diagnosis.
5. Re-visit the diagnosis in light of investigations and treatment responses.
6. Above all, do this consciously with a thought-provoking monologue so people around you can correct any faulty models of thinking.

1.5 ASSESSING SEVERITY OF ILLNESS

Over the years I have learnt that there are four kinds of patients: well, ill, very ill, and dying. There is a fifth kind – 'dead,' but really we are trying not to get there. How do I come to this conclusion? I'll give you a simple yet comprehensive way of assessing patients to tailor your history taking and examination and come up with a diagnosis or reasonable differential – all in a timely fashion. Oh, you are in for a treat.

The trick in assessing how ill a person is, is to look at the individual physiological parameters. The greater the deviation of the physiological parameters from the mean, the sicker the patient is. Then match this to the end-of-the-bed look of the person to get a fuller picture. This tells you if they are well, ill, very ill or dying.

Picture a bleep from a staff nurse on the wards. She informs you that her patient has a heart rate of 150 bpm. This is grossly abnormal. However, on arrival to the ward if you find said patient sat reading a newspaper, he is 'well' (relatively speaking). You have time to find out why he is tachycardic, take a history, examine him, and get some tests. Conversely, if you find him feeling lightheaded with a slightly low BP (100/70) you class him as 'ill.' You will have to be a bit quicker here, but you still have time.

On the other hand, if you find him lying in bed looking grey and complaining of chest pain, he is 'very ill' and if you don't act quickly, will soon be 'dying.' Eliciting that he is

Severity of illness	Time for assessment (rough guide) (min)
Well	30
Ill	20
Very ill	15
Dying	30

very ill gives you the severity of illness. It tells you to be very quick, take a focused history, do a targeted examination and get an urgent ECG *whilst* you are doing the aforementioned. So, you see vital signs or even history taken out of context can be misleading. Until and unless you have cast an eye on the patient, you cannot say how ill this person is.

A subtle component of this end-of-the-bed-o-gram is to assess the functional impact of the symptoms. This is most helpful when you do not have a set of observations guiding you – as in General Practice. Daily symptom burden impacting activities of daily living would class the person as ill or very ill depending on the degree of functional impairment. This is something I would like you to start doing. Try classing every patient you come across into either of these categories just by their end-of-the-bed appearance. This is a very subjective assessment, but comprehensive nonetheless. Used on its own it can be fatal, but if used in conjunction with other data, it is priceless.

Okay, now for some questions:

What's the first physiological parameter that goes off when someone is ill (I mean ill due to any reason)? Hazard a guess? No peeking….

Activity 1.1

(Allow few seconds)

Positive LR = sensitivity/1 – specificity.
Negative LR = 1 – sensitivity/specificity.

The 'test' in this case is a clinical sign.

1. Prevalence ~ pre-test probability prior to clinical assessment.
2. Pre-test odds = pre-test probability/(1 – pre-test probability) = 0.035/1 – 0.035 = 0.036.
3. Post-test odds = pre-test odds × LR$_1$ × LR$_2$ × LR$_3$ × ….LR$_n$ = 0.036 × 2.4 = 0.087.
4. Post-test probability = post-test odds/ (1 + post-test odds) = 0.087/1 + 0.087 = 0.08 which is 8%.

Respiratory rate.

Two unique things about respiratory rate – it's the only sign under voluntary control and the only parameter which is measured manually, and most likely to be left out. So, all those calls from nurses which say 'I do not like the look of him,' may have an underlying sign of clinical instability where the respiratory rate is abnormal (normal range 8–18).

1.6 THE SCIENCE IN THE ART OF MEDICINE

A 60 year old man sees his GP in the UK with a one week history of fever and cough. The clinician wishes to exclude the possibility of community acquired pneumonia (CAP) and takes a history and performs a clinical examination to increase or decrease their suspicion of CAP. The prevalence of CAP in the general population in the UK is 0.035 (British Lung Foundation data 2012). In practical terms, if no clinical assessment is carried out, the disease prevalence is equivalent to the pre-test probability of the disease in question (Figure 1.4). However, it is important to remember that this varies with the context in which this patient is seen. In Primary Care, the pre-test probability is lower than in a hospital where the population has been filtered.

During clinical assessment, each clinical finding (sign or symptom) increases or decreases the probability of CAP – some more so than others. The degree to which this suspicion is shifted can be measured quantitatively using the likelihood ratio (LR). LR is a measure of the diagnostic weight each finding carries. Disease prevalence does not affect sensitivity and specificity, but disease severity does (Parikh et al. 2009). Since LR is derived from sensitivity and specificity, it is unaffected by disease prevalence. Figure 1.4 conceptualises how LRs shift the post-test probability towards or away from CAP.

For instance, the positive LR for pyrexia is 2.4, raising the post-test probability of CAP to 8% (see opposite for calculation (Parikh et al. 2009)) or use a nomogram (Fagan 1975)). If

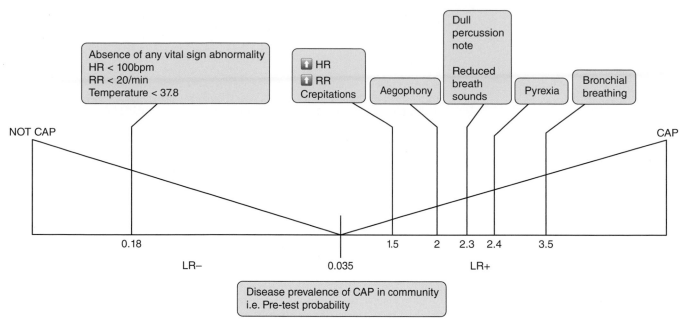

Figure 1.4 Likelihood ratios as diagnostic weights (not to scale)

the clinician gives undue importance to finding crackles alone (LR 1.6), the post-test probability then rises to 12%, which is still low to justify using antibiotics.

From literature, the LRs of all the clinical signs of CAP are as shown in Figure 1.4 (Metlay et al. 1997). Incorporating all these into the assessment will raise the post-test probability to 91.5%. In this scenario, even if the CXR does not show consolidation, we would go ahead and treat. Indeed, studies have shown that if the initial CXR is normal, consolidation can often 'blossom' following rehydration, becoming visible in the next day or two (Feldman 1999).

Let us say, the post-test probability following clinical assessment was 50%, the clinician can now choose to order a CXR. Once again, tests have sensitivity and specificity and therefore a LR. The LR for CXR is 6.21 (Self et al. 2013). If the CXR shows consolidation, the post-test probability rises to 86% from 50% helping us make treatment decisions. Remember, *tests do not make the diagnosis* – they merely increase or decrease the probability of the disease in a similar fashion to clinical assessment.

Conversely, if there is no abnormality in the vital signs, the post-test probability of CAP is <1% making it unnecessary to get a CXR (Gennis et al. 1989).

These calculations are individualised to the context in which the patient is encountered, providing truly personalised medicine. Seasoned clinicians often do all of the above intuitively without resorting to formal calculations, but even they can sometimes err in quantifying the true disease prevalence.

Cooper and Frain (2017) have simplified the approach to memorising the change in diagnostic probability according to the value of the LR. A LR of 1 implies no change in the diagnostic probability of the disease in question. The higher the LR, the greater is the probability of the disease. LRs of 2, 5, and 10 correspondingly increase the disease probability by 15%, 30%, and 45%. Similarly, by inverting the numbers 2, 5, and 10 we get LRs of 0.5, 0.2, and 0.1, which reduce the disease probability by 15%, 30%, and 45%. A positive LR implies that the clinical finding is present, whilst a negative LR implies it is absent. One limitation of a LR, is that it cannot be calculated unless the disease has a conclusive technological diagnostic standard (in this instance, a CXR).

There are several online databases showing prevalence of diseases, as well as giving LRs for common clinical findings/tests in various diagnoses. You can easily incorporate them into your practice using apps too. At the very least, they can be useful in grey cases where there is diagnostic dilemma.

Another concept to understand is the predictive value of a test. If a positive test is able to pick up everyone with disease, it has a high positive predictive value (PPV). Similarly if a negative test is able to exclude everyone without the disease, it has a high negative predictive value (NPV). However, these values vary with disease prevalence, e.g. the lower the disease prevalence, the lower the PPV. In other words, if the pre-test probability of disease is low, no matter how good a test, a positive result is less likely to rule in disease. This is why 'fishing tests' without knowing what the diagnosis is, do not give us the answer.

1.7 STRUCTURE OF THE BOOK

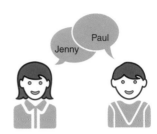

With my thinking cap on, I imagined various methods in which I could enable your learning. Everything seemed to be a drag but one. The best way of going about it was to imagine a couple of students in front of me to whom I would teach the art of clinical reasoning. Better still, what if I were to materialise two students right now? Meet Jenny and Paul, two fourth-year medical students henceforth known as J and P. They are going to be learning the basic principles of clinical reasoning, and you are most welcome to join us. Who knows, I might be able to help you and if I do I shall consider myself to be very privileged.

My aim is to paint as real a picture as possible, mirroring the real world. That includes all the inaccuracies, complexities, and fun that real life would present to us. I have assumed a fair amount of background knowledge in clinical diagnoses for you to be tackling the content of this book. If you fancy, you could have a quick revision in the Common Clinical Conditions section before tackling the rest of the book.

As we walk along, there will be plenty of space to record your thoughts and I hope you will avail of this. Feel free to use the margins in the text to record your reactions (clear, unclear, need more examples, diagrams, etc.) as you go along.

I shall begin by introducing new concepts through case based scenarios, showing my thought processes in brackets. My conversations with Jenny and Paul will be in 'CronosPro,' whilst they will converse in '*italicised CronosPro*.' The conversations with you (the reader) will be in 'Times New Roman.' I hope that the principles learnt here will be applied elsewhere in other specialties and not limited to Medicine.

The activity boxes are designed to give you a pause in your reading, allowing you to engage with the material. They are a resource in themselves and have a valid rationale. The time needed to complete them has been indicated, giving you the choice of doing them or not depending on how stretched you are. Some of these activities have no specific answers. This is done deliberately to make you think broadly, and is a reflection of clinical practice where there is often no single best answer, and entertaining several possibilities will ensure you do not miss diagnoses.

I can sense some of you are getting impatient and wondering if I'm ever going to start. I can't stop you from skipping parts of this book, and I don't intend to – you are an independent individual and are free to use this book the way you want. Once you have completed the book you can use the accompanying Reflective Action Guide. Print out the sections relevant to your placement and take them to the wards, hopefully transferring your learning into practice.

Enjoy!

References

British Lung Foundation. 2012. *Pneumonia Statistics* [Online]. United Kingdom. Available at: https://statistics.blf.org.uk/pneumonia [Accessed: 19 August 2018].

Cooper, N. and Frain, J. 2016. *ABC of Clinical Reasoing (ABC Series)*. 1st ed. BMJ Books.

Croskerry, P. (2002). Achieving quality in clinical decision making: cognitive strategies and detection of bias. *Academic Emergency Medicine: Official Journal of the Society for Academic Emergency Medicine* 9 (11): 1184–1204.

Fagan, T.J. (1975). Letter: Nomogram for Bayes theorem. *The New England Journal of Medicine* 293 (5): 257.

Feldman, C. (1999). 'Pneumonia in the elderly. *Clinics in Chest Medicine* 20 (3): 563–573.

Gennis, P., Gallagher, J., Falvo, C. et al. (1989). 'Clinical criteria for the detection of pneumonia in adults: guidelines for ordering chest roentgenograms in the emergency department. *The Journal of Emergency Medicine* 7 (3): 263–268.

Kassirer, J.P. and Kopelman, R.I. (1991). *Learning Clinical Reasoning*, 2e. Baltimore: Williams and Wilkins.

Metlay, J.P., Kapoor, W.N., and Fine, M.J. (1997). Does this patient have community-acquired pneumonia? Diagnosing pneumonia by history and physical examination. *Journal of the American Medical Association* 278 (17): 1440–1445.

McAulay, V., Deary, I.J., and Frier, B.M. (2001). Symptoms of hypoglycemia in people with diabetes. *Diabetic Medicine* 18 ((9)): 690–705.

Norman, G. (2005). 'Research in clinical reasoning: past history and current trends. *Medical Education* 39 (4): 418–427.

Parikh, R., Parikh, S., Arun, E., and Thomas, R. (2009). Likelihood ratios: clinical application in day-to-day practice. *Indian Journal of Ophthalmology* 57 (3): 217–221.

Self, W.H., Courtney, D.M., McNaughton, C.D. et al. (2013). 'High discordance of chest x-ray and computed tomography for detection of pulmonary opacities in ED patients: Implications for diagnosing pneumonia. *American Journal of Emergency Medicine* 31 (2): 401–405.

PART I
Respiratory Medicine

2 History Taking: A Breath of Fresh Air

▼

This chapter outlines a bird's eye view of little tricks and treats to get you started and take a history from a lung perspective

▲

Welcome to your respiratory placement. For those of you who need a quick overview of the basics, the following sections have been designed to give you a brief insight into assessment of the Respiratory System. They are the proverbial tip of the iceberg – just so you have something to hang your hat on. These tricks and treats will be put into action in the ensuing chapters, which will explain things much better.

I have also introduced pictorial interpretations of concepts using what we call Concept Maps (Torre et al. 2013). These tend to follow what's inside my head, but are far easier to read than thick black print. Try to develop your own concept maps and have a template of your understanding on paper. Trust me, it becomes a lot easier to understand things when you lay out whatever's inside your head in front of you.

Concept maps are diagrams that start from generalized ideas at the top and work down to more specific ideas represented in circles or boxes called 'nodes.' The nodes are connected to each other with 'linking words' that show relationships between the concepts. A simple example is illustrated opposite (Figure 2.1).

Concept maps are unique to the person who makes them. In other words, my concept map on breathlessness will be different from yours, reflecting the way we understand things. You can make concept maps on anything: history taking, diseases, pathophysiology, or treatments. Remember they are not algorithms or flow charts, although they look like them. They are meaningful representations of learning on paper and the linking words in particular, offer them 'meaning.' The more you understand something the more intricate the links are, especially the cross-links which run horizontally, connecting concepts on either end of the map, as opposed to the usual vertical ones. You can see them change as you progress too and they are a fun way of learning. Get into the habit of creating them, as they are an integral part of learning to think like a doctor.

Most of the concept maps in this book are fully formed, but others will be signposted as skeletons. You will have to flesh them out as you go through the book. You can add new extensions to the maps as you begin to understand new concepts on the wards or even better, make your own concept maps from scratch. They are also available on the companion website from where you can print those relevant to your placement. Remember, they are a work in progress and not gospel that can't be changed. With time, you will see how they evolve to reflect the greater in-depth understanding you will acquire.

Figure 2.1 An example of a concept map

The Hands-on Guide to Clinical Reasoning in Medicine, First Edition. Mujammil Irfan.
© 2019 John Wiley & Sons Ltd. Published 2019 by John Wiley & Sons Ltd.
Companion website: www.wiley.com/go/irfan/clinicalreasoning

The art of medicine dictates that you start assessing a patient even before they tell you their story. Part of this relies on having keen observational skills, which is exactly what objective structured clinical examinations (OSCEs) demand – where you observe what is around the patient and go through the motions (sometimes without giving it much thought). In exams, you pick up on oxygen, inhalers, and nebulisers around the patient. In real life you tend to pick up on subtle clues like tobacco use (tar stains on fingers), muscle wasting (cachexia), or cushingoid appearance (e.g. chronic steroid use), Horner's – small pupil and ptosis on the same side (due to perhaps an upper lobe lung tumor) etc. Remember that this non-verbal exchange is occurring in the opposite direction too – patients are ascertaining their doctor's demeanor and willingness to listen. This can make all the difference in arriving at the right diagnosis and concordance with treatment than just your assessment of what you want to hear or see.

Some patients however, may not be able to give you a history for various reasons ranging from inability to point out the most important symptom/-s, confusion or unconsciousness. In the first scenario, a guided approach to hone in on relevant symptoms/symptom clusters may work. Sometimes asking 'If there was one thing you would like to be fixed today what would it be?' might get you there. In the latter scenarios you will have to get collateral history from carers, paramedics, care home staff or if nothing else, their medication list.

2.1 THE IMPORTANCE OF EXERCISE TOLERANCE IN HISTORY TAKING

Exercise tolerance is an indirect way of assessing someone's cardiopulmonary reserve. A clear documentation of this is essential in making decisions regarding escalation of care (to ITU or not) in the event of clinical deterioration. This is because pre-morbid physiological reserve is a good prognostic marker of recovery from acute illness. Asking something along the lines of 'how many yards can you walk on a good day, on the flat, at your own pace before you get out of breath' and 'how many flights of stairs can you manage before you have to stop for breath,' will give you a rough indicator of their reserve. This can also be used in follow-up to assess whether a condition is worsening or improving with treatment.

2.2 APPROACH TO HISTORY TAKING

The starting point of good history taking is a concise understanding of the aetiologies of symptoms. Each symptom can be understood in terms of its anatomical or pathophysiological basis. The symptom of chest pain has been used as an example to illustrate this (Figure 2.2).

This list is not exhaustive, but rather a way of thinking about symptoms. You can do the same for other symptoms. Once this clear, history taking becomes easier. You start with introducing yourself and ask the open–ended question 'what brought you to see me?' You let them speak whilst listening to the main symptoms that have been bothering them – breathlessness, cough, fever, etc. Then, once you've delineated their main symptoms you ascertain each of their duration and temporal occurrence e.g. breathlessness for four days, cough and fever for two days. Each symptom then needs to be explored in its own context. The follow-up questions you ask depend not only on the answer to the previous one but also on the provisional diagnosis/-es you have arrived at – as explained in the previous chapter. The severity of illness dictates the order of impetus you give to each of the provisional diagnoses as outlined in the next page.

Using the pattern of thinking described thus far, I have produced a history taking template that can be used in medicine (Figures 2.3 and 2.4). This is by and large reproducible and works well for most situations, although there will be exceptions.

As you can see, the questions asked vary with context, provisional diagnoses and the severity of illness.

The figures that follow show the aetiologies of the remaining respiratory symptoms (Figures 2.5–2.7). Skeletal concept maps illustrating the keywords (italicised in bold) in history taking will be outlined for some of the respiratory symptoms in the following chapters. For now, remember to start with the aetiologies of specific symptoms and then use the history taking template to ask relevant questions in light of the context, provisional diagnoses and the severity of illness.

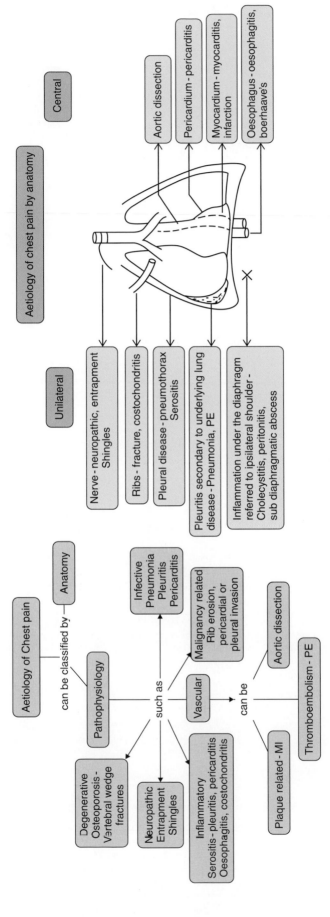

Figure 2.2 Aetiology of chest pain

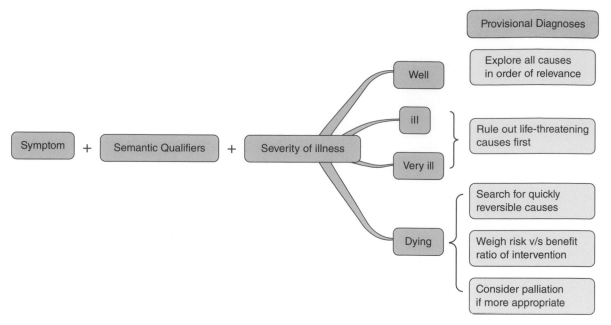

Figure 2.3 History taking template

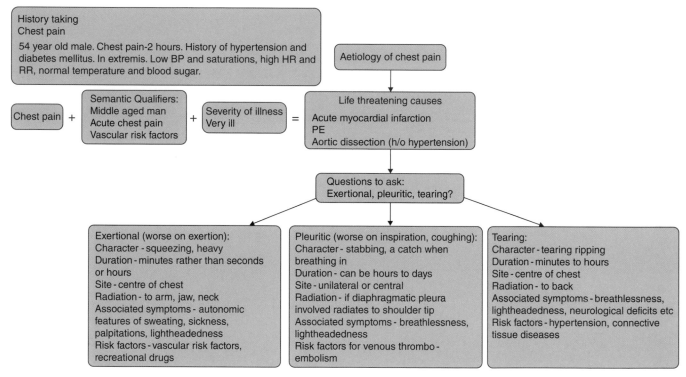

Figure 2.4 History taking template for chest pain

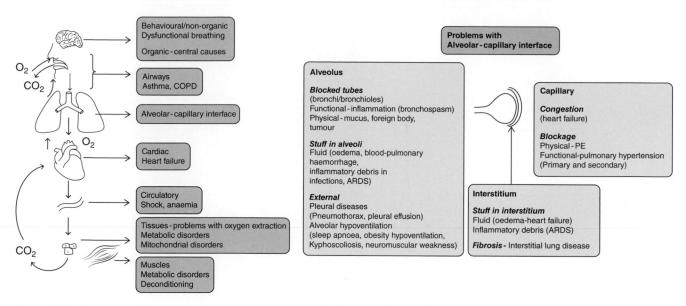

Figure 2.5 Aetiology of breathlessness based on respiratory cycle with the alveolar-capillary interface magnified

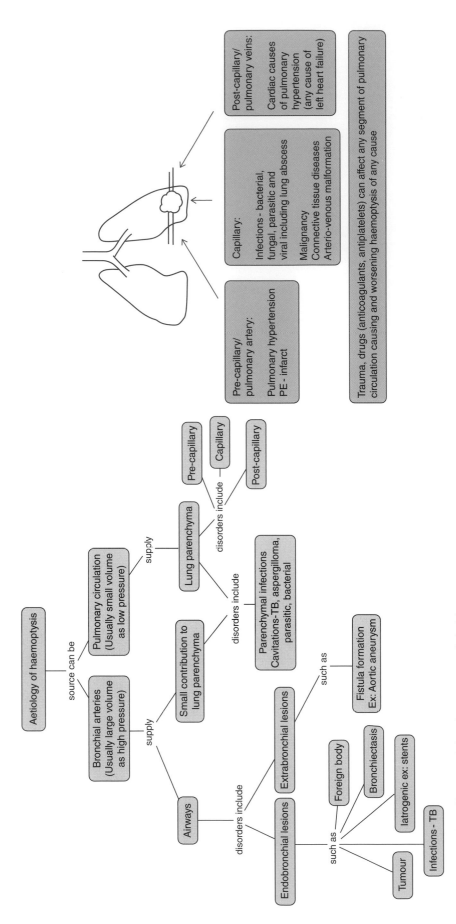

Figure 2.6 Aetiology of haemoptysis based on anatomy and physiology

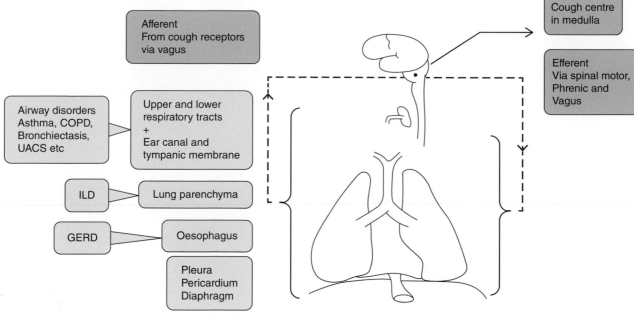

Figure 2.7 Aetiology of cough

Reference

Torre, D.M., Durning, S.J., and Daley, B.J. (2013). Twelve tips for teaching with concept maps in medical education. *Medical Teacher* 35 (3): 201–208.

3 Clinical Examination: The Rustle of Leaves

▼
Focussing on relevant clinical features and their interpretation from a respiratory perspective
▲

'Interpretation of clinical signs should start with the clinical examination,' such a simple yet profound statement which most of us tend to forget. For the purpose of this chapter you should first familiarise yourself with the common respiratory conditions that you encounter on a daily basis. Back that up with relevant applied anatomy, pathophysiology, basic principles of physics and some imagination and you'll find yourself interpreting the signs in no time.

Take the example of right middle lobe consolidation (Table 3.1). Looking at the right lung from the side, the upper lobe is mostly in the front, the middle lobe in the infra-axillary region and the lower lobe lies largely at the back (Figure 3.1a). Hence all the clinical signs are found in the infra-axillary region. The same applies to the lingula on the left. The pathological definition of consolidation is solidification of the lung. In other words, air filled alveoli are replaced by alveoli filled with inflammatory debris (Figure 3.1c). The resonant percussion note of air filled alveoli is replaced by the dull note of a solidified lung.

Now for some physics: sound travels better in solids > liquids > air. It follows that vibrations from the vocal chords through the central airways (and spoken '99') are better conducted straight to the chest wall through solidified lung than air filled lung, hence the bronchial breathing, increased vocal resonance and aegophony. Since air is not getting into this lobe easily, the breath sounds themselves are reduced. As for the added sounds, crepitations, or crackles, these occur in consolidation as the fluid filled terminal bronchioles snap open with every breath. They usually occur in the late inspiratory phase. Small airways disease (e.g. chronic obstructive pulmonary disease (COPD)) causes early inspiratory crepitations and alveolar disease causes late or pan-inspiratory crepitations.

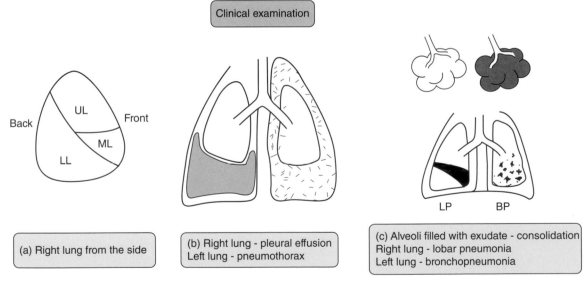

Clinical examination

Back — Front
UL
ML
LL

LP   BP

(a) Right lung from the side

(b) Right lung - pleural effusion
Left lung - pneumothorax

(c) Alveoli filled with exudate - consolidation
Right lung - lobar pneumonia
Left lung - bronchopneumonia

Figure 3.1 Understanding clinical examination using anatomy, physiology and physics

The Hands-on Guide to Clinical Reasoning in Medicine, First Edition. Mujammil Irfan.
© 2019 John Wiley & Sons Ltd. Published 2019 by John Wiley & Sons Ltd.
Companion website: www.wiley.com/go/irfan/clinicalreasoning

Table 3.1

Clinical condition	Inspection	Palpation	Percussion	Auscultation
Right middle lobe pneumonia	Chest wall expansion Bilaterally equal	No mediastinal shift: trachea central	Dull in the right infra-axillary region	Reduced breath sounds/Medium late or pan-inspiratory crepitations/Bronchial breathing/Increased vocal resonance

The latter can be fine (interstitial lung disease-ILD), medium (consolidation, left ventricular failure-LVF) or coarse (bronchiectasis).

Activity 3.1

(Allow five minutes)

Now it's your turn to apply these principles and think through the signs that you would expect to find in the diagnoses listed in Table 3.2 Remember things that pull or push the mediastinum thereby causing tracheal shift and apical impulse deviation as well as things that squash the lung away from the chest wall. Use the pictures to rekindle your imagination (Figure 3.1b).

Don't worry if you don't get this the first time, they will all be encountered in subsequent chapters.

Table 3.2 Clinical examination findings in various respiratory diseases. Please fill in the missing information to make this your own.

Clinical condition	Inspection	Palpation	Percussion	Auscultation
Asthma				Bilateral wheeze often expiratory but can also occur in inspiration
Left pleural effusion				
Right pneumothorax				
Right upper lobe collapse				
COPD with a large bulla in the right upper lobe				
Interstitial Lung Disease				

4 Interpretation of Chest Radiographs: The Light Through the Tunnel

▼
Having a framework to hang things on
▲

CXR interpretation needs a systematic check list that you can work with. It could be anything from reading it inside-out (mediastinum, hila, lungs, chest wall, and bones), vice-versa or using the letters of the alphabet (A-I) as a mnemonic. As long as you don't miss anything any system will do the job. Ensure that you don't miss the 'lawyer's zones' (apices, diaphragms, behind the heart, soft tissue shadows like the breasts and the bones) which are the most often missed areas on a CXR.

General principles of CXR interpretation:

1. Interpret the radiograph in the context of the working diagnosis.
2. There are two lungs – use them to compare each other.
3. Always compare with a previous radiograph if you have access to it.
4. Whenever the air in the alveoli is expelled for any reason the air-solid interface on a CXR is lost i.e. heart borders, diaphragms, and aorta (Figure 4.1c).
5. Once you have identified a striking abnormality don't stop, look further for both confirmatory and contradictory abnormalities and refine the radiographic diagnosis.

From a lung perspective there are a few major diagnoses that we need to discuss. For the purpose of simplicity I have classified them into:

White areas or opacifications – atelectasis, airspace shadowing (e.g. consolidation), pleural effusions (Figures 4.2, 4.3b, and 4.4).

Atelectasis results in loss of volume on the same side which pulls the mediastinum towards it. Upper lobe collapse pulls the trachea and lower lobe collapse pulls the heart and great vessels. The ipsilateral hemidiaphragm, related fissures and hilum get pulled towards the collapsed lobe. Lastly there is crowding of the ribs on the affected side i.e. the intercostal spaces get narrowed. These features though not always present are common to all atelectases regardless of the lobe involved (Figure 4.1).

Airspace shadowing/filling implies that air in the alveoli has been replaced by fluid or other processes making them more opaque to the x-ray beam. However, there is no destruction of the underlying lung parenchyma (Tuddenham 1984). If the pathological process spreads to the adjacent alveoli, airspace shadowing can coalesce resulting in larger opacifications like consolidation or more diffuse patterns like the bat's wing pattern of pulmonary oedema. Although air-bronchograms are commonly seen in consolidation they are also found in airspace shadowing of any cause.

Ground glass change is another pattern of airspace filling. One can often see the broncho-vascular markings through the haze as in seeing through 'ground glass,' compared to consolidation where it's opaque. Causes: stuff in alveoli - blood (pulmonary haemorrhage), inflammatory debris (pneumocystis carinii pneumonia (PCP), hypersensitivity pneumonitis, sarcoid – anything can happen in sarcoid), fluid (pulmonary oedema, acute respiratory distress syndrome (ARDS)) and tumour (bronchioloalveolar carcinoma).

Diagrams that follow are self-explanatory. Please do study them in detail.

The Hands-on Guide to Clinical Reasoning in Medicine, First Edition. Mujammil Irfan.
© 2019 John Wiley & Sons Ltd. Published 2019 by John Wiley & Sons Ltd.
Companion website: www.wiley.com/go/irfan/clinicalreasoning

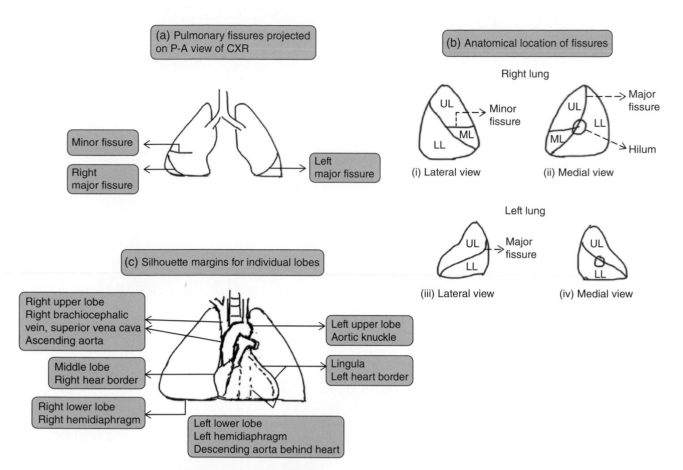

(a) Pulmonary fissures projected on P-A view of CXR

Minor fissure

Right major fissure

Left major fissure

(b) Anatomical location of fissures

Right lung

UL

ML

LL

Minor fissure

(i) Lateral view

UL

LL

ML

Major fissure

Hilum

(ii) Medial view

Left lung

UL

LL

Major fissure

(iii) Lateral view

UL

LL

(iv) Medial view

(c) Silhouette margins for individual lobes

Right upper lobe
Right brachiocephalic vein, superior vena cava
Ascending aorta

Middle lobe
Right hear border

Right lower lobe
Right hemidiaphragm

Left upper lobe
Aortic knuckle

Lingula
Left heart border

Left lower lobe
Left hemidiaphragm
Descending aorta behind heart

Figure 4.1 Anatomy as an aid in understanding chest radiographs

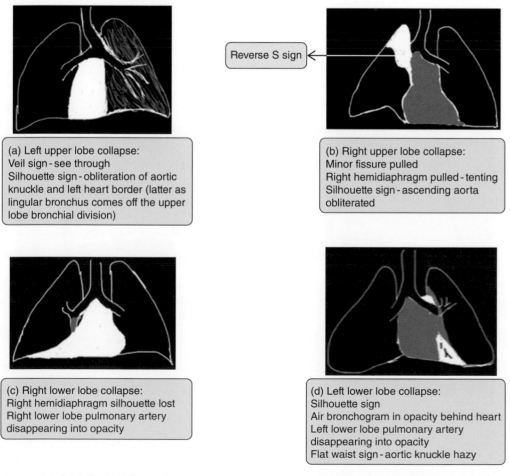

(a) Left upper lobe collapse:
Veil sign - see through
Silhouette sign - obliteration of aortic knuckle and left heart border (latter as lingular bronchus comes off the upper lobe bronchial division)

Reverse S sign

(b) Right upper lobe collapse:
Minor fissure pulled
Right hemidiaphragm pulled - tenting
Silhouette sign - ascending aorta obliterated

(c) Right lower lobe collapse:
Right hemidiaphragm silhouette lost
Right lower lobe pulmonary artery disappearing into opacity

(d) Left lower lobe collapse:
Silhouette sign
Air bronchogram in opacity behind heart
Left lower lobe pulmonary artery disappearing into opacity
Flat waist sign - aortic knuckle hazy

Figure 4.2 Lobar collapse on chest radiographs

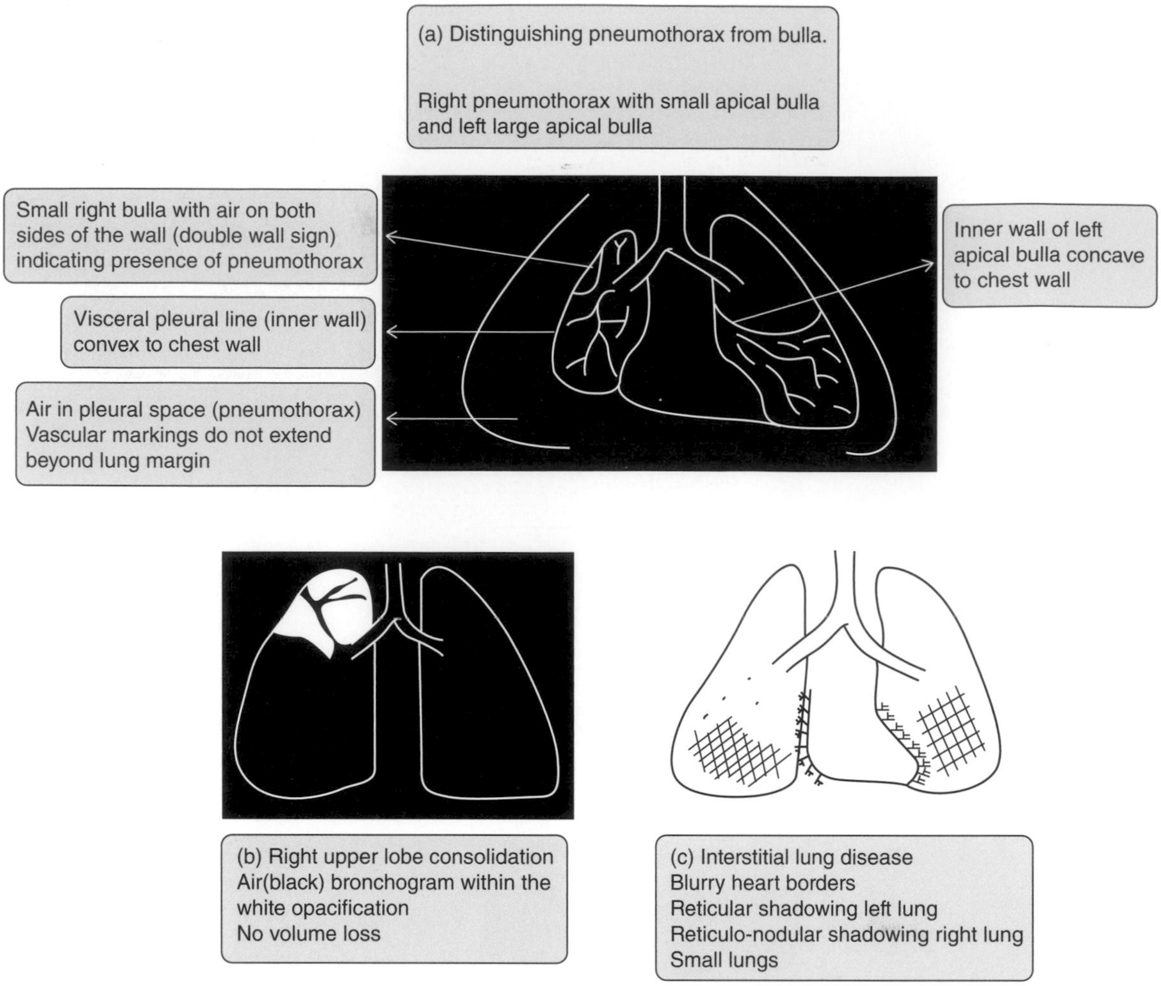

(a) Distinguishing pneumothorax from bulla.

Right pneumothorax with small apical bulla and left large apical bulla

Small right bulla with air on both sides of the wall (double wall sign) indicating presence of pneumothorax

Inner wall of left apical bulla concave to chest wall

Visceral pleural line (inner wall) convex to chest wall

Air in pleural space (pneumothorax) Vascular markings do not extend beyond lung margin

(b) Right upper lobe consolidation
Air(black) bronchogram within the white opacification
No volume loss

(c) Interstitial lung disease
Blurry heart borders
Reticular shadowing left lung
Reticulo-nodular shadowing right lung
Small lungs

Figure 4.3 Chest radiographic interpretation in a) Distinguishing pneumothorax from a bulla. b) Right upper lobe consolidation and c) Interstitial lung disease

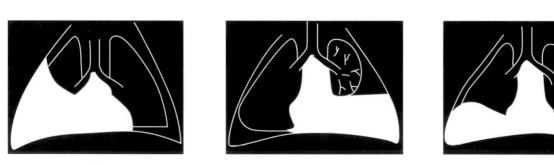

(a) Right pleural effusion:
Appears white on CXR
Meniscus
Costo-phrenic angle obliterated
Silhouette sign - right heart border and right hemidiaphragm obliterated

(b) Left hydro-pneumothorax:
Straight line indicates air and fluid in pleural space

(c) Right sub-pulmonic pleural effusion:
Apparently elevated hemidiaphragm
Lack of pulmonary markings behind right diaphragm
Lateral peaking of hemidiaphragm
Obliteration of costophrenic angle

Figure 4.4 Chest radiographic interpretation in a) Right pleural effusion. b) Left hydro-pneumothorax and c) Right sub-pulmonic pleural effusion

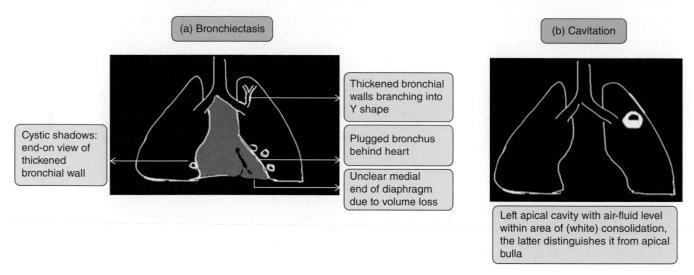

Figure 4.5 Examples of ring shadows and cysts on chest radiographs

Other white areas: line shadows and bands, ring shadows and cysts (Figure 4.5).

Black areas (compared to the other/same lung) – usually because of more air (air-trapping) or less blood e.g. pneumothorax, bullae (Figure 4.3a).

Interstitial changes - reticular, nodular, reticulo-nodular Figure 4.3c).

Table 4.1 shows the differences between the major white shadows.

Table 4.1 Major white shadows on chest radiographs

	Consolidation	Atelectasis/collapse	Pleural effusion
Unique feature (relatively speaking)	Air bronchogram (air-filled patent bronchus surrounded by airless lung parenchyma)	Pulling surrounding structures (hila, fissures, diaphragm, mediastinum)	Meniscus and loss of costo-phrenic angle
Effect on volume of the hemithorax	No effect	Reduced lung volume and hemithorax	Increase in volume of hemithorax but lung collapsed.
Similarities	Silhouette sign (Figure 4.1c) – any lesion arising from the lung, pleura or mediastinum that touches the border of the heart, diaphragm, or aorta obliterates that border.		

Reference

Tuddenham, W.J. (1984). Glossary of terms for thoracic radiology: recommendations of the nomenclature Committee of the Fleischner Society. *American Journal of Roentgenology* 143 (3): 509–517.

5 Interpretation of Arterial Blood Gases and Pleural Fluid Results: Needling it Out

▼

Having a framework to work with

▲

The ABG gives a lot of information on acid–base balance, oxygenation and ventilation (Figure 5.1). It is an objective measure of the physiology churning inside. Any disturbances in physiology will readily get reflected in the ABG.

5.1 ACID–BASE BALANCE

ABG interpretation starts with the pH (Figure 5.2). The normal range is 7.35–7.45. If it's lesser than 7.35 it is acidosis, and if it's more than 7.45 it is alkalosis.

The next parameter to check is the $PaCO_2$ (partial pressure of carbon dioxide). CO_2 is an acidic gas. Say the pH is acidic, check to see if the $PaCO_2$ is high. If it is, then it's respiratory acidosis. If it isn't then check the HCO_3^- (bicarbonate). HCO_3^- is a base, a naturally occurring buffer in the body. If the HCO_3^- is low then it's in keeping with the acidosis hence it is metabolic acidosis.

Say the pH is alkalotic. Check the $PaCO_2$ – if it's low, it is respiratory alkalosis. If it isn't low then check the HCO_3^-: If the HCO_3^- is high then it's metabolic alkalosis.

The base excess is a poor man's lactate. The base excess tells you the status of tissue perfusion. If the base excess is more negative than −4 (metabolic acidosis) then they more often than not need fluids to correct the hypoperfusion.

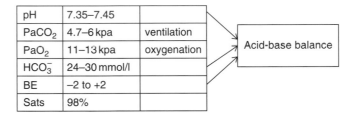

pH	7.35–7.45		
PaCO₂	4.7–6 kpa	ventilation	
PaO₂	11–13 kpa	oxygenation	Acid-base balance
HCO₃⁻	24–30 mmol/l		
BE	−2 to +2		
Sats	98%		

Figure 5.1 Normal ABG on air (FiO_2 21%)

5.2 ALVEOLAR-ARTERIAL OXYGEN GRADIENT (A-a GRADIENT = PAO₂ – PaO₂)

It is the difference between the oxygen concentration in the alveoli (PAO_2) and the oxygen concentration in the arterial blood (PaO_2). Normally there is a step down in oxygen concentration in the blood when oxygen diffuses from the alveoli into the capillaries. This is due to a physiological V/Q (ventilation/perfusion) mismatch which means the amount of oxygen and the amount of blood is not the same (i.e. not matched) throughout the lungs owing to gravity (more oxygen at the top and more blood at the bottom of the

The Hands-on Guide to Clinical Reasoning in Medicine, First Edition. Mujammil Irfan.
© 2019 John Wiley & Sons Ltd. Published 2019 by John Wiley & Sons Ltd.
Companion website: www.wiley.com/go/irfan/clinicalreasoning

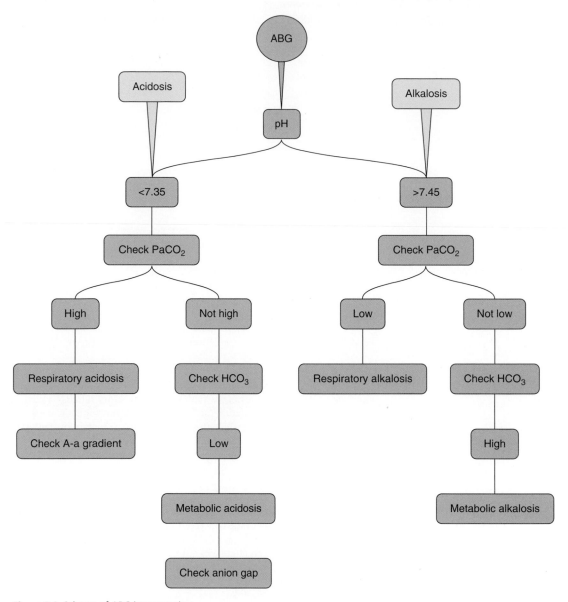

Figure 5.2 Schema of ABG interpretation

Alveolar gas equation:
PAO$_2$ (alveolar oxygen) =
(FiO$_2$ − 1) − 5/4(PaCO$_2$) in kpa

Gas 1

FiO$_2$	21%
pH	7.25
PaCO$_2$	10
PaO$_2$	7
HCO$_3^-$	32.8

A-a gradient 0.5 kpa.

Gas 2

FiO$_2$	21%
pH	7.25
PaCO$_2$	7
PaO$_2$	6
HCO$_3^-$	23

A-a gradient 5.2 kpa.

Both these gases have respiratory acidosis (type 2 respiratory failure) as the primary abnormality. However, the low PaO$_2$ in gas 1 is due to ventilatory failure needing NIV whilst the low PaO$_2$ in gas 2 is due to oxygenation failure needing oxygen and invasive intubation and ventilation.

lungs). Hence normal A-a gradient is 1–2 kpa in young and 2–3 kpa in the elderly (Figure 5.3a).

You can calculate the PAO$_2$ by the alveolar gas equation. There are innumerable 'apps' which can calculate the A-a gradient for you – use them.

5.3 OXYGENATION

Rule of thumb for PaO$_2$ (partial pressure of oxygen): The predicted PaO$_2$ for a given FiO$_2$ (fraction of inspired oxygen) is FiO$_2$-10 in kpa.

Example: If you are breathing room air, the FiO$_2$ is 21%. The predicted PaO$_2$ on the ABG if you have a healthy pair of lungs is 21–10 = 11 kpa. If breathing 35%, the predicted PaO$_2$ is 35–10 = 25 kpa.

Oxygenation means getting oxygen across the alveolar-capillary interface. Any problems with this interface – the PaO$_2$ on your ABG will drop.

The A-a gradient gives you a sneak peek into oxygen diffusion across the alveolar-capillary interface. If the A-a gradient is high there is something wrong with this interface i.e. lung failure.

Treatment follows: failure of oxygenation (type 1 respiratory failure) – oxygen +/− intubation and ventilation (if they are getting tired).

Oxygenation problems often result in the person eventually getting tired, to the point that their ventilation starts getting affected (Figure 5.3b). The first response to hypoxia is an increase in the minute ventilation (respiratory rate RR × tidal volume TV). As a result of this hyperventilation the PaCO$_2$ drops. Unfortunately, the RR is capped around 30 per minute beyond which the body is unable to sustain the high RR. As the body starts to get tired, not only does the RR drop but also the TV. Now the ventilation is starting to get affected. As a result, the PaCO$_2$ starts climbing; it initially normalises then rises above normal (Figure 5.3b).

In the beginning it is all type 1 respiratory failure (hypoxaemic) and towards the end they are in what looks like type 2 respiratory failure (hypoventilatory) but a wide A-a gradient gives the clue that this was failure of oxygenation to start with (Gas 2). The treatment is not NIV in this instance, because this is oxygenation failure. At this point oxygen alone will not work and you end up intubating and ventilating to rest their respiratory muscles and get the oxygen in. This reduces their work of breathing and corrects the hypoxia. Hence normalisation of the PaCO$_2$ is the first sign that the person is getting tired. So you see, presentation depends on where you catch them on their trajectory.

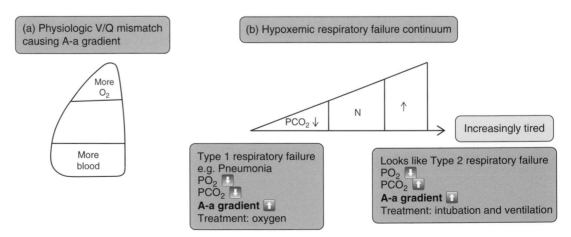

Figure 5.3 Importance of A-a gradient in recognising hypoxemic respiratory failure

5.4 VENTILATION

Ventilation involves moving air into and out of the lungs. Oxygen diffuses across the alveolar-capillary interface more readily than CO_2. Hence the first gas that accumulates in failure of ventilation is CO_2.

Failure of ventilation (type 2 respiratory failure) – treatment is ventilation, often this is by non-invasive ventilation (NIV).

If the ventilation is so bad that you are not moving any air into and out of your lungs, the PaO_2 on your ABG will also drop. How can you distinguish this from hypoxaemic respiratory failure? Well, you can turn to your friend the A-a gradient for help in this instance. In the scenario where the PaO_2 has dropped because the ventilation is so poor, the A-a gradient will be normal suggesting that it is all ventilatory failure and not failure of oxygenation (Gas 1).

Table 5.1 summarises the differences between hypoventilatory (type 2) and hypoxaemic (type 1) respiratory failure.

Table 5.1 Differences in types of Respiratory Failure

Respiratory failure	Hypoventilatory (type 2)	Hypoxaemic (type 1)
PaO_2	Low	Low
$PaCO_2$	High	Low (becomes high when tired)
Minute ventilation (RR × TV)	Low	High
A-a gradient	Normal	Increased

5.5 PLEURAL FLUID ANALYSIS

A pleural fluid pH < 7.2 (done in a blood gas machine) in the right context of suspected empyema is often an indication for chest drain insertion. Normal pleural fluid pH is 7.6. Light's criteria are used to classify pleural effusions into transudates and exudates. An exudate is defined as any one of:

- Pleural fluid protein/serum protein ratio > 0.5
- Pleural fluid LDH/serum LDH ratio > 0.6
- Pleural fluid LDH > 2/3 of the upper limit of normal serum LDH for your laboratory.

Pleural fluid triglycerides >2.8 mmol l^{-1} points to a chylothorax.

6 Chronic Cough

▼

This chapter tells you how to approach chronic cough using pathophysiologic basis of airway disorders, parenchymal disorders, and gastro-oesophageal reflux disease

▲

'Ah! Cough, woe to thee!'

Although this sounds dramatic, cough can be a very disabling symptom that affects life on a daily basis for some individuals. Having a systematic approach to deciphering it and enabling effective therapy would be the ideal goal that many a patient will thank you for.

Patients usually get referred from General Practitioners (GPs) with a chronic cough. Often they would have had a working diagnosis and treatment initiated which may or may not have helped in ameliorating their symptoms. When I see patients in the clinic, I start with their symptoms that originally made them see their GP. This is not because I do not trust the assessment of my colleagues but because often I would have information available to me that may not have been forthcoming on their initial assessment. Symptoms might have changed with or without treatment. There is always the advantage of hindsight and in the fullness of time the diagnosis may have declared itself. So, instead of jumping into treatments and investigations I start with the basics.

Although this chapter talks about chronic cough in the clinic setting, it is by no means limited to it. You would certainly see patients presenting in acute admissions with a worsening of their 'chronic' cough. We then face the dual challenge of not only diagnosing the aetiology of their chronic cough but also that of their acute problem. Often these would have a single underlying diagnosis but there will be occasions when there will be two separate pathologies causing their presentation. Remember, not to close your mind to different possibilities.

Dictum: 90% of immuno-competent, non-smokers, not on an ACE inhibitor, and a non-localising CXR, who present with chronic cough have one of three diagnoses as shown in Figure 6.1.

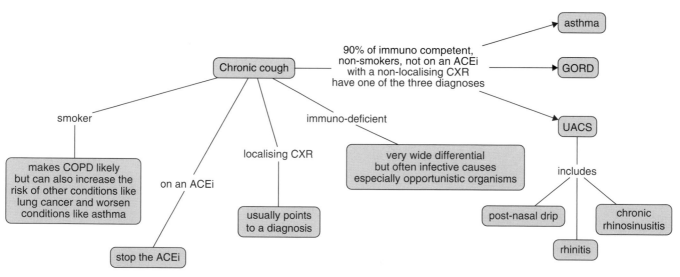

Figure 6.1 Dictum of chronic cough

The Hands-on Guide to Clinical Reasoning in Medicine, First Edition. Mujammil Irfan.
© 2019 John Wiley & Sons Ltd. Published 2019 by John Wiley & Sons Ltd.
Companion website: www.wiley.com/go/irfan/clinicalreasoning

Example 6.1

> GP referral letter:
>
> Thank you for seeing Mr A, a 23-year-old gentleman who has been troubled with a three month history of cough following an episode of chest infection. This was treated with amoxicillin to good effect but unfortunately the cough has failed to clear. He also has hay fever and eczema and he has never smoked. His medication includes cetirizine prn and emollients. A recent CXR was normal. I would appreciate your opinion regarding his diagnosis and further management.

Let's start with the SQs

J: *SQs would be young man, chronic cough, and atopy.*

CONTEXT: Epidemiologically speaking a young man presenting with chronic cough on a background of atopy would certainly raise the possibility of allergic respiratory disorders i.e. asthma. We know from the letter that he has never smoked; hence COPD would be very unlikely although not impossible (α1 anti-trypsin deficiency).

            What other possibilities can you think of?

P: *Could this be post infective cough?*

            Any particular infections that you have in mind?

P: *Viral or bacterial infections like whooping cough.*

J: *Tuberculosis (TB)?*

            Good, TB can certainly present this way and assessing risk factors would be key in this scenario. Any bacterial infection can be followed by a post infective cough. More often it is atypical infections like mycolpasma pneumonia and chlamydophila pneumoniae. However, post-infective cough is a diagnosis of exclusion. In this case it is prudent to exclude asthma in the first instance.

            Asthma (called cough-variant asthma in this case) is high on the cards whichever way you look. I would now like to draw your attention to the dictum for chronic cough. Mr A is satisfying all the criteria for it to be applicable, bringing in gastro-oesophageal reflux (GORD) and upper airway cough syndrome (UACS) into the differential.

            Provisional diagnoses: asthma, UACS, and post-infective cough.

> Mr A walks into the clinic with no objective signs of breathlessness. He reports that his exercise tolerance is unlimited. What do you think his severity of illness is?

P: *Well*

            Good. Can you give me a concept map of the questions that you would like to ask him at this juncture?

J: *Here it is:*

Risk Factors for TB

Personal history of TB or exposure to TB

Immigration from a TB-endemic country

Impaired immunity e.g. HIV

Cough

can be
duration can be
can be
associated with

Acute
Chronic >8 weeks
Other symptoms

Dry
Productive
Sub-acute 3–8 weeks
Episodic
Constant

could have

Diurnal Variation
Seasonal variation
Postural Variation

Figure 6.2 An example of a concept map of history taking in cough

Activity 6.1

(Allow three minutes)

Looks fairly comprehensive! The clinical correlates of asthma have been shown in line with their underlying pathology below:

Airway hyper-responsiveness – episodic symptoms (breathlessness and cough) with acute exacerbations precipitated by triggers.

Variable airflow obstruction – normal or near normal (exercise tolerance and symptoms) in between exacerbations

Airway inflammation – may or may not have sputum, often good response to oral steroids.

Which features of the concept map do you think will fit in with asthma? (Remember to flesh out the concept map in Figure 6.2, from a history taking perspective as you read along. You can print it from the website too.)

J: *The episodic nature of symptoms with diurnal and seasonal variation would be key.*

> Mr A reported episodic cough, which was worse at night and early in the morning. Triggers included cold air, perfumes, and dust. There were no features of UACS or GORD. He denied any recent chest infections and had no risk factors for TB.
>
> He had a normal clinical examination (which can often be the case with asthma given its episodic nature).

Would you confirm the diagnosis with further tests or would you start treatment?

Activity 6.2

(Allow a minute)

Although I cannot peek into your answer I would be happy as long as it includes confirmation of asthma as the diagnosis with objective tests given that he is well. This is particularly essential to help define treatment objectives and expectations – both yours and the patient's.

On the contrary historical information pointing to asthma might be sufficient if you were dealing with an ill or a very ill patient. In this case you would use asthma as a 'working diagnosis' based on which you would initiate treatment. This would then serve to confirm your diagnosis if the patient gets better.

Decisions to investigate and treat are not always text book directed, they are primarily dictated by the clinical urgency of treatment and patient choice. You could still order tests whilst they are on treatment but their interpretation would be difficult and will have to be done in light of their symptoms.

> He had a mannitol challenge test four weeks later which confirmed the diagnosis of asthma, and was started on inhalers.

All clinical encounters do not have such a happy ending. For instance, if you had not found any pointers towards asthma, UACS or GORD you would have proceeded to identify other causes of cough using the concept map and clues you found in the history and clinical examination.

Example 6.2

> A 56 year old woman presents with a six month history of cough with occasional sputum. There is no history of hay fever or eczema.

Write down the SQs and provisional diagnoses?

Activity 6.3

(Allow three minutes)

Epidemiologically a smoker (>20 py (pack years)), aged >35 years with chronic cough and breathlessness is likely to have COPD.

LVF can present with cough.

Inhaled recreational drugs can cause COPD.

J: *SQs- middle-aged woman, chronic cough, intermittently productive. No atopy.*

CONTEXT: Problem seems to be localised to the lung given the productive cough. Epidemiologically it could be COPD, chronic airway inflammation + damage as in bronchiectasis or ischaemic heart disease (IHD) related left ventricular failure (LVF) (clue: middle aged), but could still be asthma, GORD, UACS, and ILD (clue for the last: aged >50 years) – a broad differential indeed.

Ruling out questions: No personal/family history of asthma. No episodic symptoms. No symptoms of IHD, GORD, UACS. No cardiovascular risk factors except smoking.

Confirmatory questions: current smoker 50 py, no recreational drugs. Associated chest symptoms- progressive shortness of breath on exertion (SOBOE) + reduced exercise tolerance (ET) 30 yards. She reported recurrent chest infections requiring antibiotics (likely chronic bronchitis phenotype of COPD but also brings bronchiectasis into focus).

I would class her as *ill* given the poor exercise tolerance and symptom burden. The progressively worsening breathlessness lends credence to the diagnosis of COPD.

J: Why did you include asthma in the differential even though she is a smoker and has no atopy?

That's because smoking is a confounding factor. It can either worsen pre-existing asthma or cause co-existent COPD on a background of asthma. Additionally, late-onset asthma although unusual can still occur in adults hence this has to be kept in the differential. Finally, lack of atopy does not exclude asthma.

Provisional diagnoses – COPD, bronchiectasis.

On examination: Lung fields – Crepitations and wheeze bilaterally. Signs of right heart failure (RHF). CXR: Signs of hyperinflation of lung fields. No signs of LVF or bronchiectasis. ECG: P pulmonale suggesting right heart strain.

Treatment was initiated before further investigations given high symptom burden, using COPD as the working diagnosis.

Follow-up: Sputum microscopy, culture, and sensitivity (MC&S) ruled out on-going bronchial sepsis. Spirometry confirmed an obstructive picture and an echocardiogram excluded LV dysfunction whilst confirming RV dysfunction.

Do you think an echo was needed in this patient? Give your reasoning.

Activity 6.4

(Allow a minute)

This lady is very likely to have cor pulmonale. As the name suggests it is RHF due to pulmonary disorders (COPD) and not due to left heart failure.

A middle-aged lady with no cardiovascular risk factors except smoking and no clinical features to suggest LVF is highly unlikely to have LV impairment. Pre-test probability of finding LV dysfunction on an echo based on the above variables can also be ascertained using Bayesian analysis. On the other hand, the most common cause of RHF is left heart failure which is easily treatable if identified early. You will have to balance the two against each other and lay it out in front of the patient. Since an echo is non-invasive and low risk it is unlikely that a patient will object to it.

The opposing view is that it is an inappropriate use of limited resources when the pre-test probability is low. This camp would argue that lack of improvement following treatment of COPD would justify an echo at that point. I shall leave you to make up your mind as both are valid arguments.

Example 6.3

A 75 years old retired civil servant was admitted for an elective hip surgery which was postponed following a presumed UTI. Whilst being discharged she reported a three week history of dry cough prompting a respiratory referral for possible CAP. She had a history of IHD, diabetes mellitus (DM), and HT.

P: SQs- elderly woman, sub-acute cough, vascular risk factors

Context: Problem seems to be localised to the lung, but 'elderly' rings alarm bells of cardiac dysfunction (note history of IHD) so I'll keep it on the top of the list. The sub-acute cough brings acute bronchitis and CAP into the picture.

What questions would you ask in her history?

Activity 6.5

(Allow three minutes)

Confirmation: On review, her cough was noted to be long-standing which was narrowed down to six months on further questioning. She denied infective symptoms. IHD was stable with no orthopnoea, paroxysmal nocturnal dyspnea (PND), or exertional chest pains. She reported exertional breathlessness with a reduced ET to half a mile six months ago. (Heart failure remains on the list owing to vascular risk factors).

Given the history of IHD she was specifically asked about ACEi which had been started roughly around the time of onset of cough (temporal association). This was stopped by the GP two months ago but the cough had persisted.

Severity of illness: *relatively well* (given low symptom burden, although symptoms are beginning to impact ET). The cough is now chronic which brings new differentials into the picture including airway disease like asthma, COPD, bronchiectasis (dry cough goes against it), and parenchymal disorders like ILD.

Exertional breathlessness keeps LVF in the picture but lack of other symptoms (orthopnoea and PND) argues against it.

Ruling out: Smoking 40 py, current; no episodic symptoms, personal or family history of asthma or atopy.

Angiotensin converting enzyme inhibitor (ACEi) induced cough can take up to four weeks to clear from the time of discontinuation of the ACEi (Yeo et al. 1995).

Significant smoking history and exertional breathlessness brings COPD to the fore.

P: *Provisional diagnoses – COPD, LVF, and ILD.*

On examination: BMI normal. RS: Reduced chest wall expansion bilaterally; fine end-inspiratory crepitations bi-basally in lung fields, which did not clear on coughing. CVS: No signs of decompensated heart failure.

ECG: Q in inferior leads, and CXR: cardiomegaly (both in keeping with history of IHD), but no signs of LVF. Lung fields showed reticular changes especially in the bases with blurred cardiac borders. Spirometry: restrictive.

Fine crepitations which did not clear on coughing bring ILD into the picture, although crepitations can also occur with LVF. However the reticular changes on the CXR and the restrictive spirometry heighten my suspicion for ILD. Of note her BMI was normal as an elevated BMI can cause a restrictive picture and just to confuse, so can LVF. (congested lungs expand less easily).

Her drug list was reviewed and it was noted that she had been on prophylactic nitrofurantoin for two years for recurrent UTIs. She was advised to stop nitrofurantoin as this was most likely causing her ILD. Urology advice was sought for alternatives to the nitrofurantoin.

An out-patient high resolution computerised tomography (HRCT) confirmed the presence of nitrofurantoin-induced pulmonary fibrosis and an echocardiogram ruled out LV dysfunction.

This example illustrates how hypotheses generation is a fluid state of affairs, varying constantly with the context and adapting to changing data.

Remember, emergence of a hypothesis that is not fully explained by prevailing data should trigger ascertaining new data that corroborates it. In other words you go looking for evidence to support your diagnostic hypothesis e.g. looking for drugs (nitrofurantoin) that can cause ILD as well as evidence that refutes other hypotheses (echo to rule out LVF).

▼

Chronic cough in an immuno-competent, non-smoker, not on an ACEi with a non-localising chest radiograph is either asthma, GORD, or UACS in 90% of the cases.

Remember to utilise the concept maps for aetiology of cough, the SQs, the provisional diagnoses and the severity of illness when trying to frame the questions in history taking.

Decisions to investigate or treat are often based on clinical urgency of treatment and patient choice.

Assessing pre-test probability of a diagnosis in question can help in deciding whether to request a test or not.

Hypothesis generation should evolve with changing data and new data should be sought to cement emerging hypotheses.

▲

Reference

Yeo, W.W., Chadwick, I.G., Kraskiewicz, M. et al. (1995). Resolution of ACE inhibitor cough: changes in subjective cough and responses to inhaled capsaicin, intradermal bradykinin and substance-P. *British Journal of Cinical Pharmacology* 40 (5): 423–429.

▼

This chapter tells you how to approach acute breathlessness using the pathophysiologic basis of the respiratory cycle

▲

Breathlessness is a unique symptom in more ways than one. For starters it is quite a complex symptom with varied aetiology arising anywhere along the cycle of respiration, as illustrated in Figure 2.4 in Chapter 2. Secondly, it can be multifactorial in origin, and lastly, it can have a significant psychological component, although this can be said of any symptom, especially pain, e.g. a patient with COPD can be breathless due to problems with the alveolar-capillary interface, deconditioning, and psychological overlay.

From a respiratory perspective breathlessness can largely be conceptualised on the model of the alveolar-capillary interface (Figure 7.1), and can either be sudden or gradual in onset. Sudden onset usually signifies rapidly evolving pathophysiologic processes like infections, exacerbations of chronic lung diseases, mechanical problems like blockage of pulmonary arteries (PE), blockage of bronchi (mucus plug) or lung collapse due to pleural diseases like pneumothorax. All other pathophysiologic processes evolve slowly, thereby presenting as gradual onset breathlessness.

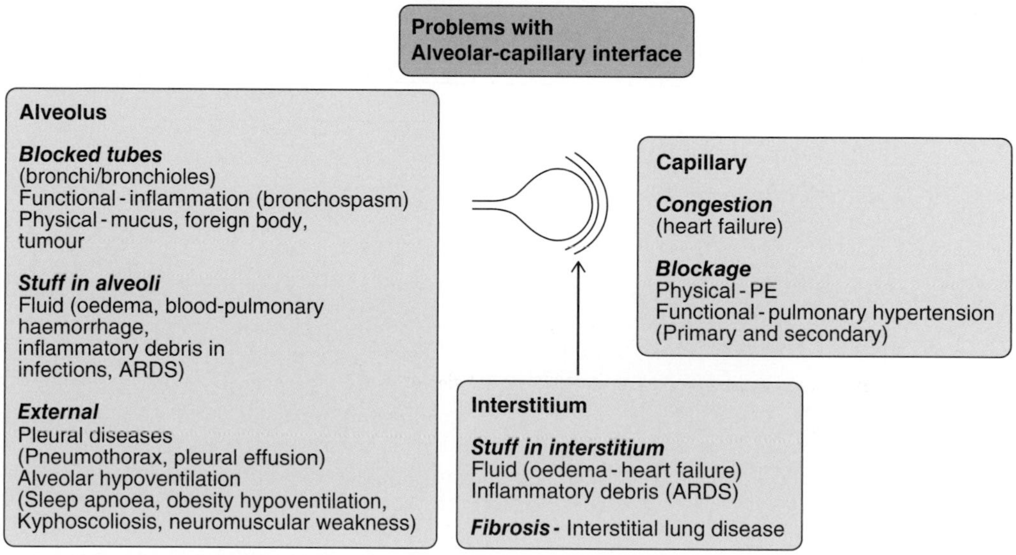

Problems with Alveolar-capillary interface

Alveolus

Blocked tubes
(bronchi/bronchioles)
Functional - inflammation (bronchospasm)
Physical - mucus, foreign body, tumour

Stuff in alveoli
Fluid (oedema, blood-pulmonary haemorrhage, inflammatory debris in infections, ARDS)

External
Pleural diseases
(Pneumothorax, pleural effusion)
Alveolar hypoventilation
(Sleep apnoea, obesity hypoventilation, Kyphoscoliosis, neuromuscular weakness)

Capillary

Congestion
(heart failure)

Blockage
Physical - PE
Functional - pulmonary hypertension
(Primary and secondary)

Interstitium

Stuff in interstitium
Fluid (oedema - heart failure)
Inflammatory debris (ARDS)

Fibrosis - Interstitial lung disease

Figure 7.1 Aetiology of breathlessness at the level of alveolar-capillary interface

If breathlessness develops over a long period of time (weeks to months) the body has time to adapt to it physiologically. Thereby the symptom burden is understated by the patient, i.e. they don't complain of breathlessness, e.g. atherosclerotic coronary artery disease, resulting in progressive LVF. Two things follow:

1. Breathlessness develops insidiously such that the patient eventually presents with an acute insult on top of this underlying problem.

The Hands-on Guide to Clinical Reasoning in Medicine, First Edition. Mujammil Irfan.
© 2019 John Wiley & Sons Ltd. Published 2019 by John Wiley & Sons Ltd.
Companion website: www.wiley.com/go/irfan/clinicalreasoning

2. People tend to limit themselves functionally to try and adapt to the symptom burden. In other words they start doing less and less with a loss of exercise tolerance (ET) over a protracted period of time. This is especially common in the elderly.

On the contrary, if breathlessness develops suddenly, the body has little time to adapt and the symptom burden is enormous. The person concerned notices this immediately, e.g. an acute coronary artery thrombosis causing a myocardial infarction resulting in LVF or a pneumothorax.

It follows that a person presenting with acute breathlessness can either have an acute insult superimposed on a chronic underlying pathology or they can have a new pathology. Your job is to tease them apart – and believe me, this is very exciting to say the least.

Example 7.1

This patient is being managed in real-time with Jenny & Paul accompanying me.

one hour from admission

> I was asked to see a 74 years old man presenting with acute shortness of breath (SOB) for two days. He is a current smoker with a H/O COPD, DM, IHD, and MI.

P: *SQs – acute SOB, elderly male, COPD, vascular risk factors, and IHD.*

Problem seems to be localised to the chest. Given H/O COPD and IHD, exacerbation of either is possible, i.e. infective or non-infective exacerbation of COPD and acute LVF (secondary to an MI or progressive heart failure with acute insult). Given the acute onset other possibilities include community acquired pneumonia (CAP), Pneumothorax (h/o COPD), and PE (presumably poor ET given COPD and IHD causing relative immobility). What questions would you ask in the history?

Activity 7.1

....

....

....

....

....

(Allow four minutes)

J: **Confirmatory questions:** *Worsening cough or SOB, change in colour, consistency or volume of sputum greater than day to day variation* (all define COPD exacerbation). *H/O exertional chest pains, orthopnea, paroxysmal nocturnal dyspnoea (PND), ankle swelling* (cardiac symptoms).

P: **Ruling out questions:** *H/O infective symptoms* (cough + sputum + fever + constitutional symptoms like loss of appetite and lethargy). *Pleuritic chest pain, risk factors for venous thrombo-embolism (VTE), symptoms of PE, deep vein thrombosis (DVT).*

one hour 15 minutes later

> Patient reported symptoms of respiratory infection (difficult to tease infective exacerbation from CAP, as symptoms overlap). No symptoms of cardiac decompensation or risk factors of VTE. Baseline ET 40 yards, now confined to bed.
>
> HR 130 bpm, BP 90/50, RR 32 per minute, Temp 38.6 °C, sats 84% on air, BMs 18 mmol l⁻¹

Severity of illness (Observations + end of the bed appearance + symptom burden): Severe sepsis (see Figure 7.2) + stress response (↑BMs) + problem with alveolar-capillary interface (↓sats) + high symptom burden (confined to bed) = Very ill.

SIRS (systemic inflammatory response syndrome) Infectious or non-infectious etiology. 2 or more of:
Temp >38.3 or <36°C
HR >90 bpm
RR >20 breaths/min
WCC >12 or <4

Sepsis = SIRS + probable or documented infection
Severe sepsis = sepsis + low BP (SBP< 90 mm of Hg or MAP < 70
Septic shock = sepsis induced hypotension not responding to adequate fluid resuscitation (30 ml/kg)
MODS (multi-organ dysfunction syndrome) =
Progressive organ specific dysfunction at severe end of sepsis

Figure 7.2 A way of thinking in sepsis

Once we have identified that he is very ill the priority is to start treatment whilst gathering further information.

Targets: Stabilise physiological derangements.

HR↑ + BP↓ → Give IV fluids, Normal saline or Hartmann's (1 L over an hour or 250 ml over three minutes) Aim: Mean arterial pressure (MAP)> 70 or Urine output >0.5 ml (kg/h)$^{-1}$. to maintain end organ perfusion.

Temp↑ → Send blood cultures and give paracetamol 1 g IV or PO.

Sats ↓ → Titrate FiO$_2$ with a venturi mask to aim for sats 88–92% in the context of COPD. Titrate flow rate in accordance with RR.

BMs↑ → Consider Insulin sliding scale as this reduces mortality in the context of sepsis.

A chest x-ray (CXR) was requested and an ABG obtained (because saturations <92% on air + sepsis evident).

RS: Right base – reduced chest wall expansion and breath sounds, crepitations, dull percussion note, and increased vocal resonance. No wheeze (focal signs + lack of wheeze makes exacerbation of airways disease less likely). CVS: no signs of heart failure. Rest of the systemic examination: normal

IV antibiotics were started in accordance with BTS guidelines/local antibiotic policy.

Activity 7.2

(Allow few seconds)

Given that we had not completed the patient work-up, do you think this was the right thing to do?

Any intervention in medicine must be viewed in terms of its risks and benefits. In this case the risks of an allergic reaction to the antibiotic, the selection of clostridium difficile in the bowels and perpetuation of bacterial resistance to antibiotics if given for the wrong

Fio$_2$	40%
pH	7.32
Na$^+$	132 mmol l^{-1}
PaCO$_2$	5 kpa
Cl$^-$	90 mmol l^{-1}
PaO$_2$	9 kpa
HCO$_3^-$	19.3 mmol l^{-1}
BE	−12
Lactate	4 mmol l^{-1}
Saturations	92%

Activity 7.3

(Allow three minutes)

reasons would be weighed against the benefits of reducing mortality. If, at the point of clinical assessment it is felt that the working diagnosis (severe sepsis) is fairly certain, the benefit of giving treatment (antibiotics) far outweighs the risk of withholding it. This is despite the fact that we do not have the results of the investigations. Remember that in the setting of sepsis, every hour of delay in administering antibiotics increases mortality by 8%.

How would you interpret the ABG shown opposite?

....

....

....

....

....

Oxygenation: Expected PaO$_2$ is 40–10 = 30 kpa, but this is grossly reduced to 9 kpa. An increased A-a gradient of 22.8 confirms our suspicions – there is a problem with the alveolar-capillary interface, and this is hypoxemic respiratory failure.

Ventilation: No problem for now.

Acid – base balance: Metabolic acidosis with a raised anion gap accounted for by raised lactate. Mechanism: sepsis → low BP → poor tissue perfusion → lactic acidosis.

CXR: right basal consolidation confirms the working diagnosis of right basal pneumonia with severe sepsis, hypoxemic respiratory failure, and metabolic acidosis.

The crucial element in these situations is to monitor the response to treatment with regular observations and clinical assessment. Discussion with seniors regarding escalation strategy to ITU or not, in the event of failure to respond to therapy should be considered earlier in the course of admission.

Example 7.2

A 42 year old lady was admitted to the surgical ward with a four day history of constant right upper-quadrant (RUQ) pain. She was a current smoker of 32 pack years. No significant past medical history.

SQs: middle-aged lady, acute RUQ abdominal pain, current smoker.

P: *Provisional diagnoses based on the anatomical site and the acute nature of the pain, would be acute cholecystitis, liver abscess or acute cholangitis. If there was anything in the history to suggest central/epigastric pain the possibility of acute pancreatitis (risk factors), peptic ulcer disease, and rupture of abdominal aortic aneurysm would have to be explored. Referred pain from the back, renal colic, or post-herpetic neuralgia would be other possibilities. The history and clinical examination can help tell them apart.*

The RUQ pain was preceded by shivers and nausea. She denied any cardiovascular risk factors or other abdominal symptoms. No pertinent travel history. O/E: localised RUQ tenderness but Murphy's sign negative. Bowel sounds present. No pulsatile mass. No tenderness in the spine or renal angle. No skin lesions seen.

P: *it seems like a gastrointestinal problem.*

Abdominal ultrasound showed a slightly thickened gall bladder wall, but no dilated intra-hepatic ducts. Bloods: bilirubin $15\,\mu mol\,l^{-1}$, ALT $50\,IU\,l^{-1}$, ALP $130\,IU\,l^{-1}$, Albumin $38\,g\,l^{-1}$; CRP $150\,mg\,l^{-1}$; WCC 14×10^9 per litre with neutrophilia; Clotting profile normal. She was treated for acute cholecystitis.

Four days into her admission, her saturations dropped to 90% on air.

Fio$_2$	0.21
pH	7.38
PaCO$_2$	5 kpa
PaO$_2$	9 kpa
HCO$_3^-$	24 mmol l^{-1}
Saturations	90%

P: *Hmm... Something has triggered the hypoxia. The relative immobility would put her at risk for a PE although she should be receiving thromboprophylaxis. She might have developed hospital acquired pneumonia (HAP).*

O/E: Reduced breath sounds in the right base of the chest but no other signs. The house officer obtained an ABG, requested a CXR, started her on supplemental oxygen, and her saturations picked up. Look at her ABG – what is your interpretation?

Activity 7.4

(Allow few seconds!)

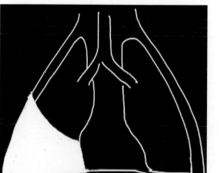

Figure 7.3 Chest radiograph

The house officer noted a widened A-a gradient of 4.7 pointing to hypoxaemic respiratory failure. He concluded that she was having a PE and started low molecular weight heparin (LMWH). The on call medical registrar was contacted.

On review, the patient denied any chest symptoms and looked rather amused at all the fuss. She looked relatively 'well.' She had no history of asthma or COPD. She was apyrexial and her CRP was settling. Clinical examination did not reveal anything new. The CXR was now available (Figure 7.3). The registrar immediately stopped the treatment dose of LMWH and understood the pathophysiologic processes that led to this lady's presentation.

How would you explain the desaturation in the context of the presenting illness?

Activity 7.5

(Allow three minutes)

The sequence of events seems to be:

Right lower lobe pneumonia presented atypically with RUQ abdominal pain due to diaphragmatic irritation. This eventually declared itself with hypoxia from a para-pneumonic effusion. Even though the hypoxia developed four days after admission this is unlikely to be HAP as the presenting symptoms indicated an incubating pneumonia which invalidates the definition of HAP.

The atypical presenting symptoms and the fact that she ended up on the surgical ward resulted in the hypothesis that she had an intra-abdominal problem. This hypothesis blinkered the clinicians into disregarding any other competing thoughts. Despite the non-conclusive blood tests (mildly elevated ALT) and an abdominal ultrasound that is quite common in middle aged women she was diagnosed with acute cholecystitis. These inconsistencies in her clinical picture should have triggered the search for an alternative hypothesis. However, this is something that we are all guilty of as clinicians.

Stepping back from the problem at hand helps. Anatomy is a good aid in such scenarios. For example, RUQ pain should trigger differentials pertaining to above the diaphragm (lungs- pneumonia etc. and heart- pericarditis and myocardial infarction) and below the diaphragm.

With regards to the ABG, this lady was no doubt at risk for a PE owing to her acute illness and the relative immobility. However, the dictum for suspecting a PE with a widened A-a gradient is in the context of a normal CXR and an appropriate history. Pleural effusion, one of the many causes that can widen the A-a gradient, does so by causing alveolar collapse from the outside (V < Q).

Example 7.3

A 60 year old gentleman had a cardiac arrest call. On assessment he was taking shallow breaths and had a cardiac output (peri-arrest). He looked grey, sweaty and was struggling to respond to questions owing to extreme breathlessness. He was two days into his hospital admission for an exacerbation of COPD.

4Hs: Hypoxia, Hypovolemia, Hypo/ hyperkalemia, hypothermia

4Ts: Tension pneumothorax, Tamponade, Thrombosis (cardiac and pulmonary), Toxins

J: *SQs – middle aged man, acute breathlessness, COPD. Severity of illness – dying. Provisional diagnoses – acute exacerbation of COPD, PE, pneumonia, pneumothorax, acute MI causing LVF.*

Good, we have made a start. Note that we did not need his observations to assess the severity of illness. In a dying patient, I tend to revert to stabilising the physiological parameters whilst looking for reversible causes in the advanced life support (ALS) algorithm (4Hs and 4Ts). It sets me on autopilot, whilst freeing my mind to look at other important issues. Remember that you are in a cardiac arrest 'team', so there will be other members to help you.

IV access, bloods, ABG, and CXR were obtained and supplemental oxygen via bag and mask was initiated owing to poor respiratory effort. He was noted to be on thromboprophylaxis. Examination: chest wall expansion and breath sounds reduced on the left with a dull percussion note anteriorly. There was wheeze on the right. Rest of the examination was normal. ECG: Sinus tachycardia.

Activity 7.6

(Allow three minutes)

J: *It can't be a PE because he is on thromboprophylaxis. Can't be an exacerbation as there are focal signs on the left. The findings are incompatible with an acute MI. Can it be a pneumonia?*

Firstly thromboprophylaxis reduces the chances of a PE but does not eliminate it. You are quite right that an exacerbation will often produce bilateral signs, i.e. wheeze bilaterally. Focal signs and normal cardiac examination argue against LVF. What signs would you get in a left sided pneumonia?

Clinical condition	Inspection	Palpation	Percussion	Auscultation
Left upper lobe consolidation				

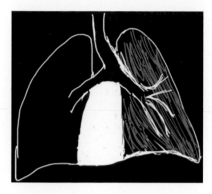

Figure 7.4 Chest radiograph

Activity 7.7

(Allow few seconds!)

J: *Reduced chest wall expansion, dull percussion note, reduced breath sounds and crepitations or bronchial breathing with an increased vocal resonance on auscultation.*

Since he is peri-arrest it would be practically difficult to assess vocal resonance. The reduced chest wall expansion and breath sounds would indicate that air is not getting into the left lung. The dull percussion note suggests that the air in the alveoli has been expelled (consolidation or collapse) or there is something between the lung and the chest wall (pleural effusion).

J: *Could there be air in the pleural space separating the lung from the chest wall?*

Air would cause the percussion note to be hyper-resonant or at least resonant not dull. Based on the explanation of the signs so far what do you think is the diagnosis?

J: *It could be a pleural effusion or collapse.*

One way of telling them apart is by the mediastinal shift. Trachea and apical impulse are pulled towards the lung that has collapsed and are pushed away from the side of pleural effusion. However a combination of the two pathologies can keep the mediastinum in the centre.

How would you interpret the CXR in Figure 7.4?

The lung field is more dense on the left with the trachea pulled towards it and the left hemi-diaphragm is elevated. This is collapse of the left lung. Lung collapse presenting with acute breathlessness in a patient with COPD is often due to mucus plugging. Underlying endobronchial lung cancer or a foreign body are other causes.

The initial CXR on admission showed features of chronic bronchitis but no collapse indicating that this was an acute process. Given the diagnosis, peri-arrest situation and a good pre-morbid status he was transferred to the intensive care unit for further management.

The intention of including this example was to illustrate how emotions can impact decision making. High emotions are a common occurrence in cardiac arrest scenarios where a purposeful calm composure is necessary to avoid heading down the wrong track. This is easier said than done.

Although it sounds insensitive, plenty of practice desensitises one to look at such situations objectively. Setting yourself on auto-pilot e.g. ALS protocols frees your mind to focus on other important issues like escalation of care and deciding when to stop resuscitation. Delegation of duties on a cardiac arrest team breaks down the enormity of the situation into manageable chunks. These are some ways in which you can mitigate the emotional impact on decision making.

▼

Breathlessness from a respiratory perspective can be conceptualised on the alveolar-capillary interface.

Any intervention in medicine should be evaluated in light of its risks versus benefits.

Anatomy is a good aid in hypothesis generation. Remember, chest pathology can present with abdominal symptoms and vice versa.

Emotions can certainly impact clinical decision making and an awareness of the same can help you exercise caution.
▼

8 Acute Chest Pain

▼

This chapter tells you how to approach acute chest pain from a respiratory perspective

▲

We are all taught to exclude life-threatening causes of chest pain as the first line of inquiry. The list typically includes MI, pulmonary embolism (PE), pneumothorax, aortic dissection, and oesophageal rupture (rare). This is a very useful strategy in the acute setting and one that I would stress. However, it is essential that once these have been ruled out, attention is directed towards finding the cause of the chest pain in a systematic manner. This is imperative as the patient concerned will still like to know why they have chest pain even if it isn't one of the life-threatening diagnoses. The concept maps for the aetiology of chest pain in Figure 2.1 would be a good starting point in this exercise.

Before we proceed I have outlined a few points worth mentioning.

1. There are no nociceptive nerve fibres in the visceral pleura and lung parenchyma. Therefore, there is no pain arising directly from them.
2. The mediastinal pleura is in direct contact with the pericardium, myocardium, and mediastinal structures including aorta and esophagus. Hence any disease process that affects these structures can indirectly involve the pleural space and vice versa.
3. Anything that inflames the pleura causes pleuritic pain.
4. Localised chest wall tenderness with pain being reproducible usually suggests musculoskeletal chest pain however there are exceptions (PE, empyema, etc.) and the context helps.
5. Chest pain lasting seconds, no matter how severe, is highly unlikely to be a myocardial infarction.

Example 8.1

A 33 year old man was referred by the GP for persistent fevers, loss of appetite and left sided chest discomfort. He had been treated for a CAP diagnosed three weeks ago.

J: *SQs – Young man + persistent inflammatory symptoms on background of CAP.*

Provisional diagnoses: Given the specific context of what appears to be 'non-resolving pneumonia' I'm thinking of its complications in the first instance, i.e. lung abscess, parapneumonic pleural effusion/empyema. Other possibilities would include:

a. wrong antibiotic
b. right antibiotic but resistant micro-organisms
c. concordance issues and
d. wrong diagnosis

Symptoms had initially subsided with antibiotics. A week later he developed pleuritic left sided chest pain which turned into a dull ache. Over the next few days the fever recurred associated with systemic symptoms of loss of appetite and nausea. He denied any breathlessness.

The Hands-on Guide to Clinical Reasoning in Medicine, First Edition. Mujammil Irfan.
© 2019 John Wiley & Sons Ltd. Published 2019 by John Wiley & Sons Ltd.
Companion website: www.wiley.com/go/irfan/clinicalreasoning

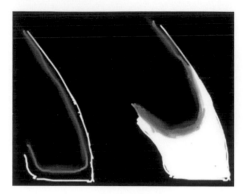

Figure 8.1 Pathophysiology of pleuritic chest pain

J: *The pleuritic chest pain suggests pleural inflammation which could be due to the underlying consolidation. I'm not sure why it turned into a dull ache.*

In consolidation, the overlying visceral pleura gets inflamed (Figure 8.1). With each breath it rubs against the parietal pleura causing the auscultatory pleural rub and the pleuritic pain. The pleura weeps due to the constant irritation/inflammation resulting in a pleural effusion. The parietal and visceral pleura now separate, and the pain disappears. Breathlessness follows due to the lung being squashed by the effusion. This can sometimes cause a dull ache. The same pathophysiology occurs in pericarditis and pericardial effusion.

On assessment he looked 'ill.' He was haemodynamically stable with saturations of 90% on air. Examination was normal. The CXR did not show any effusion and was felt to be normal. Given the hypoxia and the normal CXR, the Consultant Physician requested a computerised tomography pulmonary angiogram (CTPA) to exclude a PE.

J: *A PE would certainly explain the pleuritic pain.*

Can you account for the systemic symptoms with this diagnosis?

Activity 8.1

(Allow three minutes)

....

....

....

....

....

A PE can cause an inflammatory response including fever, raised CRP, and WCC. Multiple ongoing showers of emboli could perhaps cause the two week history of systemic symptoms with some stretch of imagination. However, this would cause significant breathlessness which was strikingly absent. An alternative would be subacute bacterial endocarditis initially presenting as CAP. The right sided vegetations showering septic emboli into the lungs but this would cause cavitation which was again absent on the CXR.

The CTPA was negative for a PE but showed a loculated left sided posterior pneumothorax with a shallow effusion. In hindsight the CXR was felt to be darker in the left hemithorax giving the clue to a posterior loculated pneumothorax. Younger patients with no co-morbidities tolerate acute insults better owing to a higher cardiopulmonary reserve which explained the lack of breathlessness.

He was referred to the cardiothoracic surgeons for further management as an ultrasound guided diagnostic pleural aspiration revealed an empyema and the locule was felt to be well organised.

It appears that the clinicians got side-tracked by the pleuritic pain and went hunting for a PE even though this diagnosis could not explain all the findings. We should always ensure that the working diagnosis explains 'all' the clinical findings, if not, search for one, or two in this case, that do.

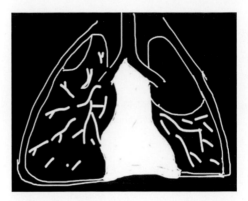

Figure 8.2 Chest radiograph

Example 8.2

A 70 year old man was assessed in A&E for a one day history of acute chest pain. He was known to have COPD and had recently been discharged from the hospital following treatment for a left pneumothorax.

P: *SQs – Elderly man + recent pneumothorax + history of COPD. Provisional diagnoses: Exacerbation of COPD, another pneumothorax, acute LVF as elderly and likely to have underlying IHD (including undiagnosed IHD), PE.*

He looked objectively breathless with saturations of 86% on air. BP 110/70, HR 90 bpm, Temp 37° C, RR 26 per minute. The A&E doctor felt that the patient looked 'ill.' He elicited reduced breath sounds on the left with a resonant percussion note and reduced vocal resonance. There was scattered wheeze bilaterally. The patient was referred to the medical registrar for a chest drain citing a diagnosis of recurrent left sided pneumothorax on the CXR.

How would you approach this patient?

Activity 8.2

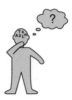

(Allow few seconds!)

P: *The signs certainly seem to be in keeping with the diagnosis. I would like to assess the patient.*

On assessment by the registrar, the patient reported sudden pleuritic chest pain on the left associated with breathlessness. He was saturating at 94% on FiO$_2$ 0.35. On examination there was nothing new. His clinical picture did not seem to match the working diagnosis of a pneumothorax as he expected the patient to be far worse. He initiated treatment for an exacerbation of COPD whilst getting an ABG and reviewed the CXR on which the diagnosis was made.

What is your interpretation of the CXR (Figure 8.2)?

Activity 8.3

(Allow three minutes)

The left upper zone is darker than the rest of the lung fields. However, the margin of the so-called 'collapsed lung' is concave to the chest wall which is against the diagnosis of a pneumothorax and favours a bulla. The best test to confirm this is to compare it with old CXRs.

The recent history of pneumothorax had coloured the vision of the A&E doctor and he put the clinical signs in this context. He fell for the confirmatory bias, i.e. he saw what he intended to see (Cook 2009). One way of avoiding it is to keep an open mind to the diagnostic possibilities and think of all conditions that can give rise to the findings. This patient nearly had a chest drain which would have been disastrous. Always take a step back when you are deciding on an invasive step in management and if you are in doubt ask a senior doctor.

Example 8.3

A 26 year old woman presented in A&E with a two day history of left pleuritic chest pain and breathlessness. She was 32 weeks into her pregnancy and had never smoked.

P: *SQs – young pregnant woman, acute pleuritic chest pain, breathlessness. Provisional diagnoses – PE, pneumothorax. I can't think of anything else.* (Other possibilities include viral pleurisy, CAP).

Exercise desaturation uncovers underlying V/Q mismatch and is found in conditions like: PE, Pulmonary hypertension, Pneumocystic carinii pneumonia and chronic lung conditions like COPD, interstitial lung disease (ILD) to name a few.

She had oesophageal reflux and took Gaviscon prn. She denied any recent infective symptoms or recreational drug use. There were no risk factors for a VTE except the pregnancy and her mum having had PE of no known cause. On examination: HR 110 bpm, BP 110/70, RR 22 per minute. The saturations dropped from 94% on air at rest to 88% after walking in the corridor. Systemic examination was normal and there were no signs of DVT. ECG showed sinus tachycardia.

P: *Severity of illness – ill. I guess PE is the working diagnosis. The Wells score would be 4.5 (moderate probability of a PE). I'm not sure if I could get a CXR as there is a risk of radiation exposure.*

Unfortunately Wells score is not validated for use in pregnancy. Although the CXR carries a small radiation risk, it can point to other diagnoses that explain the findings, e.g. effusion, pneumothorax or a consolidation. An abdominal shield can help reduce fetal irradiation. Moreover, a normal CXR implies normal ventilation (V) which radiologists use in conjunction with the perfusion (Q) component of the V/Q scan.

The CXR was normal, WCC 12×10^9 l, CRP 30 mg l^{-1}, and the PaO$_2$ was 9 Kpa on air. The junior doctor requested a D-dimer arguing that a negative test would exclude a PE. The D dimer was negative.

P: *Well, that rules out a PE!*

Unlike the non-pregnant population, a negative D-dimer in pregnancy only modestly lowers the possibility of a PE (To et al. 2008). This is especially important in our patient who has a high pre-test probability of a PE and there are no other alternatives that explain her clinical findings.

Armed with this information, would you start anticoagulation in this patient before getting a definitive test? Give your reasons.

Activity 8.4

(Allow three minutes)

....
....
....
....
....

Remember the risks v/s benefits ratio. Mortality for untreated PE is 30% (Goldhaber et al. 1999; Laporte et al. 2008). If the pre-test probability of a diagnosis (PE in this case) is high, withholding treatment would be harmful.

The possibility of a PE was discussed with the patient and the small risk of fetal toxicity with a V/Q scan and maternal breast and lung irradiation with the CTPA were explained. She was started on anticoagulation for a presumed PE. Since the CXR was normal a V/Q scan was performed as per the guidelines with the patient's consent.

The V/Q scan was reported as showing high probability of a PE with large peripheral unmatched bilateral perfusion defects. Anticoagulation was continued for three months.

Treatment decisions are based on risks versus benefits ratio. This will also include an appraisal of the risks of anticoagulation against the risks of untreated PE which in this case are tipped in favour of anticoagulation.

▼

Remember the differentials for non-resolving pneumonia.

Ensure that the working diagnosis explains all clinical findings.

Avoid the trap of confirmatory bias.

Remember the pitfalls of PE in pregnancy.

Treatment decisions are based amongst other considerations on an appraisal of risks of treatment against the risks of no treatment.

▲

References

Cook, C. (2009). Is clinical gestalt good enough? *Journal of Manual & Manipulative Therapy* 17 (1): 6–7.
Goldhaber, S.Z., Visani, L., De Rosa, M. et al. (1999). Acute pulmonary embolism: clinical outcomes in the international cooperative pulmonary embolism registry (ICOPER). *The Lancet* 353 (9162): 1386–1389.
Laporte, S., Mismetti, P., Décousus, H. et al. (2008). Clinical predictors for fatal pulmonary embolism in 15 520 findings from the Registro Informatizado de la Enfermedad. *Vascular Medicine* 1711–1717.
To, M.S., Hunt, B.J., and Nelson-Piercy, C. (2008). A negative D-dimer does not exclude venous thromboembolism (VTE) in pregnancy. *Journal of Obstetrics and Gynaecology: The Journal of the Institute of Obstetrics and Gynaecology* 28 (2): 222–223.

9 Acute Haemoptysis

▼

This chapter tells you how to approach acute haemoptysis

▲

Example 9.1

A 72 year old woman with stage IIB non-small cell lung cancer, two months post-lobectomy presents with a two days history of haemoptysis.

J: *SQs – elderly woman, surgically treated lung cancer, acute haemoptysis. Provisional diagnoses – bleeding recurrent endobronchial lung cancer, infection like acute bronchitis or pneumonia, pulmonary embolism (PE).*

I would first confirm if this was truly haemoptysis, i.e. blood on coughing. Any recent nose bleeds or infective symptoms. Amount of blood seen, any clots (signifies large volume), was it mixed with phlegm (implying infection) or not, risk factors for VTE and any other treatment received for lung cancer.

Husband reported a recent course of antibiotics for acute bronchitis. No residual infective symptoms or nose bleeds. Finished last cycle of adjuvant chemotherapy two weeks ago. Small volume haemoptysis with no clots. Blood was on its own. Relative immobility owing to recent surgery. No other risk factors for VTE. History of COPD, on inhalers. Normal ET 300 yd now reduced to room to room.

O/E: Looks poorly. HR 120 bpm, BP 100/60, RR 26/minutes, Saturations 84% on air, Temperature 37° C. Scattered wheeze bilaterally. No signs of DVT. Rest of the examination was normal. PaO_2 8 kpa with A-a gradient of 23.8 kpa on FiO_2 0.4. CXR – right post upper lobectomy changes.

J: *Severity of illness – very ill. It could still be infection induced although there are no residual infective symptoms. A bleeding endobronchial lung cancer cannot explain the significant hypoxia. PE would be on top of the list now. Wells score is eight (high probability). I would start anticoagulation after explaining to the patient and her husband and request a CTPA. There is no point in getting a D-dimer as it is a high probability PE and it would be up anyway because of the recent surgery.*

Excellent! I couldn't have done it any better. The only thing to point out is that significant blood in the alveoli from any cause can drown the lungs resulting in hypoxia which is the mode of death in these cases. However, in this scenario the CXR did not show any new changes, so PE is the working diagnosis.

WCC $12 \times 10^9 l^{-1}$, neutrophils $8 \times 10^9 l^{-1}$, CRP 30 mg l^{-1}. Na^+ 134 mmol l^{-1}, K^+ 3.6 mmol l^{-1}, urea 11 mmol l^{-1}, creatinine 120 μmol l^{-1}. LFTs normal except ALT 50 IU l^{-1}. The CTPA confirms a large saddle embolus at the bifurcation of the pulmonary artery. Her BP on return from the CT scanner drops to 80/60. ECG shows right ventricular strain (T wave inversion in right sided leads – $V_1 – V_3$). She is started on IV fluid bolus to improve her BP and the consultant is contacted.

The Hands-on Guide to Clinical Reasoning in Medicine, First Edition. Mujammil Irfan.
© 2019 John Wiley & Sons Ltd. Published 2019 by John Wiley & Sons Ltd.
Companion website: www.wiley.com/go/irfan/clinicalreasoning

Would you consider thrombolysis for this patient? Explain your reasons.

Activity 9.1

(Allow three minutes)

....

....

....

....

....

This is a difficult situation. However, the answer as usual lies in risk v/s benefit and patient choice. Remember the four principles of ethical decision making. If the patient is unable to participate in discussions, the next of kin will have to be involved. Obviously informing your seniors and letting them make such decisions is imperative but it helps to know their thinking processes.

The mortality in massive PE is up to 50%. Since the lung cancer has been surgically treated this would have little effect on the life expectancy at this point assuming the resected lung margins were clear. Thrombolysis in massive PE reduces all-cause mortality (Chatterjee et al. 2014). These benefits will have to be balanced against the risks of bleeding which are higher in the elderly. Since the surgery was greater than two weeks ago this would not be a contraindication to thrombolysis (Condliffe et al. 2014).

I'm not saying that you need to know all these figures, those will come in time; but I do want you to understand the principles behind decision making. As you can see there is no right or wrong answer but only shades of grey especially in an evidence-free zone. We must learn to accept this uncertainty and individualise treatment in such scenarios.

As the BP failed to improve with medical management the consultant discussed with the husband and opted for half dose thrombolysis given her reasonable physiological reserve. However, the poor prognosis and risks were highlighted. The patient stabilised over the next three days and was discharged in a week back to her home. She received long-term anticoagulation thereafter.

Example 9.2

A 62 year old man was referred from A&E to the medical team with angioedema. Serum tryptase levels were sent and he was given hydrocortisone and chlorphe-niramine. A CXR was documented as being normal.

P: *SQs – middle aged man, angioedema. Provisional diagnoses – exclude anaphylaxis, hereditary angioedema. I would ensure that the airway is protected, and this is not anaphylaxis as the treatment is epinephrine. I would then ask about allergens (food, insect stings), drugs and exclude hereditary angioedema.*

An additional differential would be underlying haematological malignancy (lymphoma, mast cell tumours).

Angiotensin converting enzyme inhibitor (ACEi) induced angioedema can be recurrent and episodic if the ACEi is not discontinued.

Angioedema can occur hours to years after starting ACEi.

Cough can occur two weeks to six months after starting ACEi.

The patient had noticed lip and tongue swelling three days ago. His GP had then stopped the ACEi that was started two weeks ago for hypertension (HT). There was no evidence to suggest anaphylaxis (no urticaria, itching, cardiovascular, respiratory or gastrointestinal manifestations). No other triggers, features of haematological malignancy, or family history of angioedema were noted.

He reported that the swelling was still evident despite receiving treatment in A&E. Recognising that these drugs do not have much effect on ACEi induced angioedema, the registrar reassured him that it takes 72 hours and sometimes longer to settle. He was admitted overnight for observation.

P: *Seems straightforward.*

The next morning, the history was reviewed and confirmed. The consultant re-assessed the CXR and noticed that the right paratracheal stripe was dense. A CT scan showed a right upper lobe mass with superior vena cava obstruction (SVCO), clot in the SVC and cervical, right paratracheal lymphadenopathy.

In the cold light of day, the patient appeared cachectic and was noted to be a heavy smoker (60py). The facial swelling was evidently secondary to SVCO. The SVC was radiologically stented after a cervical lymph node fine needle aspiration was sent. He was started on LMWH for the clot seen in the SVC.

P: *I'm utterly surprised at this turn of events. What made the consultant think of SVCO?*

The ACEi in this case was a red herring. The context of smoking history and cachexia seems to have triggered the possibility of a mimic and the lack of resolution of swelling despite discontinuation might have pushed him into reviewing the CXR. This can only be guessed but the lesson is to always think of other conditions that present with similar clinical features and not get bogged down by someone else's thinking, the latter is called diagnosis momentum.

He re-presents in two months with haemoptysis.

P: *Would you start with SQs again?*

I would, as framing the right context from the very beginning is essential and this is a new presentation.

P: *SQs – middle aged man, haemoptysis on a background of lung cancer, SVCO and clot in SVC, HT. Provisional diagnoses – PE, progression of lung cancer, infection.*

Questions would be along the lines of small volume or large volume haemoptysis, infective symptoms, risk factors for VTE, any treatment received for lung cancer.

I would add a differential of chemotherapy induced clotting disorders, i.e. low platelets, LFT dysfunction (from lung cancer progression or chemotherapy) causing prolonged PT or DIC due to lung cancer.

He had been diagnosed with small cell lung cancer and received chemotherapy, the last of which was two weeks ago. He reported large volume haemoptysis with clots which had now settled. Denied any infective symptoms, chest pain or breathlessness. Had no other risk factors for VTE. He had continued to lose weight and was feeling very poorly.

O/E: HR 100 bpm, BP 110/70, RR 20/minutes, Saturations 92% on air and temperature 36.6 °C. Reduced breath sounds in right upper zone. No signs of pulmonary hypertension. The swelling in the face had gone down and there were no signs of DVT. Rest of the examination was normal.

P: *So far there is nothing to suggest propagation of clot from SVC into pulmonary artery, i.e. PE. I think this is progression of lung cancer.*

Bloods: Hb 90 g l^{-1}, WCC 14 × 10^9 l^{-1}, Platelets 30 × 10^9 l^{-1}, clotting profile normal. CRP 40 mg l^{-1}, U&Es normal, LFTs normal except albumin 26 g l^{-1}. CXR: The right upper lobe mass had increased in size. ECG: No right ventricular strain. Sinus tachycardia. The LMWH was stopped.

Would you have stopped the LMWH? Give your reasons.

Activity 9.2

(Allow three minutes)

....

....

....

....

....

Again, use the risk vs. benefit ratio and ethical principles of decision making. The working diagnosis at this point is progression of lung cancer. The risk of further bleeding is higher if LMWH is continued especially since the platelets are low. This will have to balanced against the risk of the stent being blocked and the possibility of PE which can be fatal. Now, you can use Bayesian analysis to derive numerical indices for the probability of each of these conditions to occur. Although numbers are useful to quote in your conversations with the patient they can be difficult to put into context. For example, say the chances of having a PE by stopping the LMWH is calculated as 50%; if the patient does go on to have one, he experiences a 100% likelihood and the mortality associated with it.

I tend to keep the overall prognosis of the patient in the backdrop, i.e. mortality from the lung cancer. Looking at the patient holistically in this manner is useful to weigh your decisions and involve the patient or relatives in the discussions. Patient choice, their outlook on life and quality of life issues weigh such decisions more heavily than statistical analyses. Each approach has its own merits and I shall leave it to you, to use one you are comfortable with.

> On transfer to the wards he had another massive bout of haemoptysis. Medical management settled the bleeding. Discussions were initiated with the family about palliation as the morbidity/mortality of a recurrent bleed was considered to be very high and the overall prognosis from the lung cancer very poor. Decision not to resuscitate in the event of cardio-respiratory arrest was made in the best interests of the patient owing to the underlying irreversibility of pathology (lung cancer). The patient had a recurrent bleed the next day which was unfortunately fatal.

▼

In the context of PE, haemodynamic instability signifies massive PE requiring thrombolysis.

Avoid the trap of diagnosis momentum.

Evidence poor areas in medicine warrant individualised treatment.

Decision making should take into account a holistic perspective of the patient and not just risks versus benefits ratio.
▼

References

Chatterjee, S., Chakraborty, A., Weinberg, I. et al. (2014). Thrombolysis for pulmonary embolism and risk of all-cause mortality, major bleeding, and intracranial Hemorrhage. *Journal of the American Medical Association* 311 (23): 2414.

Condliffe, R., Elliot, C.A., Hughes, R.J. et al. (2014). Management dilemmas in acute pulmonary embolism. *Thorax* 69 (2): 174–180.

PART II
Cardiovascular Medicine

▼
This chapter outlines a bird's eye view of little tricks and treats to get you started in Cardiovascular Medicine and take a history from this perspective
▲

As before, we start with a quick overview of cardiovascular assessment. This is followed by examples that illustrate the clinical reasoning processes in diagnosis, as well as investigational and therapeutic choices in this context.

Cardiovascular disease is the most prevalent noncommunicable disease on a global scale. It includes:

- Ischemic heart disease (IHD)
- Cerebrovascular disease (strokes)
- Peripheral vascular disease (PVD)
- Atherosclerosis induced aortic aneurysms, peripheral atheroembolism, and dissection.

The common theme that binds them together is the pathological process of atherosclerosis and its complications. Hence disease in one vascular bed is a harbinger of disease elsewhere.

Risk factors that increase the likelihood of cardiovascular disease include:

- Increasing age
- Male gender (higher mortality)
- Hypertension
- Obesity
- Hyperglycaemia (diabetes mellitus)
- Dyslipidaemia
- Tobacco smoking
- Alcohol excess
- Chronic kidney disease and
- Family history of premature vascular disease (first degree relatives <55 in men and <65 in women).

Whilst going through this chapter, remember that the cardiovascular system is not a stand-alone organ system. It interacts with the rest of the systems to cause holistic morbidity and mortality, a point that will be illustrated through various examples.

Concept maps on aetiology of breathlessness and chest pain have been omitted from this chapter as they have already been presented. However, it would be prudent to point out the characteristics of chest pain that point to cardiac ischaemia:

- Central chest pain radiating to the neck, arms or shoulders, lasting for several minutes (usually >20 minutes). Corollary: no matter how severe, any chest pain lasting a few seconds is not cardiac in origin.
- 'Heavy,' 'squeezing' in nature. 'Sharp' pain often reported by patients refers to the intensity rather than the nature, something worth clarifying.

The Hands-on Guide to Clinical Reasoning in Medicine, First Edition. Mujammil Irfan.
© 2019 John Wiley & Sons Ltd. Published 2019 by John Wiley & Sons Ltd.
Companion website: www.wiley.com/go/irfan/clinicalreasoning

- Associated with autonomic features like sweating, sickness, palpitations.
- Often exertional but, cardiac sounding pain at rest signifies unstable angina.
- Relieved by rest (indicates stable angina). Relief by GTN is not specific to cardiac ischaemia.

Counterintuitively, cardiovascular risk factors do not increase the likelihood of acute myocardial infarction but certainly predispose to development of coronary artery disease (Goodacre et al. 2003).

Breathlessness worse in supine position (orthopnoea) and paroxysmal nocturnal dyspnoea are two unique manifestations of breathlessness in cardiac disease although not limited to it. This is due to redistribution of fluid from the peripheries back into the central circulation aided by gravity in the supine position. You have to quantify the orthopnoea in the number of pillows that they use, to sleep comfortably. It helps in objective assessment of disease evolution.

Here are a few terms that will be used frequently in this section.

Structural heart disease: Is roughly translated as an anatomical abnormality of the heart in this book. This could be due to muscle not moving enough (dying/ischaemia) or not moving at all (dead/infarction), valve or pericardial disease.

Ischaemic heart disease: Is a disease of the heart that results from reduced blood supply (coronary artery disease) to the heart muscle.

Transient loss of consciousness (TLOC): Anything that causes poor blood supply to the brain (cerebral hypoperfusion), chemical imbalance (metabolic disturbance, e.g. hypoglycaemia) or generalised electrical disturbance (epilepsy) in the brain can result in TLOC (Table 10.1).

Syncope (Figure 10.1): Anything that causes cerebral hypoperfusion will result in syncope and if the cerebral hypoperfusion is long enough it can result in myoclonic jerks or even hypoxic seizures erroneously diagnosed as epilepsy. Hence history is very important.

Remember: Unexplained syncope + history of significant structural heart disease → cardiac arrhythmia unless proven otherwise.

Table 10.1 Primary differentials of TLOC

Primary differentials of TLOC	Vasovagal syncope	Cardiac syncope	Fits/epilepsy
Pre-episode	Pre-syncopal symptoms e.g. nausea, feeling faint, sweating, vision turning dark.	No warning	May have an aura: visual, olfactory, gustatory.
During episode	TLOC (seconds-minutes) If prolonged can result in twitching or myoclonic jerks.	TLOC (seconds) If prolonged can result in twitching or myoclonic jerks.	TLOC (minutes) Either tonic, clonic movements or, in complex partial seizures, automatisms: lip smacking, grimacing, chewing, repeating words or phrases.
Post-episode	Pallor, sweating may persist. (If prolonged, can result in post-episode fatigue lasting minutes-hours).	Clear-headed immediately upon regaining consciousness.	Lateral tongue biting, urinary incontinence. Post-ictal phase: Fatigue and confusion lasting minutes-hours.

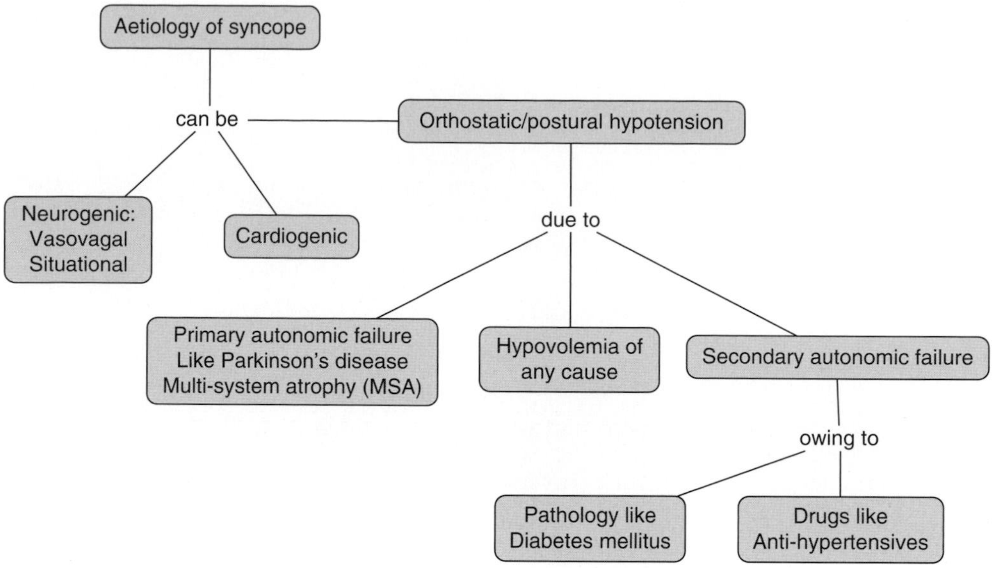

Figure 10.1 Aetiology of syncope

Palpitations (Figure 10.2)

- Anxiety can cause chest pain, dizziness, palpitations, and breathlessness. However, anxiety can also arise as a consequence of organic palpitations, i.e. underlying arrhythmias. A case of chicken and egg.
- Chest pain occurring before palpitations signifies ischaemia induced arrhythmias.

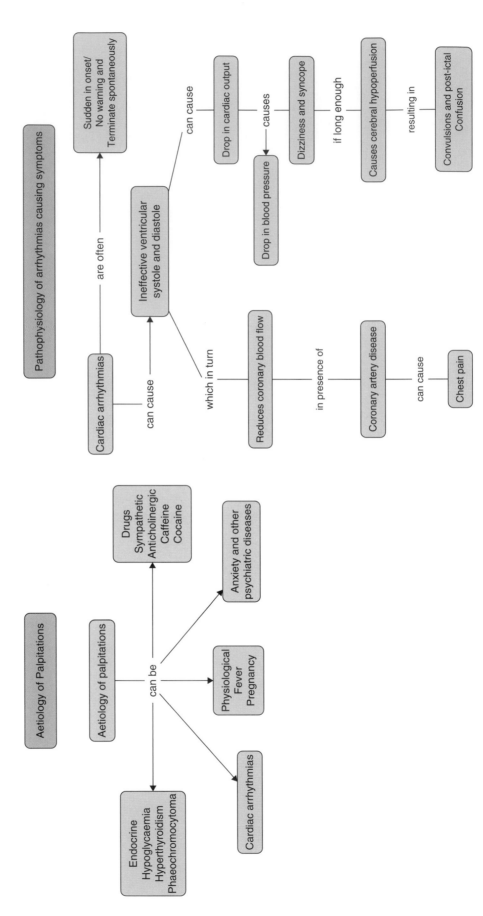

Figure 10.2 Aetiology of palpitations and its pathophysiology from a cardiology perspective

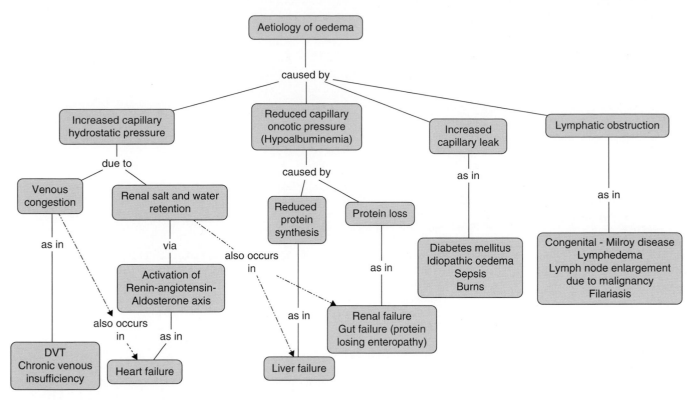

Figure 10.3 Aetiology of oedema based on pathophysiology

Oedema (Figure 10.3):
- Pitting oedema is seen in all failures, hypoalbuminaemia of any cause, venous congestion, and salt and water retention (pathological states and drugs).
- Dependent oedema in the absence of the above causes should trigger the possibility of restrictive cardiomyopathy [infiltrative conditions (sarcoid, amyloid, haemochromatosis, cancer) and fibrosis] and pericardial disease causing restriction. Pathogenesis – restriction of diastolic filling of the heart causes back pressure (venous congestion) and oedema.
- Non-dependent oedema (peri-orbital and facial) is often seen in renal failure, myxoedema, angioedema, superior vena cava syndrome, dermatomyositis, and drugs.
- Dependant oedema in the elderly who sit for prolonged periods of time is due to reduced venous emptying owing to gravity. It is a diagnosis of exclusion. Diuretics do not help as it is not due to volume overload. Mobilisation and elevation of legs when immobile is helpful.
- Non-pitting oedema is seen in lymphedema and pre-tibial myxoedema of hyperthyroidism.

Unilateral leg oedema is often due to localised causes such as:

DVT
Cellulitis
Ruptured Baker's cyst
Compartment syndrome
Extrinsic compression of venous return by enlarged lymph nodes or pelvic tumours.
Secondary lymphoedema due to tumour, radiation, infection (filariasis).

Reference

Goodacre, S.W., Angelini, K., Arnold, J. et al. (2003). Clinical predictors of acute coronary syndromes in patients with undifferentiated chest pain. *QJM: Monthly Journal of the Association of Physicians* 96 (12): 893–898.

11 Clinical Examination: The Orchestra of Sounds

▼

Focusing on relevant clinical features and their interpretation from a cardiology perspective

▲

At first glance, cardiovascular examination can look daunting but the realization that most clinical signs are based on a mechanical model of cardiac function, will immediately alleviate the distress. Looking at the patient as a whole will provide several clues in unraveling the underlying cardiac diagnosis.

Starting with the age, younger individuals should make one think of congenital heart conditions including arrhythmias. Increasing age (>50 years) increases the chances of underlying IHD and its accompanying mechanical problems ranging from a big baggy heart (dilated cardiomyopathy) to arrhythmias requiring insertion of an implantable cardioverter defibrillator (ICD) or a PPM, all clues to underlying IHD in the right age group.

Scars can tell you a lot if you listen to them (Figure 11.1).

Corneal arcus, xanthelasmata around the eyelids and tendon xanthomas, plucked chicken skin appearance in axillae (pseudoxanthoma elasticum) all predispose to IHD. Clubbing

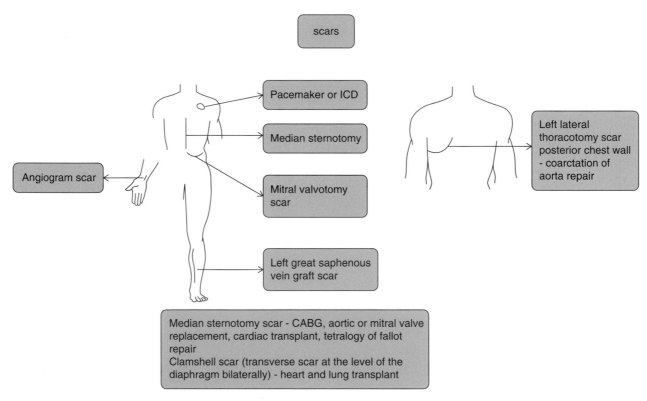

Figure 11.1 Scars giving clues in cardiovascular examination

The Hands-on Guide to Clinical Reasoning in Medicine, First Edition. Mujammil Irfan.
© 2019 John Wiley & Sons Ltd. Published 2019 by John Wiley & Sons Ltd.
Companion website: www.wiley.com/go/irfan/clinicalreasoning

often points to congenital heart disease. Bruises on the skin point to anticoagulation with warfarin and its indications of AF, prosthetic metallic valves and PE.

The radial arterial pulse gives you information about the heart rate and rhythm. Radio-radial inequality in timing and volume (corroborated by difference in systolic blood pressure in the two arms) implies aortic dissection in the right context or more commonly atherosclerotic narrowing of the subclavian artery on one side. Radio-femoral delay indicates coarctation of aorta. An irregularly irregular pulse points to AF as one possibility, which again increases in prevalence with age. AF should also make one think of atrial dilatation and all its causes from a cardiac perspective, the most common being left sided valvular heart lesions and cor pulmonale.

Central pulses like the brachial and ideally the carotid arteries give information on volume and character. The pulse pressure, systolic blood pressure - diastolic blood pressure, normal being 40, gives you a cheat sheet for the volume of the pulse. Pulse pressure >40 implies a high volume pulse and vice versa.

The jugular venous pressure (JVP) is an in-built manometer of right atrial pressure and is a reflection of right sided heart problems. In other words, left heart failure does not cause an elevated JVP.

However, hepato-jugular reflux gives you an indication of elevated left atrial end-diastolic pressure and will be positive in left heart failure. Imagine the left heart is failing; the left atrial wall gets stiff because of higher pressures → high pulmonary artery pressure → high right heart pressure. Now the extra volume of blood you have squeezed by pressing on the right upper quadrant cannot be accommodated in the right heart owing to the high pressures. Where does this column of blood go? It goes the only way it can – up into the internal jugular vein thereby raising the JVP.

The superior and inferior vena cavae (SVC and IVC respectively) and the atria are thin walled. Hence intra-thoracic pressures are easily transmitted to the blood contained within them.

11.1 A FEW CONCEPTS TO NOTE

Pressure overload: implies higher pressure in the ventricles. This often happens in outflow tract obstruction leading from the right and left ventricles (RV and LV, respectively). Common causes include, aortic and pulmonary stenosis, systemic and pulmonary hypertension and HCM (the last affects LV). These result in LV or RV hypertrophy and stiffening of the ventricular walls in order to overcome the high pressure in the outflow tract.

Volume overload: implies higher volume in the ventricles. These result in LV or RV dilatation to accommodate the higher volume of blood. Examples include regurgitant valvular lesions. Dilated cardiomyopathy caused by IHD results in dilatation of the mitral and tricuspid annuli resulting in functional (because the leaflets themselves are normal) mitral regurgitation and tricuspid regurgitation which results in volume overload.

The apical impulse is the outermost palpable counterpart of the cardiac apex. Its location is practically more useful than its subjective characteristics like 'tapping,' 'thrusting' etc. Lateral displacement along the fifth ICS is indicative of pressure overload whilst a 'down and out' displacement to the sixth ICS and lateral to the mid-clavicular line is indicative of volume overload.

S1: Closure of mitral and tricuspid valves. Timed just before the carotid upstroke.
S2: Closure of aortic and pulmonary valves. Timed just after the carotid upstroke. Note that the carotid upstroke coincides with ventricular systole.
S3: Is a ventricular filling sound heard in volume overload conditions which enlarge the ventricles.
S4: Is an atrial 'kick' sound heard in pressure overload conditions. Imagine the ventricles in diastole – the first 75% of blood enters the LV by passive flow from the LA when the mitral valve opens. The last 25% of blood is 'kicked' out of the LA by atrial contraction. When this ejected blood drops onto a thickened ventricular wall (pressure overloaded conditions) it produces the S4. It follows that when atrial contractility is chaotic (AF or atrial flutter) you would lose 25% of your cardiac output as well as the S4. The chaotic atrial contractility is the reason why S1 is of variable intensity in AF.

11.2 HEART FAILURE

Let us use the mechanical model of cardiac function and anatomy to explain the findings in cor pulmonale or secondary right heart failure (Figure 11.2). All you do is backtrack against the anatomical direction of blood flow and you will be able to predict the signs that manifest. You can then use this model to explain left heart failure and other valvular heart problems.

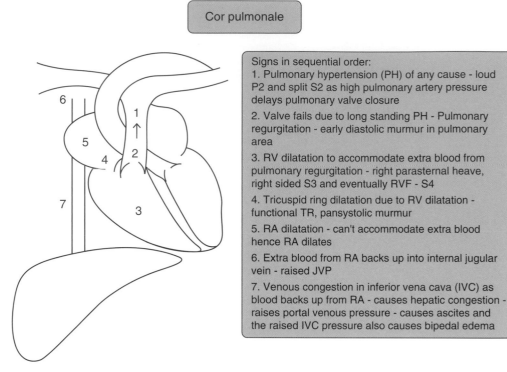

Cor pulmonale

Signs in sequential order:
1. Pulmonary hypertension (PH) of any cause - loud P2 and split S2 as high pulmonary artery pressure delays pulmonary valve closure

2. Valve fails due to long standing PH - Pulmonary regurgitation - early diastolic murmur in pulmonary area

3. RV dilatation to accommodate extra blood from pulmonary regurgitation - right parasternal heave, right sided S3 and eventually RVF - S4

4. Tricuspid ring dilatation due to RV dilatation - functional TR, pansystolic murmur

5. RA dilatation - can't accommodate extra blood hence RA dilates

6. Extra blood from RA backs up into internal jugular vein - raised JVP

7. Venous congestion in inferior vena cava (IVC) as blood backs up from RA - causes hepatic congestion - raises portal venous pressure - causes ascites and the raised IVC pressure also causes bipedal edema

Figure 11.2 Clinical signs of cor pulmonale explained by pathophysiology

11.3 CARDIAC AUSCULTATION

They say that you should be able to deduce a differential diagnosis before you put the stethoscope on the heart! Obviously there would be surprises but that is not the rule. For instance, having deduced that the patient has cardiovascular risk factors with symptoms of left heart failure, you go in search of left sided S3 and S4 ± functional MR with a pansystolic murmur and crepitations at the lung bases. If you do not find these signs you will have to revise the diagnosis.

Here's an analogy that I would like you to consider. Imagine listening to a song with your earphones on. If you wanted to, you could blank out all the sounds of other musical instruments to concentrate on one particular instrument. Now apply the same prowess of your beautiful mind to focus on just the S1 and S2 to start with, timing them in relation to the carotid upstroke, no matter where you put the stethoscope on the praecordium. You then do another round of the praecordium listening intently to the added sounds (S3, S4, clicks, and snaps) and a last round just listening to murmurs. This way there is no danger of missing signs.

Have a look at Figure 11.3 which points out all the relevant areas for auscultation and the best place to listen to a particular sound.

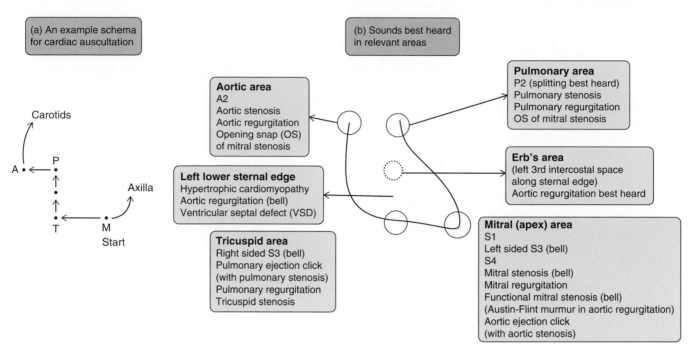

(a) An example schema for cardiac auscultation

Carotids

A • ← P
↑
• ↑
• ↑
T ← M
Start

Axilla

(b) Sounds best heard in relevant areas

Aortic area
A2
Aortic stenosis
Aortic regurgitation
Opening snap (OS)
of mitral stenosis

Left lower sternal edge
Hypertrophic cardiomyopathy
Aortic regurgitation (bell)
Ventricular septal defect (VSD)

Tricuspid area
Right sided S3 (bell)
Pulmonary ejection click
(with pulmonary stenosis)
Pulmonary regurgitation
Tricuspid stenosis

Pulmonary area
P2 (splitting best heard)
Pulmonary stenosis
Pulmonary regurgitation
OS of mitral stenosis

Erb's area
(left 3rd intercostal space
along sternal edge)
Aortic regurgitation best heard

Mitral (apex) area
S1
Left sided S3 (bell)
S4
Mitral stenosis (bell)
Mitral regurgitation
Functional mitral stenosis (bell)
(Austin-Flint murmur in aortic regurgitation)
Aortic ejection click
(with aortic stenosis)

Figure 11.3 Cardiac auscultation

11.4 VALVULAR HEART DISEASE

Valves are uni-directional in the normal state of affairs. Turbulence in stenosed (narrowed) lesions occurs in forward flow i.e. normal anatomical flow. Turbulence in regurgitant (leaky) lesions occurs in backward flow i.e. not anatomical. It follows that stenotic lesions produce a murmur in forward flow and regurgitant lesions in backward flow.

Take aortic stenosis for instance. The name says it is a stenotic lesion of the aortic valve which sits between the LV and the aorta. We know that stenotic lesions produce a murmur in forward flow, i.e. LV → aorta. The only phase of the cardiac cycle when this would happen is ventricular systole, making it a systolic murmur.

Mitral regurgitation: the name says it is a regurgitant lesion of the mitral valve which sits between the LA and LV. The normal direction of blood flow across this valve is LA → LV. Regurgitant lesions produce a murmur in backward flow, i.e. LV → LA. The only phase when this can happen is ventricular systole making it a systolic murmur.

Mitral stenosis: stenosis of mitral valve which sits between LA and LV. Normal direction of blood flow LA → LV. Stenotic lesions produce a murmur in forward flow which is LA → LV. The only phase when this can happen is ventricular diastole making it a diastolic murmur.

Use this thinking process to come up with the murmurs that you hear in the following conditions: mitral and aortic regurgitation, pulmonary and tricuspid stenosis and regurgitation and fill in the relevant boxes in Table 11.1.

The phase of systole or diastole when the murmur is most prominent can be deciphered based on the phase when there is maximum pressure difference between the two participating compartments. For example, in aortic stenosis, the maximum pressure difference exists in the beginning of ventricular systole when the LV is contracting against a narrowed aortic orifice. Hence it is an ejection systolic murmur.

Table 11.1 Clinical features of valvular heart disease. Fill in the missing information to make it your own

Valvular lesion	Volume/Pressure overload from ventricular perspective	Apical impulse position	Heart sounds	Added sounds (snaps, clicks)	Direction of turbulent blood flow (forward/ backward)	Primary murmur (systolic/ diastolic)
Aortic stenosis	Pressure overload	Lateral displacement	Soft S2, S4 if severe	Ejection click	Forward	Systolic
Aortic regurgitation	Volume overload		Left sided S3 S4 if in LVF	None		Diastolic
Mitral stenosis	None	Not displaced		Opening snap	Forward	Diastolic
Mitral regurgitation		Down and out	Left sided S3 S4 if in LVF		Backward	
Tricuspid regurgitation			Right sided S3 S4 in RVF			
Tricuspid stenosis						
Pulmonary stenosis						
Pulmonary regurgitation						
Hypertrophic cardiomyopathy	Pressure overload	Lateral displacement	Left sided S4		Forward	Systolic

Mitral regurgitation: The pressure difference remains elevated between the high pressure LV and the low pressure LA throughout systole making it a pansystolic murmur.

Mitral stenosis: The LA pressure builds up until it snaps open (opening snap) the mitral valve followed by a mid-diastolic trickling murmur.

Aortic regurgitation: The pressure difference is at its maximum in early diastole when the ventricle has just begun to relax and nearly empty making it an early diastolic murmur.

11.5 HAEMODYNAMIC ACCENTUATION MANOEUVRES

Since murmurs are caused by turbulent blood flow, having a greater volume of blood in the heart will increase the turbulence/intensity of the murmur and vice versa. The only exceptions to this rule are MVP and HCM. Manoeuvres that increase blood volume are squatting and leg raising, whilst standing and valsalva manoeuvres decrease blood volume. Inspiration increases venous return to the right heart (and therefore accentuates right sided murmurs) and expiration does the opposite. Sustained hand grip (20–30 seconds) increases arterial pressure and LV volume. It reduces the intensity of the murmur in aortic stenosis and worsens it in mitral regurgitation.

Let us summarise everything we have learnt so far in a tabular fashion (Table 11.1). I have got you started with aortic stenosis. Use the principles learnt to fill in the rest.

12 Interpretation of Chest Radiographs: Let There Be Light

▼
Having a framework to hang things on
▲

Although we will be discussing chest radiograph interpretation from a cardiology perspective this does not imply scrutinising it in isolation from the lungs and the surrounding structures. In reality you will be blending everything into one when you look at a CXR.

The heart lies rotated in the chest, i.e. the right side of the heart lies in front of the left side with a slither of left atrium and left ventricle peeping on the left. The mediastinal silhouette on a CXR will thus have to be interpreted in this light. Figure 12.1 illustrates this.

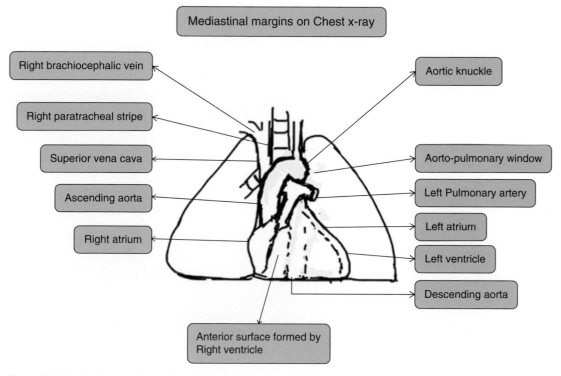

Figure 12.1 Mediastinal margins on chest radiograph

12.1 PULMONARY OEDEMA

Pulmonary oedema can be cardiogenic (Figure 12.2) or non-cardiogenic. The pathophysiology of cardiogenic oedema is: raised left ventricular filling pressures (end-diastolic pressure) → raised left atrial pressure → raised pulmonary venous pressure (upper lobe blood diversion) → raised capillary hydrostatic pressure → fluid leaks into the pulmonary interstitium (septal lines, subpleural oedema, bronchial wall thickening, hilar haze, lamellar oedema) → then floods the alveoli (alveolar oedema – bat's wing pattern). Of note, it is hypothesised that peri-bronchial interstitial oedema causes 'cardiac asthma' with wheezing.

The Hands-on Guide to Clinical Reasoning in Medicine, First Edition. Mujammil Irfan.
© 2019 John Wiley & Sons Ltd. Published 2019 by John Wiley & Sons Ltd.
Companion website: www.wiley.com/go/irfan/clinicalreasoning

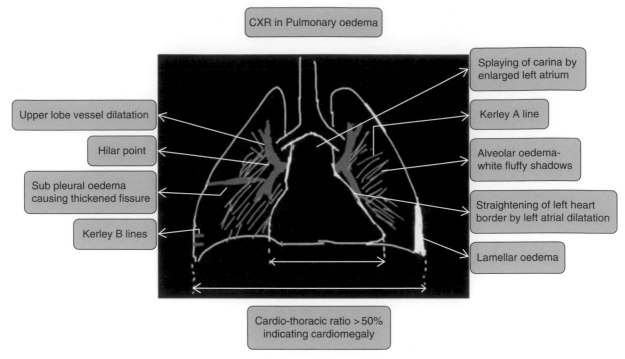

CXR in Pulmonary oedema

Splaying of carina by enlarged left atrium

Upper lobe vessel dilatation

Kerley A line

Hilar point

Alveolar oedema- white fluffy shadows

Sub pleural oedema causing thickened fissure

Straightening of left heart border by left atrial dilatation

Kerley B lines

Lamellar oedema

Cardio-thoracic ratio > 50% indicating cardiomegaly

Figure 12.2 CXR in pulmonary oedema

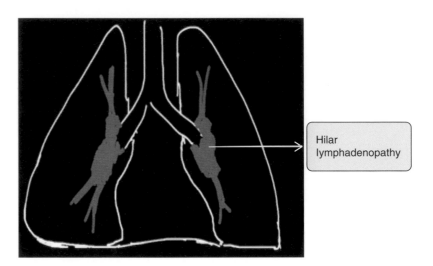

Hilar lymphadenopathy

Figure 12.3 Bilateral hilar lymphadenopathy

Unlike consolidation where radiographic change lags behind clinical features, hydrostatic pulmonary oedema usually induces rapid changes on CXR which clear with similar rapidity on treatment. Similarly, the changes can be positional. Although bat's wing/ butterfly pattern is classically defined as bilateral perihilar shadowing with sparing of outer lung fields, asymmetric changes are common. This is especially in the presence of background lung disease which indirectly affects pulmonary vasculature in diseased lobes.

A few features in Figure 12.2 need explanation: Lamellar oedema is subpleural oedema, so called because of its shape. Kerley A lines are deep septal lines seen in upper and middle zones stretching 4 cm from the hila to the middle of the chest. Kerley B lines are interlobular septal lines in the lower zones, <1 cm in length at right angles to the pleura and running parallel to each other. The hilar point is the angle between the superior pulmonary vein and the inferior pulmonary artery (Ellis and Flower 2006). It helps in assessing vascular congestion as the pulmonary vein would be engorged. It is also useful in detecting hilar lymphadenopathy as the concave angle is filled resulting in a convex margin (Figure 12.3).

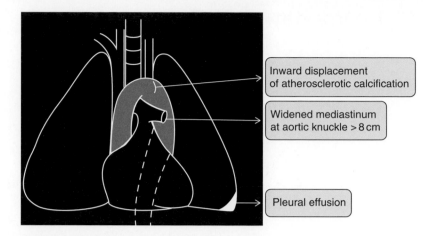

Figure 12.4 Aortic dissection

Presence of pacemaker, implantable cardiovertor defibrillator, prosthetic valves, and median sternotomy wires from coronary artery bypass graft (CABG) all point to cardiogenic pulmonary oedema in the right context. Lastly, mediastinal widening in the appropriate clinical context suggests aortic dissection (Figure 12.4).

Reference

Ellis, S. and Flower, C. (2006). *The WHO Manual of Diagnostic Imaging*. World Health Organization. ISBN: 9241546778.

13 Interpretation of Electrocardiograms: The Rhythm of Life

A complete treatise on ECG interpretation is out of the scope of this book. A practical approach to common clinical problems is what we will be aiming for.

The sino-arterial (SA) node is the intrinsic pacemaker of the heart. Waves of depolarization spread from the SA node towards the apex and are followed by waves of repolarisation. As this wave spreads, an electrical current (electrical dipole) is generated that flows from the depolarized regions of the heart to the polarised (resting) areas of the heart which is recorded in the shape of ECG complexes. One such complex has been illustrated in Figure 13.1.

A few concepts that will help in understanding the ECG:

1. Resting cardiac myocyte has a negative charge inside the cell relative to the ECF, i.e. membrane potential (V_m) is $-90\,mV$. Influx of positive charge causes depolarization, thus V_m becomes more positive (closer to zero). Therefore, depolarization is a positive vector and repolarisation is a negative vector.
2. A positive vector moving towards a positive lead causes an upward deflection and vice versa.

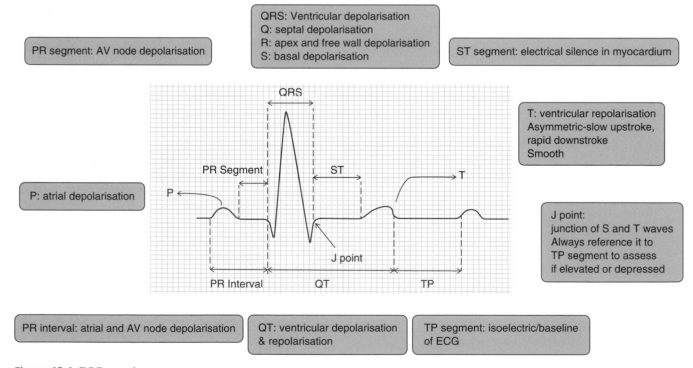

PR segment: AV node depolarisation

QRS: Ventricular depolarisation
Q: septal depolarisation
R: apex and free wall depolarisation
S: basal depolarisation

ST segment: electrical silence in myocardium

P: atrial depolarisation

T: ventricular repolarisation
Asymmetric-slow upstroke, rapid downstroke
Smooth

J point:
junction of S and T waves
Always reference it to
TP segment to assess
if elevated or depressed

PR interval: atrial and AV node depolarisation

QT: ventricular depolarisation & repolarisation

TP segment: isoelectric/baseline of ECG

Figure 13.1 ECG complex

The Hands-on Guide to Clinical Reasoning in Medicine, First Edition. Mujammil Irfan.
© 2019 John Wiley & Sons Ltd. Published 2019 by John Wiley & Sons Ltd.
Companion website: www.wiley.com/go/irfan/clinicalreasoning

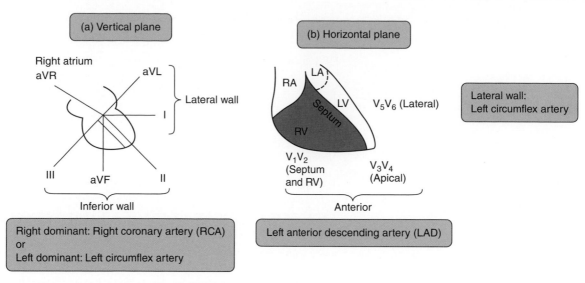

Figure 13.2 Anatomical and physiological orientations of ECG leads

3. The heart lies rotated in the chest, i.e. the right side of the heart is in front of the left side such that the left atrium is the posterior-most part of the heart. The interventricular septum lies in the frontal plane with the right ventricle (RV) in the front and left ventricle (LV) behind it. So V1 and V2 look at both RV and the septum (Figure 13.2b).
4. The interventricular septum depolarizes from left to right causing the R (positive) in V1 and physiological q (negative) in V5, 6.
5. The ventricular muscle depolarizes from endocardium to epicardium and repolarises in the reverse order. This is because the contracting ventricular muscle wall squeezes the subendocardial coronary vessels more than the subepicardial ones. Hence the subepicardial region repolarises faster than the transiently blood starved subendocardial region.
6. Repolarisation is a negative vector. A negative vector moving away from a positive lead causes a net positive deflection. Therefore, the normal T wave is upright in all leads except aVR and V1.
7. The TP segment is the isoelectric line of the ECG.

13.1 ECG COMPLEX

ECG tracings have time on the X axis and voltage (mV = millivolts) on the Y axis. The standard speed at which the paper rolls under the recording stylus is 25 mm/second. The ECG paper has 1 mm square boxes in a grid and 1 mm horizontally = 0.04 seconds and 10 mm vertically = 1 mV on the Y axis.

Heart rate: Regular rhythm – heart rate = 300/number of large boxes between two successive R waves. Irregular rhythm – heart rate = number of QRS complexes on the rhythm tracing of lead II at the bottom X 6. This is because a standard 12 lead ECG records for 10 seconds.

P: Three small squares in length and 2½ small squares in height. The first part of the P wave is RA depolarization and the second part is left atrial (LA) depolarisation. Biphasic P wave in V1- Depolarization of the right atrial (RA) towards V1 causes the initial positive deflection in the P wave and the wave moving to the LA posteriorly, away from V1 causes the negative deflection. The same logic causes the P wave to be tall in RA enlargement (takes longer for RA to depolarize) and wide in LA enlargement (takes longer for LA to depolarize).

PR interval: 3–5 small squares.

PR segment: atrial repolarisation (atrial ST) is normally masked within the PR segment. In pericarditis, the PR segment is depressed especially in lead II reflecting atrial current of injury similar to the current of injury seen in MI causing ST elevation.

Q: any Q waves in V2, V3 or Q in other leads roughly ≥1 small square in height and width signify prior MI (Thygesen et al. 2012).

QRS: up to 3 small squares. >3 small squares signify bundle branch block.

ST segment: electrical silence in myocardium between depolarization and repolarisation.

QT interval: includes the QRS complex, therefore can be prolonged in bundle branch blocks which widen the QRS duration. Always consider this when QT is prolonged. Varies with heart rate and is therefore corrected ($QT_c = QT \div \sqrt{RR}$ interval (respiratory rate)). Normal range – men <0.44 seconds and women <0.45 seconds.

T: is smooth and asymmetric. Any bump on the smooth surface of T implies an embedded P.

13.2 ECG CHANGES IN MYOCARDIAL ISCHEMIA AND INFARCTION

A 12-lead ECG consists of six limb leads and six chest leads as shown in the Figure 13.2. The limb leads look at the heart in a vertical plane and the chest leads in a horizontal plane. The orientation of individual leads and their combination looking at the different walls of the left ventricle has also been shown. These walls are supplied by coronary artery territories as indicated.

ST depression on its own often signifies ischemia rather than necrosis. It is of three types: horizontal/planar, downsloping, and upsloping. The first two are ischemic in origin, whilst upsloping for instance, can occur with digoxin.

In subendocardial infarction, the current of injury flows away from the ECG leads (epicardium → endocardium) causing ST depression. These ECG changes are common to both unstable angina (UA) and non-ST elevation myocardial infarction (NSTEMI). A positive troponin result (indicating necrosis) in NSTEMI alone distinguishes it from UA.

ECG criteria for diagnosis of ST elevation myocardial infarction (STEMI) (Thygesen et al. 2012):

ST elevation ≥1 mm in two or more contiguous leads in all leads except V2 and V3.

In leads V2 and V3 – ST elevation ≥2 mm in men ≥40 years or ≥ 2½ mm in men <40 years or ≥ 1 ½ mm in women.

Note: J point elevation is referenced to TP segment when assessing ST elevation. Contiguous leads are leads grouped according to the wall they face as shown in Figure 13.2. ex: II, II, and aVF are contiguous.

Time course of ECG changes in MI:

1. Hyperacute T waves (minutes) – tall, symmetric. Signify ischemia rather than necrosis.
2. Early Q waves (within six hours) in leads **with ST elevation** in some cases which disappear with reperfusion. Therefore, Q waves on ECG with chest pain in right context demand reperfusion therapy. Do not assume it is an old MI. (Nable and Brady 2009).
3. ST elevation – signifies necrosis. ST segment is normally electrically silent. The necrosed myocardium repolarises (more negative intracellularly) faster than healthy surrounding myocardium. The ECF around the necrosed myocardium is thus positive compared to the surrounding myocardium. A 'current of injury' flows from negative (depolarised) to positive (repolarised), i.e. healthy myocardium → necrosed region (towards the ECG leads) causing an ST elevation.

4. Reciprocal changes in mirror image leads are the same ST elevations seen from the opposite wall as ST depressions. These are an important component in the diagnosis of STEMI (Brady et al. 2002). In general, anterior STEMI causes reciprocal changes in inferior leads and vice versa.
5. T wave inversion – signifies epicardial infarction in the setting of STEMI.
6. Normalisation of ST segment – when the affected tissue dies there are no currents of injury and ST elevation settles.
7. Late Q waves – transmural infarct acts as a window through which the ECG lead gets a direct view of the opposite wall. The posteriorly directed depolarisation wave on the opposite wall results in a negative deflection, i.e. Q wave.

Posterior wall infarction: Whenever you see ST/T changes in inferior leads think of posterior wall infarction (left dominant circulation) or right ventricular infarction (right dominant circulation). Posterior wall infarction – reciprocal changes of ST depression/T wave inversion are seen in V1, V2 which look at the posterior wall from the front. Right ventricular infarction is suggested by ST elevation in V1.

STEMI mimics are best distinguished with history, examination and comparison with old ECGs if available:

LV aneurysm (lack of reciprocal ST depression), LBBB, pericarditis and Brugada syndrome are few examples.

13.3 OTHER COMMON ECG ABNORMALITIES

Left ventricular hypertrophy (LVH): more electrical activity in muscular LV causes taller and wider QRS complexes in lateral leads (V5, 6, I and aVL) with left axis deviation. Lateral T wave inversion or ST depression in leads with tall R waves reflecting relative subendocardial ischemia because of more muscle mass. Voltage criteria: S in V1 + R in V5 or $6 \geq 35$ mm.

Right ventricular hypertrophy (RVH): more electrical activity in muscular RV causes tall and wide (incomplete RBBB) QRS complexes in right sided leads (V1 and V2) with right axis deviation. ST depression and T wave inversion in right ventricular leads V1 and V2.

Right bundle branch block (RBBB): wide QRS > 3 small squares in width in right praecordial leads V1 and V2. RSR[1] or 'M' pattern in V1 and V2. RSR[1] – initial positive R from left to right septal depolarisation, negative S from LV depolarisation and another positive R[1] by the depolarisation wave from LV towards RV as right bundle has blocked. Cannot interpret ST, T wave changes of MI in right sided leads in presence of RBBB.

Left bundle branch block (LBBB): wide QRS > 3 small squares in width and broad or notched R wave in lateral leads. Cannot interpret ST, T wave changes of MI in presence of LBBB.

First degree heart block: PR interval > 5 small squares in duration.

Second degree heart block: Type 1 – progressively lengthening PR interval with dropped QRS. Type 2 – infra-Hisian (below bundle of His), therefore PR interval constant and QRS widened but occasional P waves can fail to be accompanied by a QRS.

Third degree heart block: No relationship between P and QRS complexes. PP interval (sinus rate) and RR interval (ventricular escape rate usually around 40 bpm) however remain constant. Type two second degree heart block and third degree heart block often need a pacemaker.

13.4 MEAN QRS AXIS

The sum total of all electrical vectors that flow through the myocardium in a vertical plane is the mean axis. In general, the wave of depolarization spreads from the SA node towards the apex and is dominated by the LV as this has the most muscle mass in a normal heart (more muscle = more electrical activity). Hence the major vector is towards leads I and II on the left.

Quadrant method to determine axis: decide if the predominant deflection of QRS complex in leads I, II, and aVF is positive or negative. See Figure 13.3 for interpretation.

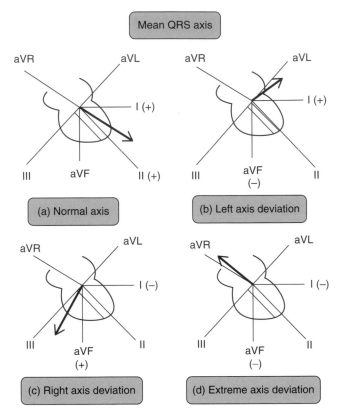

Figure 13.3 Quadrant method to determine mean QRS axis on ECG

References

Brady, W.J., Perron, A.D., Syverud, S.A. et al. (2002). Reciprocal ST segment depression: impact on the electrocardiographic diagnosis of ST segment elevation acute myocardial infarction. *The American Journal of Emergency Medicine* 20 (1): 35–38.

Nable, J.V. and Brady, W. (2009). The evolution of electrocardiographic changes in ST-segment elevation myocardial infarction. *The American Journal of Emergency Medicine* 27 (6): 734–746.

Thygesen, K., Alpert, J.S., Jaffe, A.S. et al. (2012). Third universal definition of myocardial infarction. *Circulation* 126 (16): 2020–2035.

14 Palpitations

This chapter tells you how to approach cardiac arrhythmias as a cause of palpitations

Any cardiac arrhythmia ranging from sinus tachycardia to ventricular tachycardia can cause palpitations. Deciphering the cause is important as this would mean a world of difference in their management. Often times the ECG is the clinching piece of evidence but the context is still key.

Example 14.1

> A 67 year old lady is referred by the GP for AF. She has a history of hypertension and diabetes mellitus for which she takes ramipril and gliclazide. Blood results on admission showed a mildly elevated highly sensitive (hs) troponin T of 20 ng l^{-1} (normal <14 ng l^{-1}).

P: SQs – AF + middle aged lady + Vascular risk factors (hypertension, diabetes mellitus) + raised troponin.

What provisional diagnoses can you think of?

Activity 14.1

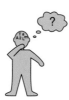

(Allow few seconds!)

A middle aged lady with vascular risk factors makes one think of incipient IHD in the first instance. Any cardiovascular risk factors with increasing age increase the risk of developing AF. We would certainly have to keep an open mind about secondary risk factors for AF like sepsis, hyperthyroidism, etc. The raised troponin should be accounted for with a targeted history (Thygesen et al. 2010).

> Upon exploring why, she went to see the GP in the first place it turned out that she had been troubled by a four month history of fatigue. The GP had then picked up AF incidentally. She was a non-smoker and her exercise tolerance was around half a mile on the flat. There were no symptoms suggestive of IHD, recent chest pain within the last two weeks, hyperthyroidism or palpitations. Her diabetes was well controlled.
>
> On examination: Pulse 140 bpm irregularly irregular, BP 130/80, Saturations 96% on air, RR 14 per minute and temperature 36.6 °C. No signs of heart failure. Rest of the systemic examination was normal.

The Hands-on Guide to Clinical Reasoning in Medicine, First Edition. Mujammil Irfan.
© 2019 John Wiley & Sons Ltd. Published 2019 by John Wiley & Sons Ltd.
Companion website: www.wiley.com/go/irfan/clinicalreasoning

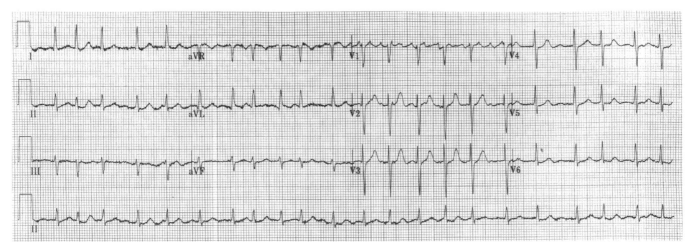

Figure 14.1 ECG

What is your interpretation of the ECG shown in Figure 14.1?

....

....

....

....

....

P: *It's narrow complex tachycardia with a heart rate of 132 bpm. There are no P waves, the RR interval is irregular, no acute ST, T wave changes. Severity of illness – ill as her pulse is 140 bpm. Working diagnosis – new onset fast AF.*

A pulse of 140 bpm taken in isolation can make you feel that she is 'ill.' However, this heart rate is asymptomatic implying a very low symptom burden. I would class her as 'relatively well' but I appreciate that everybody has their own threshold.

Hb 130, WCC 12, CRP 20. U&Es, LFTs and TFTs were normal. The admitting doctor started bisoprolol 2.5 mg to control the heart rate and treated her for acute coronary syndrome (ACS) in view of the raised troponin. A CXR done later was normal.

P: *There doesn't seem to be any obvious cause for the AF like dehydration or sepsis. I agree that this is an MI especially with the raised troponin.*

MI rarely presents with AF alone. If the history was more suggestive of ischemic sounding chest pain or there were ischemic changes on ECG one could certainly consider an MI. Fast AF can however cause type 2 MI with a raised troponin (demand supply imbalance inducing ischemia – see common clinical conditions) but this is not amenable to antithrombotic therapy or coronary intervention as the primary pathology is not atherosclerotic plaque rupture. In this case reducing the heart rate alleviates the ischemia.

An echocardiogram can also help rule out myocardial necrosis by assessing regional wall motion abnormalities (ischemic muscle part moves slowly and abnormally – dyskinesis and infarcted muscle part does not move at all – akinesis).

Repeat troponin 12 hours later was normal and ACS treatment was stopped. Since the duration of AF was unknown she was advised to have an echocardiogram with a view to cardioversion in three weeks whilst on anticoagulation if the echo was normal. Pros and cons of anticoagulation were explained and long-term warfarin was started as the CHA_2DS_2-VASc score was four (high risk of embolic stroke).

The raised troponin was wrongly ascribed to ACS. If one were to turn this around and ask, what was the pre-test probability of an MI in this context; the raised troponin could then have been evaluated in this light. If doubt persists one can treat ACS if benefits outweigh the risks. However, continuing with a systematic approach when a test result throws us off the track ensures that the correct diagnosis is reached.

Example 14.2

An on call doctor was fast-bleeped to the ward to review a 54 year old lady for tachycardia and a sudden drop in BP.

J: *SQs – middle aged lady + undefined tachycardia + hemodynamic instability. Provisional diagnoses: There is a wide differential for the tachyarrhythmia. Middle aged lady does make me think of underlying IHD.*

On arrival, the nurses reported a BP of 70/40, Pulse 160 bpm, RR 30 per minute, Temperature 38 °C, saturations 90% on air and capillary blood glucose 12 mmol l⁻¹. The patient looked grey and sweaty. She appeared confused and responded with groans.

J: *Severity of illness – very ill. Would you call this a peri-arrest situation?*

Yes, definitely.

J: *I would put out a crash call for the cardiac arrest team. I don't know where to begin though!*

The cardiac arrest team leader assigned IV access and bloods to one of the team members, ABG to another and the anaesthetist took over control of the airway. A 12 lead ECG and a CXR were requested. Oxygen and IV fluid bolus were started with an aim to stabilise the physiological parameters. The rhythm strip is shown in Figure 14.2. What is your interpretation?

Activity 14.3

(Allow three minutes)

....

....

....

....

....

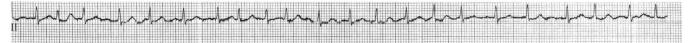

Figure 14.2 Rhythm strip

J: It shows a narrow complex tachycardia, irregular RR interval with no discernible P waves. Looks like AF.

Great! So, how would you proceed?

J: Not sure. Would you give her something to slow down the heart rate?

Without complicating things why don't we look at the observations again.

J: She has a tachycardia causing low BP with low saturations indicating a problem with the alveolar-capillary interface and pyrexia. I wonder if the low BP and tachycardia are due to sepsis.

That might be the aetiology but focus on the sudden onset AF with a drop in BP. You could qualify this further as narrow complex tachycardia causing haemodynamic compromise and symptoms (confusion, breathlessness). What does the Advanced Life Support (ALS) protocol advise in this scenario?

J: Shock! I mean cardioversion.

Perfect!

The notes revealed a persistent tachycardia of around 130 bpm over the last 10 days since admission. She had a history of psychiatric disorder and depression. She was originally admitted with an acute bronchitis on a background of ongoing weight loss of 10 kg over three months. She then developed a presumed urinary tract infection for which she was on antibiotics. She had had a CT scan of the chest, abdomen and pelvis to help identify a cause for her weight loss but these were unremarkable.

O/E: She looked emaciated and breathless. RS – Bibasal crepitations, CVS – Irregular rhythm and no other signs of heart failure. Rest of the systemic examination was normal.

Since there was no response to the IV fluid bolus she was electrically cardioverted under sedation. She reverted to sinus rhythm.

J: I would continue with IV fluids as she appears to be septic.

CXR showed pulmonary oedema and the ABG revealed hypoxemic respiratory failure with metabolic acidosis. She then reverted back to AF albeit at a rate of 120 bpm and a BP of 110/70. ECG showed AF and lateral ischemic changes.

J: Given that there is no haemodynamic compromise, rate control would be better especially since sepsis seems to be driving the AF.

She was given IV metoprolol 2.5 mg and frusemide 40 mg IV. IV fluids were stopped and low molecular weight heparin (LMWH) was started to prevent embolisation in the short term. The junior doctor in the team felt that TFTs were indicated given the new onset AF.

J: Two questions – Would you continue with long term anticoagulation and secondly, would you treat her for ACS?

Long term anticoagulation depends on the CHA$_2$DS$_2$-VASc score, the underlying cause of the AF and informed patient choice. Since AF resulted in pulmonary oedema with ischemic changes on the ECG, ACS will have to be ruled out and treated in the interim.

The TFTs showed hyperthyroidism. She was started on propylthiouracil and propranolol via a nasogastric tube having been diagnosed with thyroid storm.

J: *Wow, I hadn't expected that it would be abnormal. Isn't that a rare cause of AF?*

If you look at the SQs with all of the information thus far the diagnosis screams out at you. Middle aged lady + weight loss + pyrexia + persistent tachycardia + new onset AF + confusion/psychiatric disorder. Although pyrexia and persistent tachycardia were attributed to sepsis these seemed to be confounding factors in the bigger picture. It is always worthwhile revisiting the SQs once more information is obtained to refine the diagnosis.

▼

Management of AF or any arrhythmia for that matter should incorporate the context.

Life-threatening arrhythmias should be managed according to Advanced Life Support (ALS) protocols.

Fast AF can cause type 2 MI which should be managed by treating the AF (rate or rhythm control) per se.

A rising ± falling troponin is essential to diagnose ACS (Thygesen et al. 2010).

▲

Reference

Thygesen, K., Mair, J., Katus, H. et al. (2010). Recommendations for the use of cardiac troponin measurement in acute cardiac care. *European Heart Journal* 31 (18): 2197–2204.

15 Worsening Breathlessness

▼
This chapter tells you how to approach breathlessness from a cardiology perspective
▲

Breathlessness from a cardiology perspective falls on the capillary side of the diagram showing the alveolar-capillary interface (Figure 7.1). In this context, pulmonary capillary congestion is by and large the most common mechanism of breathlessness.

Example 15.1

A 26 year old post-partum lady was admitted in the early hours of the morning for a three week history of worsening breathlessness since childbirth.

P: *SQs – young woman + subacute breathlessness + post-partum. Provisional diagnoses – PE, anaemia, acute bronchitis to start with.*

The gradual onset of breathlessness had made it difficult to climb stairs. She had a normal vaginal delivery with no complications. Denied infective symptoms or symptoms of anaemia. There was no past medical history or risk factors for a PE other than the recent delivery. The A&E doctor notes a pulse of 100 bpm and no signs of DVT. He refers her in as possible PE.

Would you treat her for a PE?

Activity 15.1

(Allow few seconds!)

P: *She has one risk factor for PE (Well's score 1.5 – low probability of PE) and there are no competing diagnoses that explain her breathlessness. On balance I would treat her for a PE until a definitive test rules it out.*

She is treated with therapeutic LMWH for presumed PE pending a computerised tomography pulmonary angiogram (CTPA). The registrar reviews her and notes that the breathlessness was gradual in onset. He specifically asks for symptoms of heart failure or recent viral illness. She denies them all except orthopnoea.

O/E: She had an elevated BMI. Pulse 100 bpm, BP 110/70, RR 20 per minute, Saturations 92% on air, Temperature 36.6 °C. Bilateral pitting ankle oedema was noted but JVP was not discernible owing to body habitus. CVS – No other signs of heart failure. RS – reduced breath sounds bibasally. Rest of the systemic examination was normal.

The Hands-on Guide to Clinical Reasoning in Medicine, First Edition. Mujammil Irfan.
© 2019 John Wiley & Sons Ltd. Published 2019 by John Wiley & Sons Ltd.
Companion website: www.wiley.com/go/irfan/clinicalreasoning

P: *Bilateral pitting oedema could be due to bilateral DVTs or clot in the IVC but bilateral DVTs are rare though. It could also mean right heart failure, renal failure or liver failure.*

What is your interpretation of the CXR (Figure 15.1)?

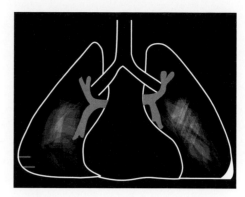

Figure 15.1 Chest radiograph

Activity 15.2

(Allow few seconds!)

The CXR showed signs of interstitial oedema and cardiomegaly. ECG showed sinus tachycardia and low voltage complexes. Urine dipstick, U&Es and LFTs were normal and serum albumin 36 g l^{-1}, Hb 140 g l^{-1}. D dimer was positive.

P: *Hmm.. So she has biventricular heart failure.*

You have rightly discarded the positive D dimer as this has poor specificity, would be expected to be positive since she is post-partum and the breathlessness has already been explained by the biventricular failure. On the contrary if she had disproportionate signs (ex: severe breathlessness at rest) that could not be accounted for by the tests (interstitial oedema alone) this would prompt a search for a second diagnosis (co-existent PE).

She has what we call peri-partum cardiomyopathy. I would certainly not expect you to know this but there are some good reasons to bring in this example.

1. A discrepancy between the working diagnosis and the signs and symptoms should compel one to explore other possibilities.
    In this case, a PE can only explain all her clinical findings if it was large enough to cause right heart failure or if it was associated with thrombus in the IVC. Either way it would imply a significant clot burden which would be so high as to compromise the pulmonary vascular bed resulting in severe breathlessness which wasn't the case.
2. You can't expect a full house of all the signs to make a diagnosis. In this example, bipedal oedema accounted for RVF and pulmonary oedema with cardiomegaly accounted for LVF.

An echocardiogram confirmed the diagnosis of peri-partum cardiomyopathy with globally reduced LV systolic function and an ejection fraction (EF) of 25%. A cautious clinician nevertheless obtained a CTPA which was negative for a PE.

Example 15.2

A 78 year old lady was admitted with a three day history of worsening breathlessness. She had a history of congestive cardiac failure (CCF), metallic aortic valve replacement, AF, hypertension, diabetes mellitus, and chronic kidney disease (CKD) stage 3.

P: *Wow! That's a lot of co-morbidities. SQs – Elderly lady + worsening breathlessness + CCF + prosthetic valve + AF + cardiovascular risk factors. Provisional diagnoses – something is making the heart failure worse. Exacerbation of CCF (myocardial infarction MI), AF, CKD, prosthetic valve incompetence, anaemia, infection (valve or acute bronchitis) come to mind.*

She reported worsening of ankle swelling, using three pillows to sleep as opposed to the usual one (orthopnoea) and waking up breathless in the middle of the night (PND) over the last week. Denied any chest pains, palpitations, syncope (due to fast AF), bleeding from any orifice or infective symptoms. She had not missed any of her medications and the INR was stable.

She was on warfarin, ramipril 5 mg od, bisoprolol 5 mg od, aspirin 75 mg od, frusemide 40 mg od, digoxin 62.5 mg od, gliclazide 80 mg a.m. and 40 mg p.m., doxazosin 2 mg od, simvastatin 40 mg od, and naproxen 250 mg prn for osteoarthritis using it up to three times a day over the last two weeks owing to worsening pain.

P: *It all seems to be down to her heart (pedal oedema, orthopnoea and PND). I can't rule out a silent MI (as she has diabetes) or valve incompetence.*

O/E: Pulse 100 bpm irregularly irregular, BP 110/70, RR 20 per minute, Temperature 37 °C, saturations 90% on air and capillary blood glucose 14 mmol l⁻¹. CVS – Left sided S3, no early diastolic murmur in aortic and Erb's area, elevated JVP, bipedal pitting oedema up to knees. RS – bibasal crepitations and reduced breath sounds. No clinical stigmata of infective endocarditis (IE). PA – Mild hepatomegaly but no ascites. Rest of the examination was normal. Urine dipstick 1+ blood and 2+ protein.

P: *Severity of illness – ill. She has decompensated biventricular failure (CCF). The urine is positive for microscopic haematuria and proteinuria. I guess we would still have to keep IE and MI in mind.*

How would you interpret her ECG (Figure 15.2)?

Activity 15.3

(Allow few seconds!)

CXR: Pulmonary oedema. ECG: AF at 60 bpm, lateral T wave inversion. Hb 120 g l⁻¹, WCC 14 × 10⁹ l⁻¹, platelets 200 × 10⁹ l⁻¹, CRP 30 mg l⁻¹, Bilirubin 32 μmol l⁻¹, ALT 50 IU l⁻¹, ALP 30 IU l⁻¹, Albumin 30 g l⁻¹, INR 4.5 (target 2.5-3.5), Na⁺ 128 mmol l⁻¹, K⁺ 3.2 mmol l⁻¹, Urea 15 mmol l⁻¹, Creatinine 150 μmol l⁻¹ (baseline 120 μmol l⁻¹), and hs Troponin T 30 ng l⁻¹. Blood cultures were sent.

P: *I'm a bit overwhelmed with this information.*

Let's break things down.
- We have established that she has decompensated CCF but there is no cause identified yet.
- The ECG does not suggest an obvious MI.

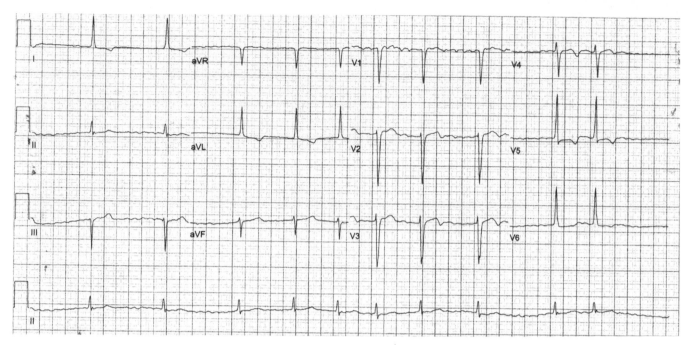

Figure 15.2 ECG

- The AF is rate-controlled and hence unlikely to be contributing to the decompensated CCF. With the acute kidney injury (AKI) and slow AF we will have to think of digoxin toxicity.
- She is not anaemic.
- Inflammatory markers (WCC and CRP) are mildly elevated. The presence of a prosthetic valve should alert us to the possibility of IE although it could just be a stress response.
- LFTs reveal a hepatitic picture. Clinical findings tied to them suggest congestive hepatomegaly (i.e. liver is congested with blood due to worsening CCF). The ↑INR is likely secondary to this as the liver produces clotting factors. Reduced synthetic function can prolong prothrombin time especially whilst she is taking warfarin.
- Renal function has worsened (AKI on background of CKD). It could be due to the lowish BP (either drug induced or due to worsening CCF) or the nephrotoxic drugs that she is on (ramipril, naproxen).
- Positive urine dipstick is due to AKI although IE should be kept in the background.
- Hyponatremia is dilutional and a poor prognostic marker in the context of CCF.
- The elevated troponin is either because of an ACS or due to CCF or CKD or a combination of the three. The only way to distinguish an ACS is by repeating the troponin in six hours to establish a rise or fall in the levels. Either way the raised troponin is also a poor prognostic marker.

Armed with this information, can you modify her drug chart to improve the haemodynamics and symptoms?

Activity 15.4

(Allow three minutes)

....

....

....

....

....

Warfarin, ramipril (low BP), digoxin (can accumulate in AKI), doxazosin, simvastatin (causes muscle damage in AKI), and naproxen (non-steroidal anti-inflammatory drug (NSAID)) – nephrotoxic and causes fluid retention were withheld. She was started on 80 mg frusemide IV and fluids were restricted to 1 litre per day. Strict fluid balance chart, daily weights, daily U&Es and close blood sugar monitoring (Gliclazide can accumulate in AKI causing hypoglycaemia) were initiated. Pre-test probability of ACS was felt to be low hence she was not treated for the same. Repeat hs Troponin T reassuringly was 28 ng l⁻¹ (>20% change is needed for it to be significant).

On day 5, she was much better with a BP of 130/70, HR 90 bpm, apyrexial and saturations 95% on air. Her pulmonary and pedal oedema improved. Repeat bloods showed improvement and warfarin, ramipril 2.5 mg od and simvastatin 40 mg od were restarted. Digoxin, doxazosin and naproxen were stopped permanently and she was discharged on co-codamol for pain relief.

The pathophysiologic sequence of this decompensation seems to have been: Naproxen → AKI on background of CKD → Fluid retention due to both AKI and direct effect of naproxen → worsening CCF.

This was a complex albeit common presentation of decompensated CCF. It illustrates the benefits of:

- adopting a logical sequence of working through various competing hypotheses of equal weight
- using tests to exclude the erroneous diagnoses and
- honing in on the final diagnosis which explains all the findings.

▼
A discrepancy between the working diagnosis and the signs and symptoms should compel one to explore other possibilities.

Drug interactions are a common cause of emergency presentations especially re-admissions (a fifth) – look for them (Davies et al. 2010; Jha et al. 2001).
▲

References

Davies, E.C., Green, C.F., Mottram, D.R. et al. (2010). Emergency re-admissions to hospital due to adverse drug reactions within 1 year of the index admission. *British Journal of Clinical Pharmacology* 70 (5): 749–755.

Jha, A.K., Kuperman, G.J., Rittenberg, E. et al. (2001). Identifying hospital admissions due to adverse drug events using a computer-based monitor. *Pharmacoepidemiology and Drug Safety* 10 (2): 113–119.

16 Vague Systemic Symptoms

▼

This chapter tells you how to approach a constellation of systemic symptoms from a cardiology perspective

▲

Any disease state (ranging from infection to malignancy) causing a systemic inflammatory response will result in systemic symptoms.

Example 16.1

A 25 year old man presented to the medical admissions unit with a two week history of increasing malaise, lethargy, loss of appetite and cough. The GP had treated him with clarithromycin for acute bronchitis a weeks ago with no impact on symptoms. He had a history of right leg DVT four years ago and asthma for which he took salbutamol and serevent inhalers.

J: *SQs – Young man + cough + subacute non-specific systemic symptoms + chronic lung disease + history of VTE. Provisional diagnoses – exacerbation of asthma (infective or non-infective).*

He reported a non-productive cough with occasional night sweats and fever. No relevant travel history or exposure to TB. On direct questioning he admitted abusing intravenous heroin, the last injection being two weeks ago into the right groin. He smoked tobacco (14 py) and drank 30 units of alcohol per week.

J: *This information brings HIV ± opportunistic infections, Hepatitis and TB into the picture.*

O/E: Unkempt appearance. Pulse 86 bpm, RR 14 per minute, BP 130/70, Temperature 38 °C, saturations 94% on air and BMs 12 mmol l⁻¹. Systemic examination was normal except intravenous needle marks in both arms and groins. There was no lymphadenopathy.

ECG normal. Hb 110 g l⁻¹, MCV 88 f, WCC 14 × 10⁹ l⁻¹, platelets 500 × 10⁹ l⁻¹, CRP 60 mg l⁻¹, ALT 60 IU l⁻¹ with ALP 350 IU l⁻¹, and albumin 32 g l⁻¹. Blood film showed thrombocytosis. Clotting normal. U&Es normal. Urine dipstick was positive for leucocytes, blood 1+ and protein 1+. CXR showed bilateral pulmonary cavitations and he was isolated for
suspected TB. HIV and viral hepatitis serology were requested with consent.

J: *Severity of illness – relatively well. Working diagnosis – Pulmonary TB.*

The lowish albumin, elevated platelets and mild normocytic anaemia seem to point towards a chronic inflammatory condition. The mild LFT dysfunction could be due to clarithromycin or viral hepatitis.

The Hands-on Guide to Clinical Reasoning in Medicine, First Edition. Mujammil Irfan.
© 2019 John Wiley & Sons Ltd. Published 2019 by John Wiley & Sons Ltd.
Companion website: www.wiley.com/go/irfan/clinicalreasoning

What other differentials can you think of in this scenario?

Activity 16.1

(Allow three minutes)

> ....
>
> ....
>
> ....
>
> ....
>
> ....

Lung abscesses (H/O alcohol and IV drug abuse), autoimmune conditions such as Wegener's granulomatosis (pulmonary cavitations, positive urine dipstick), malignancy (although the relatively acute onset makes this unlikely).

A respiratory consult uncovered a pansystolic murmur in the tricuspid area. Given that he was an IV drug user with microscopic haematuria on the urine dipstick, the presence of a regurgitant murmur lent credence to infective endocarditis. An echo was suggested as the pulmonary cavities were suspected to be secondary to septic emboli showering off from the tricuspid valve into the pulmonary circulation.

The echo confirmed tricuspid valve vegetation and blood cultures grew *Staphylococcus aureus*. He was treated with intravenous antibiotics and discharged. The HIV and viral hepatitis tests were negative and the LFT dysfunction was blamed on the clarithromycin.

Why do you think, you got side tracked to pulmonary TB when you knew about the intravenous drug abuse and the risk of infective endocarditis?

J: *I guess pulmonary cavities made me immediately think of TB. Moreover, he abused both intravenous drugs and alcohol which triggered TB and HIV.*

Both are valid points, but I think you went with the availability heuristic i.e. the most common and plausible explanation for cavitation (Tversky and Kahneman 1974). The admitting team honing in on TB did not help as this seemed to give further proof that this was the diagnosis. This is something that often happens in clinical practice. It takes a fresh mind to disregard previous opinions and approach the task with a clean slate. One can enable this by stopping for a moment to think of all the possible causes that can explain the clinical presentation as demonstrated above. This approach always pays off to the advantage of the clinician and the patient.

Example 16.2

A 54 year old lady was referred to the Respiratory physicians with a left sided pleural effusion. She was a 40 py ex-smoker who stopped smoking after an myocardial infarction (MI) six weeks ago requiring coronary stent insertion.

P: *SQs – middle aged lady + unilateral pleural effusion + recent MI + ex-smoker. Provisional diagnoses – malignant pleural effusion (lung and elsewhere), infection – e.g. empyema.*

Establishing if it is a transudate (e.g. heart failure secondary to recent MI) or an exudate would be a good starting point as this will dictate the differentials.

She developed severe left sided pleuritic chest pain and fever a week ago followed by breathlessness which led to the admission. O/E: Temperature of 38 °C, saturations 92% on air, pulse 100 bpm, BP 130/70 and RR 20 per minute. Clinical features were in keeping with a left pleural effusion.

Blood tests – WCC 18×10^9 per litre and CRP 80 mg l^{-1}. U&Es, LFTs normal. CXR confirmed a small left pleural effusion. ECG –sinus rhythm with Q waves in anterior leads (recent MI) but no ST/T changes. Given the inflammatory marker response it was felt that she might have an empyema and she was given a broad-spectrum antibiotic.

P: *Severity of illness – ill. There is certainly a possibility of CAP and parapneumonic effusion with the inflammatory response.*

A diagnostic pleural aspiration by the cardiology team revealed an exudate with negative microbiology and no malignant cells. The pH was 7.3. Her inflammatory markers seemed to settle by day 3 and the cardiologists wanted her effusion drained.

P: *It has responded to the antibiotics. Would you drain it?*

It depends on the working diagnosis. If it is a para-pneumonic effusion, then a small effusion with clinical improvement on antibiotics would not warrant draining. pH of 7.3 also diminishes the possibility of an empyema. If it is malignancy, leaving the effusion alone for entry by thoracoscopy would be essential.

Respiratory review noted no red flag symptoms of malignancy and opined that this was likely to be Dressler's syndrome (post-cardiac injury syndrome, PCIS). However, they suggested excluding a PE.

An echo showed normal LV function and a trace of pericardial effusion. Since she had improved clinically the team discharged her. She re-presented with similar symptoms and blood tests a week later. The pleural effusion was now moderate sized. CTPA was negative for PE and there was no suggestion of malignancy. The Cardiology team were again concerned about an empyema or malignancy and re-referred the patient to their Respiratory colleagues.

Would you carry on testing or would you treat at this point?

Activity 16.2

(Allow a minute)

The pleural effusion was drained to relieve the breathlessness and colchicine was started to help with pain. She was discharged with a diagnosis of PCIS. On follow-up two weeks later, she had improved dramatically with no recurrence of effusion.

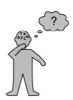

Once again I do not expect you to know about Dressler's syndrome but it is the clinical reasoning issues that need attention. This example illustrates the point at which one has to decide on initiating treatment or persist with investigations. These two decisions are not separate. Often, the severity of illness, symptom burden and informed patient choice become the factors in helping us decide. In other instances, the degree of certainty of the working diagnosis will have to be weighed against the risks of the test including sensitivity and specificity, and the risk/benefit ratio of the treatment. For example, if you are fairly certain that the patient has disease 'x' and the test 'y' is risky and lacks specificity with treatment 'z' being fairly safe you could opt for the treatment without subjecting the patient to further tests.

This thinking process can be applied to the scenario where there are no confirmatory tests and the diagnosis is one of exclusion. How many competing diagnoses will you have to exclude before you start treatment? The simplistic answer is to exclude life-threatening conditions and those that are easily treatable.

PCIS is a diagnosis of exclusion. Antimyocardial antibodies can sometimes be positive but are not specific to PCIS (Hoffman et al. 2002). The echo and CTPA had excluded major diagnostic possibilities and the case for PCIS was strengthened by the presence of pleuropericardial effusions and an inflammatory response. Treatment in this case would also serve as a therapeutic trial in confirming the diagnosis with a lack of response signalling the need for further tests.

▼

Unusual presentations of common diagnoses are more common than rare diagnoses.

Be wary of availability heuristic and approach clinical problems with an open mind.

Understand the point at which one decides to stop investigations and start treatment.

▲

References
Hoffman, M., Fried, M., Jabareen, F. et al. (2002). Anti-heart antibodies in postpericardiotomy syndrome: cause or epiphenomenon? A prospective, longitudinal pilot study. *Autoimmunity* 35 (4): 241–245.
Tversky, A. and Kahneman, D. (1974). Judgment under uncertainty: heuristics and biases. *Science (New York, N.Y.)* 185 (4157): 1124–1131.

17 Acute Chest Pain

▼

This chapter illustrates clinical reasoning in acute chest pain from a cardiology perspective

▲

Aetiology of chest pain from a cardiac perspective includes both myopericardial and vascular disease.

Example 17.1

An 85 year old previously fit and well man presented with central chest pain which started two hours ago. This was associated with sweating, nausea and light headedness. He described it as a squeezing sensation before he passed out.

J: *SQs – elderly man + cardiac sounding chest pain + syncope. Provisional diagnoses – MI (IHD is high on the list as he is elderly), aortic dissection or PE although the 'squeezing' sensation does not agree with the last two. The syncope suggests an arrhythmia or infarction in a large territory causing reduced output.*

One hour later

The paramedics brought him into A&E post-intubation, following thrombolysis with alteplase and per rectal aspirin. How would you interpret the ECG (Figure 17.1)?

J: *It shows sinus bradycardia, ST elevation in II, III and aVF, V1 and V2 and reciprocal ST depression in lateral leads. Taken together with the history this is an inferior wall MI.*

Good! You are supposed to have sympathetic activation and tachycardia in MI. Why do you think he is bradycardic?

Activity 17.1

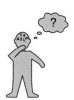

(Allow a minute)

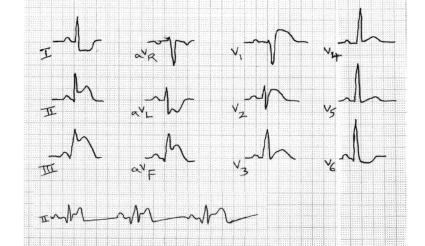

Figure 17.1 Representative ECG

The Hands-on Guide to Clinical Reasoning in Medicine, First Edition. Mujammil Irfan.
© 2019 John Wiley & Sons Ltd. Published 2019 by John Wiley & Sons Ltd.
Companion website: www.wiley.com/go/irfan/clinicalreasoning

J: *I'm not sure.*

The additional ST elevation in V1 in the context of inferior wall MI suggests right ventricular myocardial infarction (RVMI). This is often associated with high vagal tone causing pallor, sweating, nausea and bradycardia (Zimetbaum 2003). On the other hand, bradycardia and heart block in anterior wall MI is due to septal necrosis involving the conducting system (atrioventricular – AV node).

One hour 15 minutes

O/E: Pulse 50 bpm, BP 60/40, saturations 99% on FiO_2 1.0, RR 14 per minute, Temperature 36.6 °C and BMs 8 mmol l^{-1}. RS: clear, CVS: JVP high, no pedal oedema, S3, S4 or murmurs. Rest of the systemic examination: normal.

J: *Severity of illness – dying. He has been thrombolysed. I would repeat the ECG to ensure resolution of ST elevation. Would you give inotropes to raise the BP?*

One hour 30 minutes

RVMI was confirmed with a right sided lead V4R showing ST elevation (also suggested by bradycardia, hypotension, raised JVP and clear lung fields) he was given IV fluid boluses to ↑ RV filling → improve forward flow into the lungs → ↑LV filling → ↑BP. He was then started on inotropes and vasopressors as BP remained low. Repeat ECG was as before.

J: *Would you give him nitrates? Oh, you can't as he is hypotensive.*

That's right nitrates and opioids are contraindicated in RVMI as both reduce RV filling. In general, nitrates would be indicated if there is ongoing ischemic pain. Non-resolving ST elevation 90 minutes post thrombolysis suggests need for rescue angioplasty.

One hour 40 minutes

He was given atropine 3 mg IV which improved the bradycardia to 80 bpm. BP initially improved and then dropped again.

J: *Would you consider rescue angioplasty?*

Firstly, the patient is too unstable to be moved and secondly, he has remained hypotensive for nearly 100 minutes despite all possible medical intervention. This would have certainly caused cerebral and other end-organ damage (kidneys, gut) by now. Where do you draw the line? Would you carry on resuscitating or stop?

J: *I would leave this to the seniors.*

Fantastic! That is the right answer from your perspective. However, it would be wise to go through the reasoning process here. You would be balancing the risk of immediate death (53% – short term mortality) against a slim chance of survival but with high degree of dependency (long term morbidity) the latter being harder to quantify (Jacobs et al. 2003). Then there is the argument of preserving dignity in death.

There is no black and white answer to this. It partly rests on individual physician views as well as patient views. Every physician has a threshold beyond which they see futility in continuing treatment. Sometimes, it is also harder for physicians directly involved in the care to be objective and a second hopefully unbiased opinion would help. Speaking with the next of kin and ascertaining the patient's views on a life albeit with significant disability is also useful.

The team discussed the patient with the Consultant on call and the relatives. Given the poor outlook he was commenced on palliative treatment and he passed away peacefully.

Example 17.2

A 65 year old man was admitted with a one week history of worsening breathlessness looking pale, clammy and lethargic. His unlimited ET had declined to room to room over the last week. He had a history of hypertension and diabetes mellitus for which he took bisoprolol 2.5 mg od and gliclazide 40 mg bd. The admitting doctor noted a BP of 100/60 and pulse 70 bpm and contacted the senior physician for review as she felt that he looked 'very poorly' although the numbers were not too bad.

P: *SQs – middle aged man + gradually worsening breathlessness + hypertension + diabetes mellitus. Provisional diagnosis – undiagnosed IHD causing LVF or PE although gradual onset does not seem to fit.*

Unresolved clots from a PE can cause gradual onset breathlessness. Other possibilities include CAP with sepsis.

O/E: JVP was elevated, a pansystolic murmur heard in the left lower parasternal edge. No pedal oedema. RS: Bibasal crepitations. Rest of the systemic examination: normal. ECG: Q waves in V1 – V4. He denied any chest pain over the last week.

What do you think is the diagnosis?

Activity 17.2

(Allow a minute)

P: *The elevated JVP and bibasal crepitations indicate biventricular failure. I'm not sure of the murmur.*

You seem to be focusing on clinical findings alone. If you re-state the SQs – old MI changes on ECG + one week of breathlessness + biventricular failure, the pathophysiologic sequence that emerges is: MI a week ago → decompensated biventricular failure. The murmur gives the clue for the cause of his decompensation. A pansystolic murmur in the context of a recent MI at the left lower sternal edge should make you think of a ventricular septal defect (VSD).

An urgent echo confirmed a VSD on a background of a missed recent antero-septal MI and he was transferred to a tertiary centre for surgical repair. Unfortunately, he died three days later despite surgery.

Two unique processes of clinical reasoning can be seen here.

1. Identification that the patient was 'very poorly' despite the vital signs being fairly normal.
2. Recognition of the relative acuteness of presentation leading to an early diagnosis of VSD through temporal sequencing of events despite incomplete data (i.e. absence of chest pain). However, caution is still advised despite the virtues of diagnosis through clinical Gestalt (Cook 2009).

Example 17.3

An 80 year old man presented to A&E with a two week history of breathlessness. He was a 40 py ex-smoker and reported a four stone weight loss over a few months. He had a history of IHD, diabetes mellitus and hypertension. He was on ramipril, metformin, aspirin and frusemide.

P: *SQs – Elderly + gradual onset breathlessness + weight loss + IHD + vascular risk factors. Provisional diagnoses – LVF, CAP, PE.*

O/E: pulse 130 bpm irregularly irregular, BP 80/60, RR 35 per minute, Temperature 36.5 °C, saturations 95% on air. Systemic examination: normal except marked cachexia. CXR: obscure left heart border and left costophrenic angle blunting with haziness in the left lower zone.

P: *Severity of illness – very ill. Left lower lobe CAP very likely but significant weight loss raises the possibility of malignancy.*

What is your interpretation of the ECG (Figure 17.2)?

Activity 17.3

(Allow a minute)

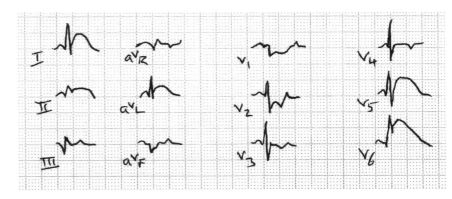

Figure 17.2 Representative ECG

P: *There is ST elevation in I, II, aVL, V5-V6. Horizontal ST depression in V1-V2.*

Repeat ECG showed no P waves with an irregular RR interval. Fast AF with lateral wall STEMI was suspected. The registrar reviewed the patient and decided not to thrombolyse. He treated the fast AF with digoxin as the BP was low.

P: *Two questions: What were the reasons for not thrombolysing and, not cardioverting the AF despite the low BP?*

If we were to assume that this was a postero-lateral STEMI, we should see reciprocal changes which are strikingly absent. More importantly looking at the whole picture it does not add up. Prior to the ECG, malignancy was included on your list which seemingly got side lined as the ECG took the spotlight.

As for the AF, the accompanying hypotension was not causing symptoms of light headedness or loss of consciousness which suggests that he ran on a lowish BP normally. Hence the decision against cardioversion.

The WCC was 13×10^9 l^{-1} and CRP 40 mg l^{-1}. Serial troponin Ts were 50 and 35 μg l^{-1} respectively. He had an echo which showed an ejection fraction of 20%, a mildly aneurysmal LV and a bright pericardium around the LV. CT confirmed a bronchial carcinoma invading the heart postero-laterally. Despite treatment the heart rate did not settle and he clinically deteriorated. He was managed palliatively and he passed away peacefully.

You have two reasons for the ST elevation here: LV aneurysm and malignant pericardial invasion. Lastly, decompensated LVF due to AF resulted in the breathlessness. The lesson here is to always look at the whole picture and not get swayed by a test result on its own.

▼
Reciprocal changes on an ECG help in confirming the diagnosis of STEMI.

MI can be complicated by electro-physiological and mechanical problems.
▲

References

Cook, C. (2009). Is clinical gestalt good enough? *The Journal of Manual & Manipulative Therapy* 17 (1): 6–7.

Jacobs, A.K., Leopold, J.A., Bates, E. et al. (2003). Cardiogenic shock caused by right ventricular infarction. *Journal of the American College of Cardiology* 41 (8): 1273–1279.

Zimetbaum, P.J. (2003). The electrocardiogram in acute myocardial infarction. *The New England Journal of Medicine* 348 (23): 2362.

18 Blurring the Margins

▼
This chapter illustrates how to tease apart competing differential diagnoses accounting for breathlessness
▲

Breathlessness as a symptom has a broad etiological basis as shown in Figure 2.4. When there are complex interacting factors causing breathlessness, our job is to tease them apart, weigh each of their contributions to the symptom burden and identify those factors that can be reversed or modified to ease breathlessness. This should be followed by patient education, as a better understanding allays fears.

Example 18.1

> A 65 year old man was seen in the chest clinic for follow up of his moderate COPD. He had a history of left sided stroke from which he had recovered, diabetes mellitus, hypertension and pulmonary embolism three years ago.
>
> He was recently hospitalised for worsening breathlessness over three months which was treated as an infective exacerbation of COPD. A lack of improvement led to an inpatient echo which demonstrated mild LV diastolic dysfunction and a raised pulmonary artery pressure of 70 mm of Hg. He was started on bisoprolol and frusemide and discharged but his breathlessness had unfortunately worsened.

> J: SQs – Middle aged man + gradually worsening breathlessness + COPD + Vascular Risk Factors + PE. Provisional Diagnoses – I'm Stuck!

What provisional diagnoses can you think of?

Activity 18.1

(Allow three minutes)

```
..............................................................................................
..............................................................................................
..............................................................................................
..............................................................................................
..............................................................................................
```

He seems to have several reasons to be breathless and listing them will help. COPD, Pulmonary hypertension, LV diastolic dysfunction are a few causes. It could be either of them getting worse over a period of time or a combination of all that is making him breathless. He reported that he had gained two stones in weight over two months and his legs had

> grown into 'tree trunks' due to swelling. His ET had reduced from 200 yards on the flat to breathlessness on getting dressed.

The Hands-on Guide to Clinical Reasoning in Medicine, First Edition. Mujammil Irfan.
© 2019 John Wiley & Sons Ltd. Published 2019 by John Wiley & Sons Ltd.
Companion website: www.wiley.com/go/irfan/clinicalreasoning

O/E: Pulse 90 bpm, BP 120/70, Saturations 92% on air desaturating to 88% on exertion in the corridor, RR 18 per minute and Temperature 37 °C. RS: scattered wheeze, CVS: raised jugular venous pressure (JVP), loud P2, pansystolic murmur over tricuspid area and pitting bilateral leg oedema up to thighs. Rest of the systemic examination: normal.

J: *Has he developed cor pulmonale secondary to COPD?*

That's certainly a possibility. The LV diastolic dysfunction could also be contributing to the right heart failure.

J: *Could it be a recurrent PE?*

Risk factors include the previous PE and relative immobility. However, the three month history is too long for an acute PE. Nevertheless, you are on the right track!

Blood tests showed no evidence of anaemia and CXR did not show any pleural effusions contributing to the breathlessness. The registrar felt that his breathlessness and right heart failure were out of proportion to the moderate COPD and mild LV diastolic dysfunction. He noted the PE three years ago and hypothesised whether he had developed chronic thrombo-embolic pulmonary hypertension (CTEPH), from unresolved clots, a complication of the previous PE.

He was referred to a tertiary centre for right heart catheterisation and a second opinion. CTEPH was confirmed and treated medically. On return to the clinic three months later he had dramatically improved to his baseline and the leg swelling had disappeared.

Breathlessness in this case was multifactorial: moderate COPD, LV diastolic dysfunction, CTEPH, Pulmonary hypertension due to all three aforementioned and weight gain, the last of which is sometimes under-estimated. Understanding that the symptoms were disproportionate to the known factors led the registrar to hypothesise another condition (CTEPH) which could explain the worsening breathlessness. This was a modifiable factor which resulted in symptom alleviation.

Example 18.2

An 86 year old man was referred by the GP for worsening breathlessness over a few months. He had a history of moderate LV impairment, severe aortic stenosis, moderate COPD, AF, right pleural effusion and liver cirrhosis from previous alcohol excess. His frusemide had recently been increased to 80 mg mane and 40 mg mid-day with no benefit. The GP wondered if draining the effusion might help.

P: *SQs – Elderly man + worsening breathlessness + significant cardiac and lung impairment + liver cirrhosis. Provisional diagnoses – It could be worsening heart or lung problems or a combination of the two.*

Figure 18.1a shows possible causes of his breathlessness and the interrupted lines show their interactions in Figure 18.1b. Note that deconditioning is caused by all the main causes of breathlessness.

He had declined CABG and aortic valve replacement five years ago owing to anaesthetic risks. He had also made an informed decision not to take warfarin for his AF. The right pleural effusion was a transudate and had remained stable over a year. He lived alone and his ET had reduced to 50 yards on the flat. He denied any recent chest pains, cough or risk factors for VTE.

(a)

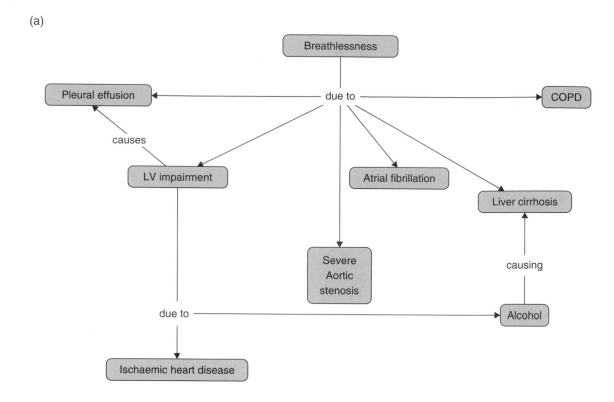

(b)

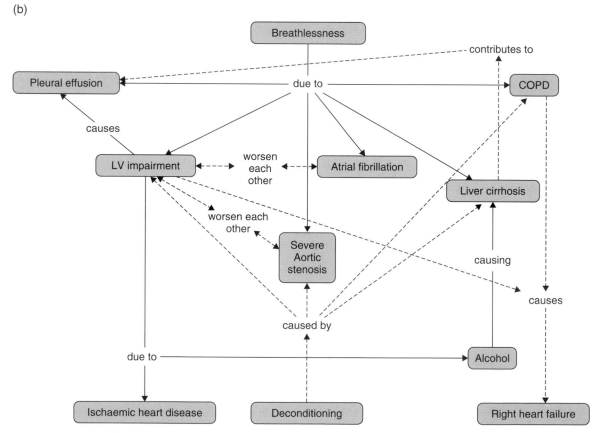

Figure 18.1 Concept map of breathlessness in our patient

Other medications: bisoprolol 2.5 mg od, losartan 50 mg od, aspirin 75 mg od, Seretide 500 inhaler 1 puff bd, tiotropium 18 mcg 1 puff od, digoxin 125 mcg od, atorvastatin 80 mg od, and salbutamol inhaler prn.

O/E: Pulse 94 bpm, BP 120/70, Saturations 94% on air which dropped to 90% on exertion, Temperature 36 °C, RR 18 minute. RS: bibasal crepitations and signs of right pleural effusion, CVS: irregularly irregular pulse with a loud ejection systolic murmur all over the praecordium, loudest over the aortic area radiating into carotids. Pansystolic murmur over mitral area. Raised JVP but no other signs of right heart failure. Rest of the systemic examination: normal.

P: *Addressing each possibility –*

- *COPD – No evidence of exacerbation and on appropriate inhalers.*
- *AF is rate controlled*
- *IHD is adequately treated as there is no active angina*

I would like to see the CXR for any increase in the pleural effusion, Hb to exclude anaemia, LFTs for any decompensation although that doesn't seem to be the main problem and echo to assess worsening LV function.

I wouldn't get an echo as detecting a deteriorating LV function is not going to change our management as he has refused surgery before. Instead, optimising medical management of his LVF should be our aim.

CXR: stable pleural effusion, ECG: rate controlled AF and no acute ischemic changes, Bloods: Hb 120 g l⁻¹, WCC 11 × 10⁹ l⁻¹, platelets 300 × 10⁹ l⁻¹. Na⁺ 134 mmol l⁻¹, K⁺ 3.2 mmol l⁻¹, Urea 8 mmol l⁻¹, creatinine 90 µmol l⁻¹, albumin 30 g l⁻¹, rest of LFTs: normal. CRP 20 mg l⁻¹.

P: *Pleural effusion is the same, he is not anaemic. The K+ is low, I would replace it.*

Even if the pleural effusion had increased there is no point in draining it, as a transudative effusion recurs especially since the underlying causes are still active. The low albumin is contributing to the effusion too. The K⁺ is low because of the frusemide, correcting it with out-patient supplements other than diet is fraught with risk of hyperkalemia.

Since the renal function had remained steady spironolactone 25 mg od was added (mortality benefit in heart failure). The side effect of hyperkalemia with spironolactone was beneficial since he was hypokalemic. Transcatheter aortic valve implantation (TAVI) and newer oral anticoagulants (NOAC) were proposed to the patient and both were declined. Limitations of medical management were stressed and social services were involved in optimising his environment to help with activities of daily living. Finally, the GP was advised to monitor U&Es.

Would you have considered offering him NOAC for AF?

Activity 18.2

(Allow a minute)

Long-term risk reduction of ischemic stroke by 2/3 (benefits of warfarin and NOACs) should be weighed against the risks of intracranial haemorrhage (ICH) (NOACs have a reduced relative risk of ICH compared to warfarin) (Friberg et al. 2012; Ruff et al. 2014). We also tend to forget that although NOACs have fewer side effects and interactions and require no monitoring compared to warfarin they are still an extra tablet to take. This brings us to the burdens of polypharmacy especially when viewed against a limited life-expectancy with all the co-morbidities. Keeping all this in mind, exploring the views of the patient and discussing this openly will help in choosing the right option.

This example illustrates the following points:

1. Recognising the limitations of medicine does not portend failure on the part of the physician. It is equally good medicine to accept and communicate this to the patient which in itself can be therapeutic.
2. The important role that the patient plays in managing his/her health cannot be stressed enough.
3. Refusal of therapy at one point in time does not preclude this forever. Re-discussion especially with recent medical advances will help in making an updated informed decision.
4. Investigations should always be chosen based on their ability to change the management of the patient.

▼

Think of CTEPH whenever there is worsening right heart failure on a background of normal LV function, especially with a history of PE.

Remember the ills of polypharmacy in the elderly and make therapeutic decisions in consultation with them.

▲

References

Friberg, L., Rosenqvist, M., and Lip, G.Y.H. (2012). Net clinical benefit of warfarin in patients with atrial fibrillation: A report from the Swedish atrial fibrillation cohort study. *Circulation* 125 (19): 2298–2307.

Ruff, C.T., Giugliano, R.P., Braunwald, E. et al. (2014). Comparison of the efficacy and safety of new oral anticoagulants with warfarin in patients with atrial fibrillation: a meta-analysis of randomised trials. *The Lancet* 383 (9921): 955–962.

PART III
Nephrology

19 History Taking: Blood in the Urine

▼

Focussing on relevant aspects of history from a renal perspective

▲

Patients with renal problems can present with specific upper or lower urinary tract symptoms. Upper urinary tract includes the kidneys and ureters whilst the lower urinary tract includes the bladder and the urethra with the prostate in the male. However, symptoms can certainly overlap in some instances.

Infective symptoms can often be localised to upper and lower urinary tracts but symptoms such as haematuria, oliguria, anuria, nocturia, and polyuria can originate anywhere in the urinary tract. Non-specific symptoms of fatigue, nausea, confusion can be secondary to uraemia or hypocalcaemia as a consequence of renal failure.

Urinary tract infection (UTI):

In general, UTIs present with systemic symptoms of fever, malaise and lethargy. In the elderly UTIs can be asymptomatic or present as delirium. In this context, UTIs are often associated with constipation which should also be treated.

Pyelonephritis (upper UTI) – rigors, loin pain, nausea, and vomiting. Pyelonephritis in the setting of renal or ureteric stones can present with colicky pain radiating from loin to groin. Blood clots in the upper urinary tract can also cause colic and fever, which can sometimes portend the diagnosis of renal cell carcinoma.

Cystitis (lower UTI) – dysuria (painful micturition), frequency, urgency, and suprapubic pain.

UTI in catheterized patients presents with systemic symptoms of fever, malaise, lethargy and delirium, the last especially in the elderly.

Benign prostatic hyperplasia (BPH):

Voiding symptoms of hesitancy, slow stream, dribbling, stopping, and starting. BPH often causes UTI like symptoms of frequency, urgency, and nocturia too.

As before, we will be discussing the aetiology of symptoms to identify the questions used in history taking.

The Hands-on Guide to Clinical Reasoning in Medicine, First Edition. Mujammil Irfan.
© 2019 John Wiley & Sons Ltd. Published 2019 by John Wiley & Sons Ltd.
Companion website: www.wiley.com/go/irfan/clinicalreasoning

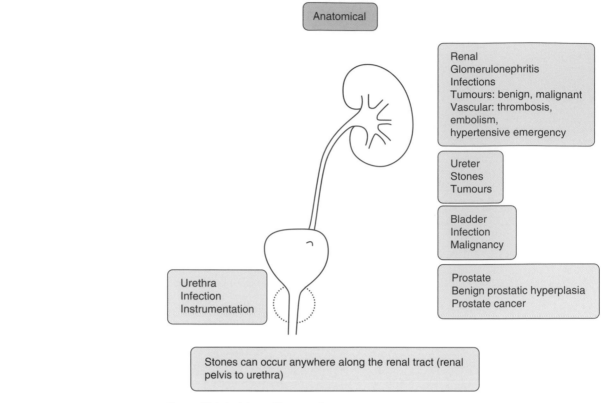

Figure 19.1 Aetiology of haematuria

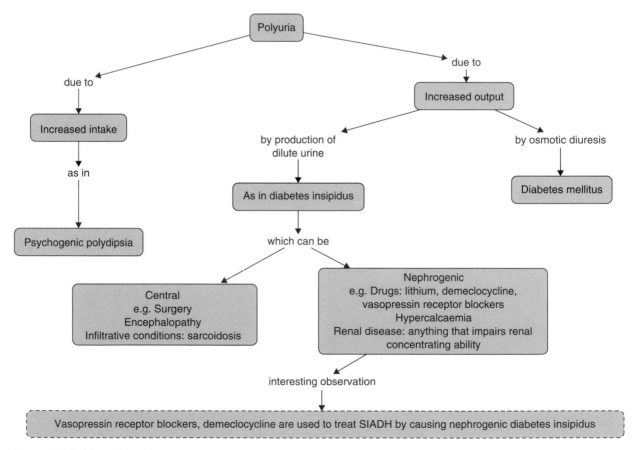

Figure 19.2 Aetiology of polyuria

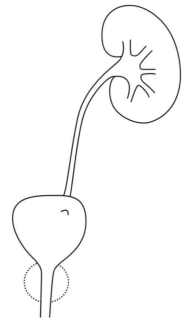

Causes of oliguria

Pre-renal:
Hypotension
Hypovolemia
Renal artery stenosis
Drugs causing a drop in GFR:
NSAIDs (afferent arteriolar constriction),
ACEi (efferent arteriolar dilatation)

Renal:
All causes of ATN

Post-renal:
Congenital

Intraluminal obstruction by
stones, blood clots,
sloughed papillae, malignancy

Extrinsic compression of ureter
(tumours, lymph nodes, fibrosis) or
urethra (benign prostatic hyperplasia,
malignancy)

Figure 19.3 Aetiology of oliguria

Haematuria in someone <40 years of age should make one think of glomerulonephritides and stones whilst >40 years of age should trigger the thought of malignancy (Figure 19.1). On the other hand, urinary tract infection causing haematuria can occur at any age. Glomerular haematuria classically does not cause clots hence clots should raise suspicion of non-glomerular downstream bleeding.

Polyuria (Figure 19.2) implies a urine output $>3\,L\,day^{-1}$. Nocturia implies frequency of urination exceeding two times per night. Nocturnal polyuria implies nocturnal voiding of urine that exceeds 35% of total urine output over 24 hours.

Oliguria (Figure 19.3) is defined as urine output $<0.5\,ml\,(kg/h)^{-1}$ and anuria as $<50\,ml\,day^{-1}$. Oliguria that persists for more than six hours is one of the criteria to diagnose acute kidney injury and predicts acute tubular necrosis in the right context. Acute tubular necrosis implies tubular epithelial cell death due to:

1. Poor perfusion
2. Toxins (drugs)
3. Tubular obstruction by proteins (myeloma, haemoglobinuria, myoglobinuria) or crystals (oxalate, urates).

Acute kidney injury – AKI (Figure 19.4):
It is defined as a rise in serum creatinine of ≥26.5 µmol l^{-1} (≥0.3 mg dl^{-1}) over 48 hours or >50% above baseline over seven days OR urine output <0.5 ml (kg/h)$^{-1}$ for >6 hours. It is important to note that AKI can be oliguric or non-oliguric, the prognosis in the latter being better.

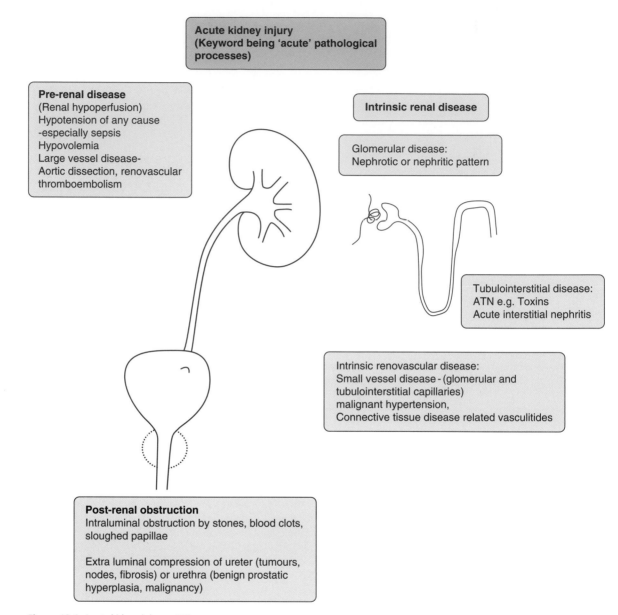

Acute kidney injury
(Keyword being 'acute' pathological processes)

Pre-renal disease
(Renal hypoperfusion)
Hypotension of any cause
-especially sepsis
Hypovolemia
Large vessel disease-
Aortic dissection, renovascular thromboembolism

Intrinsic renal disease

Glomerular disease:
Nephrotic or nephritic pattern

Tubulointerstitial disease:
ATN e.g. Toxins
Acute interstitial nephritis

Intrinsic renovascular disease:
Small vessel disease - (glomerular and tubulointerstitial capillaries)
malignant hypertension,
Connective tissue disease related vasculitides

Post-renal obstruction
Intraluminal obstruction by stones, blood clots, sloughed papillae

Extra luminal compression of ureter (tumours, nodes, fibrosis) or urethra (benign prostatic hyperplasia, malignancy)

Figure 19.4 Acute kidney injury – AKI

Chronic kidney disease – CKD (Figure 19.5):

CKD is defined as abnormalities of kidney structure or function for ≥3 months. Markers of structural kidney damage can be histopathologic or radiologic abnormalities or history of renal transplantation. Markers of functional kidney damage include eGFR <60 ml/min/1.72 m², albuminuria (ACR ≥ 30 mg per 24 hours), urinary sediment abnormalities, or electrolyte and other abnormalities due to tubular disorders.

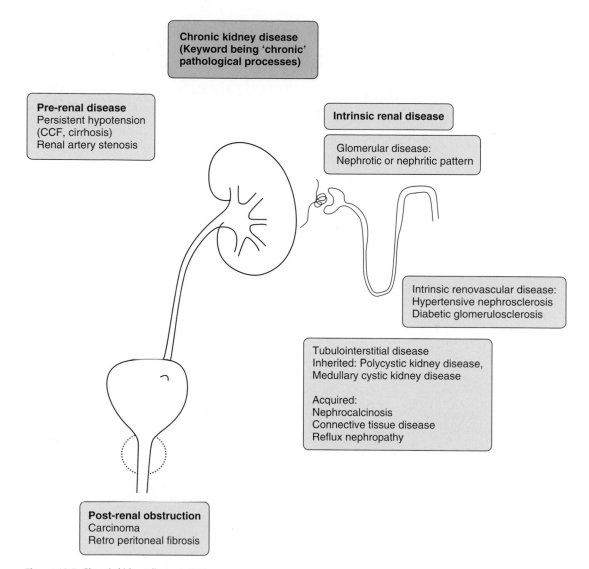

Figure 19.5 Chronic kidney disease – CKD

Non-specific symptoms of renal failure (Figure 19.6):

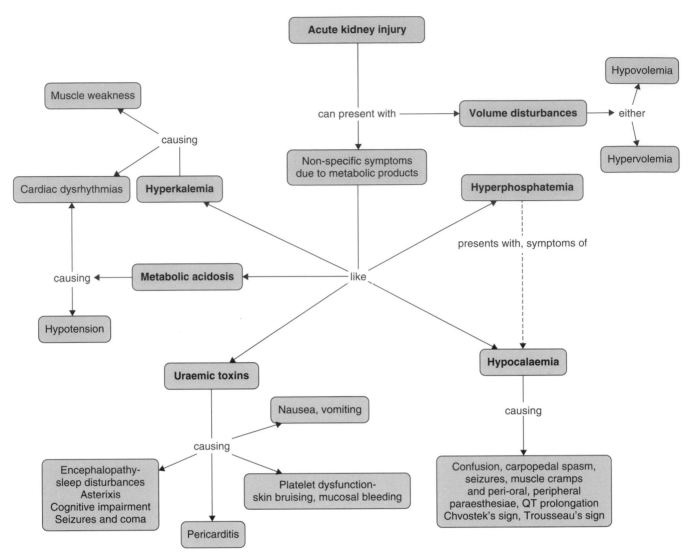

Figure 19.6 Non-specific symptoms of renal failure

▼
Focussing on relevant clinical features and their interpretation from a renal perspective
▲

Historically renal examination has been part of abdominal examination. However, it is worth focusing on renal examination in its own right to facilitate a quicker assessment in the right clinical context. For the sake of simplicity one could classify renal examination into two contexts: AKI and CKD. In both these scenarios the common theme is to identify the cause of the renal problem, assess complications arising out of renal failure and identify the need for renal replacement therapy. This entails examining other organ systems outside the abdomen. Obviously not all renal pathologies fall neatly into these two categories hence clinical judgement should be exercised.

Nephrology is also unique in that tests often do not follow clinical examination in a sequential manner. Often there is backward and forward thinking logic that is used in the evaluation of AKI and worsening CKD. For instance, AKI can first come to light when blood results become available. In these instances re-taking the history and re-examining the patient with a focus on the renal system will yield valuable insight into further management.

Figure 20.1 shows the concept map for clinical examination in AKI and Figure 20.2 shows the same in CKD.

A renal mass is distinguished from splenomegaly on the left and hepatomegaly on the right by its vertical movement on respiration, ballotability, ability to palpate the upper border, not crossing the midline (as opposed to splenomegaly) and a resonant percussion note over the mass as the kidney is a retroperitoneal organ that lies behind gas filled bowel. Always look for a left sided varicocele in males upon encountering a renal mass on the left. This often implies a renal cell carcinoma causing renal vein thrombosis and left varicocele as the left testicular vein enters the renal vein on the left. The right testicular vein drains into the inferior vena cava.

Renal angle tenderness or costovertebral angle tenderness is elicited at the angle between the 12th rib posteriorly and its vertebral body. Tenderness here implies renal capsule inflammation, e.g. pyelonephritis.

Renal artery bruits are best heard on either side of the midline in the epigastrium above the umbilicus and a systolic-diastolic bruit is more significant for renal artery stenosis than one which is evident in systole alone (Turnbull 1995).

A transplanted kidney is often found in an iliac fossa as a mass under a surgical scar. Three things need to be elicited upon encountering a transplanted kidney–

- Is it palpable? Non-palpable kidney under the scar implies a failed graft, i.e. chronic graft rejection.
- Is it tender? Tenderness implies inflammation from acute graft rejection or infection.
- Can you hear an arterial bruit over the mass? This implies that there is no impediment to its vascular supply.

The Hands-on Guide to Clinical Reasoning in Medicine, First Edition. Mujammil Irfan.
© 2019 John Wiley & Sons Ltd. Published 2019 by John Wiley & Sons Ltd.
Companion website: www.wiley.com/go/irfan/clinicalreasoning

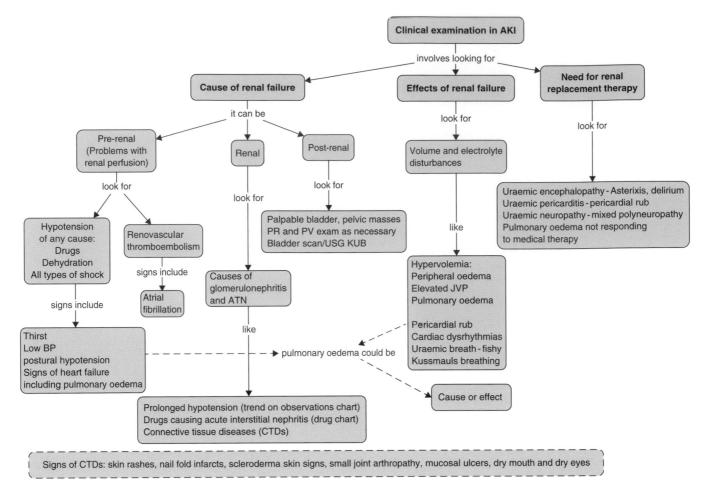

Figure 20.1 Clinical examination in acute kidney injury (AKI)

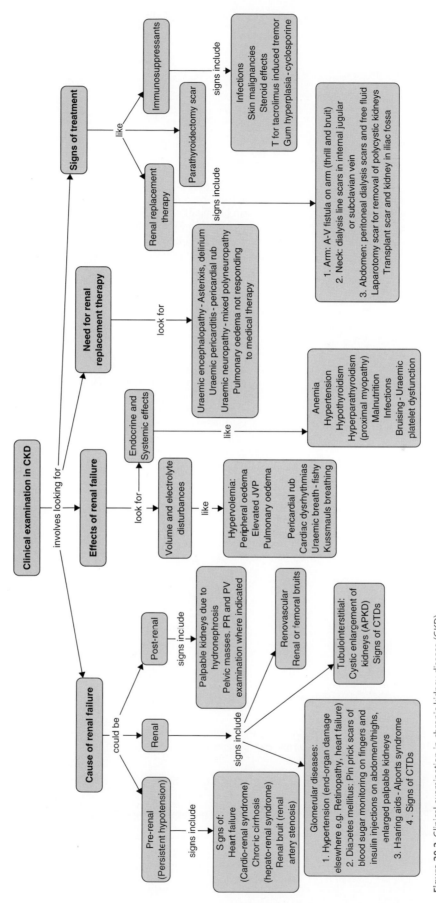

Figure 20.2 Clinical examination in chronic kidney disease (CKD)

Reference

Turnbull, J.M. (1995). The rational clinical examination. Is listening for abdominal bruits useful in the evaluation of hypertension? *JAMA* 274 (16): 1299–1301.

21 Renal Investigations: The Case of the Frothy Urine

▼

This chapter describes interpretation of urine dipstick, radiological scans, and arterial blood gases (ABGs) from a renal perspective

▲

Figure 21.1 shows the sequence of events that occur during the evolution of renal dysfunction. It clearly shows how symptoms lag far behind the actual loss of nephrons. The same can be said of serum creatinine as this lags behind glomerular filtration rate (GFR). In fact serum creatinine only begins to rise above upper limit of normal when the GFR has dropped by at least 50%. This is because of hyperfiltration in the remaining nephrons and increased proximal tubular secretion of creatinine. An active urinary sediment, e.g. albuminuria indicates glomerular damage as do dysmorphic red cells, red cell casts, and lipiduria.

Hypertension in this context can be perceived as the 'cry of the dying kidneys'. When glomeruli are starved of blood supply (e.g. ischemic regions in scarred areas of the kidneys) the drop in the GFR activates the renin-angiotension-aldosterone axis. The resulting hypertension raises the intraglomerular pressure (even in the normal areas of the kidneys) thus maintaining the GFR. Appropriate treatment of hypertension drops the intraglomerular pressure and the GFR. Counter-intuitively this slows down the progression of renal dysfunction by protecting the capillaries from high pressures which would ultimately lead to pathological sclerosis. This is especially true in patients who have diabetes mellitus and hypertension – two conditions that are most prevalent from an epidemiological stance. Angiotensin converting enzyme inhibitor/angiotensin receptor blocker (ACEi/ARB) therapy followed by nondihydropyridine calcium channel blockers (diltiazem, verapamil) have the most antiproteinuric effect (Kunz et al. 2008; Bakris et al. 2004).

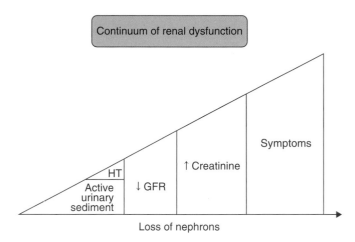

Figure 21.1 Continuum of renal dysfunction

21.1 URINALYSIS

A complete urinalysis includes gross inspection of urine, a urine dipstick, and microscopy. Figure 21.2 shows the different components of urinalysis.

The Hands-on Guide to Clinical Reasoning in Medicine, First Edition. Mujammil Irfan.
© 2019 John Wiley & Sons Ltd. Published 2019 by John Wiley & Sons Ltd.
Companion website: www.wiley.com/go/irfan/clinicalreasoning

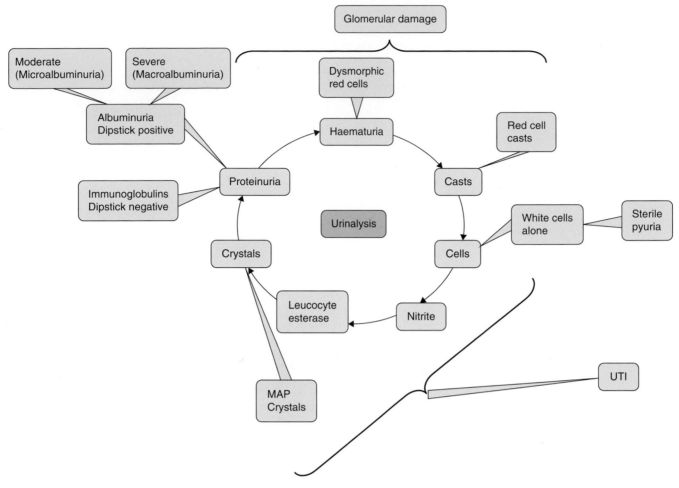

Figure 21.2 Interpretation of urinalysis

It is important to appreciate that various combinations of these components point to specific pathological states and these findings should always be correlated to the clinical context. For example, a clinical diagnosis of UTI can be cemented by finding white cells in the urine with a positive leucocyte esterase and nitrite. One can also find trace protein and haematuria, the latter especially in cystitis. However, nitrites can only be positive when the causative organism produces nitrate reductase (e.g. enterobacteriaceae). Again, a short dwell time in the bladder prevents bacteria from multiplying, making the test falsely negative. Finding renal stones with magnesium ammonium phosphate crystals (triple phosphate) lends credence to the possibility of Proteus UTI as this alkalinizes the urine crystallising triple phosphate out. Use your imagination to justify finding any of these components in various pathological states. I have got you started in Figure 21.2. Scribble alongside the diagram to make it your own.

21.2 PROTEINURIA

Urine dipsticks can only detect albuminuria and that too when it is greater than 300 mg per day (normal upper limit 150 mg per day). This is called overt proteinuria/severe albuminuria or macroalbuminuria. Any other protein in the urine is dipstick negative. This includes immunoglobulin light chains in myeloma, hence the need for testing Bence Jones protein in this setting. If moderate albuminuria (known as microalbuminuria previously) is suspected, either in the context of diabetes mellitus or glomerular disease of other aetiology, a spot urine albumin-creatinine ratio (ACR) will be helpful. An ACR of 30–300 mg g^{-1} or 3.4–34 mg mmol^{-1} indicates moderate albuminuria whilst an ACR > 300 mg g^{-1} or 34 mg mmol^{-1} indicates severe albuminuria.

21.3 HAEMATURIA

Figure 21.3 shows a concept map for haematuria from a urinalysis perspective. Read this in conjunction with the Figure 19.1 showing aetiology of haematuria in Chapter 19. Glomerular bleeding implies that red cells are squeezing through glomerular basement membranes and getting disfigured in the process (dysmorphic). They develop protrusions and are called acanthocytes. Clots are absent and glomerular bleeding is often accompanied by proteinuria. The red cells squeezed through the basement membranes get trapped in Tamm-Horsfall protein (tubular epithelial mucus) and appear as red cell casts akin to a fossilised insect trapped in amber. Non-glomerular bleeding does not have any of these features.

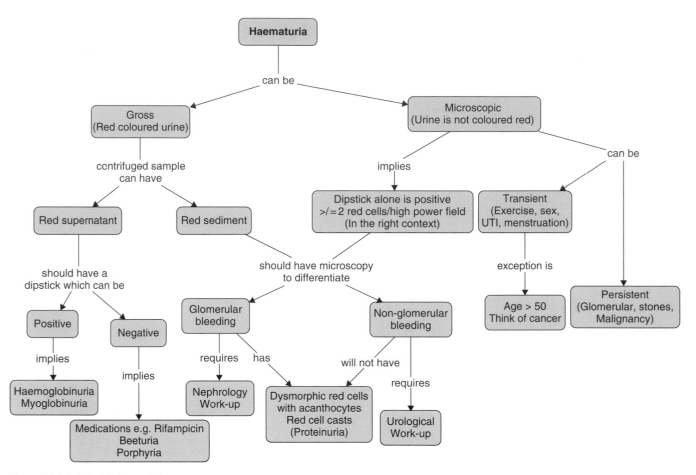

Figure 21.3 Urinalysis in Haematuria

21.4 CASTS

As mentioned above, a cast is essentially proteinaceous mucus which is normally produced by the tubular epithelium. Any cells that enter the tubule whilst the mucus is being secreted get trapped within it. Hence cellular casts imply intra-renal origin. Red cell casts point to glomerulonephritis or acute interstitial nephritis (AIN). White cell casts often imply AIN as there is inflammatory infiltration into the tubular epithelium. Tubular epithelial casts would mean that tubular epithelial cells have been shed into the tubule which often happens in acute tubular necrosis, AIN or proliferative glomerulonephritis. Too much of protein (immunoglobulin light chains) can obstruct tubules causing cast nephropathy as seen in myeloma.

21.5 CRYSTALS

In the setting of AKI finding crystals in the urine can point to its aetiology. For example, ethylene glycol ingestion causes calcium oxalate crystals and AKI. Uric acid crystals are seen in tumour lysis syndrome.

21.6 ABGs IN RENAL DYSFUNCTION

ABGs provide insight into acid–base balance in which the kidneys and lungs play a central role. An in-depth analysis of an ABG can often reveal the cause of AKI, e.g. lactic acidosis can point to inadequate tissue perfusion that concomitantly causes AKI. On the other hand, renal failure by itself can cause metabolic acidosis.

$$AG = (Na^+ + K^+) - (HCO_3^- + Cl^-)$$

Normal range = $12 \pm 4\,mmol\,l^{-1}$. If K^+ is included in the calculation then it is $16 \pm 4\,mmol\,l^{-1}$. Remember to check the normal range in your laboratory as this varies.

21.7 ANION GAP (AG)

When an ABG shows metabolic acidosis, the AG can help narrow down the causes. The concept of AG is based on the fact that molecules have electrical charges. Anions are negatively charged whilst cations are positively charged. Normal serum has more unmeasured anions (albumin, organic acids such as sulphates and phosphates) than unmeasured cations (K^+, Ca^{2+}, and Mg^{2+}).

Figure 21.4a shows that the AG is actually unmeasured anions (UAs) minus unmeasured cations (UCs). Since we cannot measure these we indirectly infer the AG by calculating it from the measured ions, i.e. Na^+, Cl^-, and HCO_3^-.

If serum HCO_3^- is lost via the kidneys (mild to moderate renal dysfunction, renal tubular acidosis) or the gut (diarrhoea) a metabolic acidemia ensues. If this drop in serum HCO_3^- is compensated by a rise in Cl^- the AG remains normal (Figure 21.4b).

Mnemonic for raised AG:
K – ketones
U – urea
S – salicylates
S – sulphates and phosphates
M – methanol, ethylene glycol, propylene glycol (common solvent for intravenous lorazepam, etc.)
A – alcohol
U – unmeasured anions
L – lactate

On the other hand, if extra acid (UA) is added to the extra-cellular fluid (ECF), HCO_3^- gets used to buffer this. The serum HCO_3^- now drops causing a metabolic acidemia. On this occasion there is no compensatory rise in Cl^- resulting in an elevated anion gap (Figure 21.4c). A high anion gap implies that there are more unmeasured anions in the blood than normal. The mnemonic 'KUSSMAUL' (see opposite) lists some of the common causes of a raised AG (Mehta et al. 2008).

In mild to moderate renal impairment, a normal AG hyperchloremic metabolic acidosis is seen, whereas end-stage renal disease produces an elevated AG metabolic acidosis (Kraut and Madias 2007, 2012). This is because in the former, tubular dysfunction predominates, resulting in a loss of HCO_3^- into the lumen. Instead of HCO_3^-, chloride gets reabsorbed causing hyperchloremia. The loss of HCO_3^- and the inability of the tubular epithelial cells to generate new HCO_3^- and secrete H^+ results in the metabolic acidaemia. In end-stage renal disease, the GFR drops to the point where no electrolytes or organic acids are being filtered, increasing the acid load in the ECF. The accumulating organic acids (sulphates and phosphates) elevate the AG.

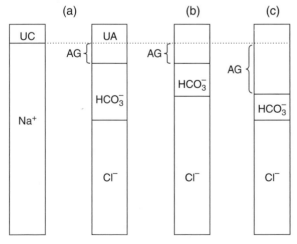

Cations = Anions

$$Na^+ + K^+ + UC = HCO_3^- + Cl^- + UA$$

$$(Na^+ + K^+) - (HCO_3^- + Cl^-) = UA - UC$$

$$(Na^+ + K^+) - (HCO_3^- + Cl^-) = AG$$

Figure 21.4 Explanation of anion gap

Calculated serum osmolality = (2 × serum sodium) + urea + glucose + (1.25 × ethanol)

Osmolal gap = measured serum osmolality – calculated serum osmolality

Normal value – 6 mOsmol l^{-1}

Raised osmolal gap >10 mOsmol l^{-1}

21.8 OSMOLAL GAP

The primary solutes in plasma that contribute to serum osmolality are sodium salts, urea, and glucose. Unexplained elevated AG metabolic acidemia in conjunction with a raised osmolal gap should make one think of volatile acid intoxication like ethylene glycol and methanol. The formula given opposite is especially useful in this setting since these solvents are commonly ingested with ethanol (Purssell et al. 2001). In fact, patients presenting in the early stages of solvent ingestion can have a raised osmolal gap alone without the elevated AG metabolic acidemia. Other causes of an elevated osmolal gap are propylene glycol (used as a solvent for lorazepam) and pseudohyponatremia which is a laboratory error secondary to co-existent hyperlipidaemia and hyperproteinaemia. Pseudohyponatremia is not accompanied by an elevated AG metabolic acidemia.

21.9 ULTRASONOGRAPHY (USG) IN RENAL MEDICINE

Ultrasound is uniquely placed in nephrology as it is a non-ionising imaging modality which does not require use of any contrast material, the latter potentially causing further problems in renal failure. In post renal failure an USG can help identify hydronephrosis which can be unilateral or bilateral depending on the level of obstruction. Post void bladder volume assessment can be useful in bladder outflow tract obstruction especially in men with prostatic enlargement.

USG can also help in discriminating AKI from CKD. Chronic kidney disease would often show small (<10 cm), echo dense kidneys with thin renal cortices. A unilaterally small kidney points to renovascular disease, i.e. renal artery stenosis on that side. The normal length of a kidney is roughly 11 cm.

Finally, an USG is useful in non-resolving pyelonephritis as it can help identify perinephric abscesses or a stone complicating the infection.

References

Bakris, G.L., Weir, M.R., Secic, M. et al. (2004). Differential effects of calcium antagonist subclasses on markers of nephropathy progression. *Kidney International* 65 (6): 1991–2002.

Kraut, J.A. and Madias, N.E. (2007). Serum anion gap: its uses and limitations in clinical medicine. *Clinical Journal of the American Society of Nephrology* 2 (1): 162–174.

Kraut, J.A. and Madias, N.E. (2012). Differential diagnosis of nongap metabolic acidosis: value of a systematic approach. *Clinical Journal of the American Society of Nephrology* 7 (4): 671–679.

Kunz, R., Friedrich, C., Wolbers, M., and Mann, J.F. (2008). Meta-analysis: effect of monotherapy and combination therapy with inhibitors of the renin angiotensin system on proteinuria in renal disease. *Annals of Internal Medicine* 148 (1): 30–48.

Mehta, A.N., Emmett, J.B., Emmett, M. et al. (2008). GOLD MARK: an anion gap mnemonic for the 21st century. *Lancet (London, England)* 372 (9642): 892.

Purssell, R.A., Pudek, M., Brubacher, J. et al. (2001). Derivation and validation of a formula to calculate the contribution of ethanol to the osmolal gap. *Annals of Emergency Medicine* 38 (6): 653–659.

22 Hypertension

▼

This chapter tells you how to approach hypertension from a renal perspective

▲

Although primary hypertension is one of the most prevalent conditions on a population-wide basis there are occasions when secondary causes need to be considered. It is worth noting that hypertension in renal disease can be either cause or effect or both.

Example 22.1

> A 38 year old man is referred by the GP for a two month history of worsening hypertension despite being on amlodipine, bendroflumethiazide, and bisoprolol. He had a 30 py history of smoking and hypercholesterolemia in the background.

> J: SQs- young man + worsening hypertension + vascular risk factors. Provisional diagnoses – all causes of secondary hypertension or concordance issues, i.e. not taking his medications.

Hypertensive emergency

Evidence of end-organ damage
Brain – encephalopathy
Eyes – Severe hypertensive retinopathy
Heart – acute heart failure
Kidneys – acute hypertensive nephrosclerosis
(microscopic haematuria)
Vessels – aortic dissection

> The GP having ensured concordance had started ramipril to help control the BP but this had worsened the renal function with a K+ of 5.5 mmol l⁻¹ and creatinine of 140 μmol l⁻¹ from a baseline creatinine of 110 μmol l⁻¹. O/E: He looked well with a BP of 180/110 mmHg. He had grade 2 hypertensive retinopathy on fundoscopy but the rest of the examination was normal with no evidence of renal bruits. There were no features to suggest an endocrine cause of hypertension. ECG showed normal sinus rhythm and LVH. Urine dipstick: 1+ protein. The admitting physician raised the possibility of renal artery stenosis and requested an ultrasound of the kidneys.

> J: severity of illness – relatively well. There is grade 2 hypertensive retinopathy and LVH on the ECG but no strong evidence of end-organ damage indicating hypertensive emergency. Renal artery stenosis does seem a possibility.

> Bloods: Hb 110 g l⁻¹, MCV 90 fl, Na+ 136 mmol l⁻¹, and urea 6 mmol l⁻¹, remaining bloods: normal. The Consultant Physician reprimanded the registrar for ordering unnecessary tests and continued the ACEi. The BP dropped to 150/90 in three days and the creatinine plateaued at 130 μmol l⁻¹.

The Hands-on Guide to Clinical Reasoning in Medicine, First Edition. Mujammil Irfan.
© 2019 John Wiley & Sons Ltd. Published 2019 by John Wiley & Sons Ltd.
Companion website: www.wiley.com/go/irfan/clinicalreasoning

Activity 22.1

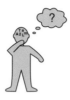

(Allow a minute)

Would you have requested the renal ultrasonography (USG)?

```



```

ACEi inhibit the action of ACE thereby reducing the levels of angiotensin II. Normally angiotensin II constricts the efferent arteriole raising the intraglomerular pressures causing a rise in GFR. ACE inhibition abolishes this action dropping the intraglomerular pressures and GFR. This inadvertently raises the serum creatinine modestly. A persistent elevation in creatinine >30% above baseline following ACEi therapy suggests renal artery stenosis (Bakris and Weir 2000). This is not the case here, making renal artery stenosis unlikely.

However, resistant hypertension in a young person should raise the suspicion of secondary hypertension with underlying endocrine and renal causes. Given the lack of features suggestive of an endocrine disorder it would be prudent to investigate the kidneys in the first instance.

The ultrasound surprisingly showed polycystic kidneys. This was confirmed with a positive family history and he was referred to the nephrologists for further management.

Although the context was rightly framed in the beginning, the admitting physician was misled by the ACEi induced rise in creatinine. Resistant hypertension especially in a young man albeit with vascular risk factors should trigger the possibility of secondary hypertension, which was overlooked by the consultant physician. In this case, an ultrasound scan done for the wrong reasons luckily gave the right diagnosis. The lesson is, to never lose sight of the context as defined by the SQs for the problem at hand.

Example 22.2

A 70 year old man was admitted with worsening breathlessness over a week. He was being treated with erythromycin for cellulitis over the last 10 days. He had a history of hypertension, diabetes mellitus, and ischemic heart disease.

P: SQs- elderly man + worsening breathlessness + cellulitis + vascular risk factors. Provisional diagnoses – infection causing decompensated heart failure, Type 2 MI due to sepsis, CAP or PE (relative immobility).

O/E: He appeared short of breath, with Pulse 110 bpm, BP 150/90, RR 28 per minute, Saturations 90% on air, BMs 21 mmol l^{-1} and Temperature 38 °C. RS: Bi-basal crepitations; CVS: Bi-pedal oedema and an elevated JVP with an S3; marked tenderness, erythema on his right leg - representing acute cellulitis. No clinical evidence of DVT or peripheral neurovascular disease was found.

CXR: Pulmonary oedema. ECG: Sinus tachycardia with old Q waves in inferior leads. An ABG revealed metabolic acidosis with a pH of 7.3, lactate 4, HCO_3^- 17, pCO_2 4 kpa and pO_2 of 9 kpa. He was started on supplementary oxygen, IV frusemide, IV benzylpenicillin, and sliding scale of insulin.

P: *Severity of illness – very ill. It seems to be straightforward cellulitis causing sepsis and metabolic acidosis. This may well be causing decompensated heart failure owing to the vascular risk factors.*

Bloods: High WCC 16×10^9 per litre, Hb $110\,g\,l^{-1}$, CRP $80\,mg\,l^{-1}$, Na^+ $136\,mmol\,l^{-1}$, K^+ $3.6\,mmol\,l^{-1}$, urea $12\,mmol\,l^{-1}$, creatinine $150\,\mu mol\,l^{-1}$. Normal LFTs, troponin I was 4. The senior house officer noted his previous U&Es were normal (creatinine $110\,\mu mol\,l^{-1}$) a month ago when checked in the diabetes clinic. She asked for a urine dipstick, which showed 2+ protein, 2+ blood, leucocytes, no nitrites. The sample was sent for microscopy and culture.

P: *He has an AKI with proteinuria and haematuria. Could it be because of sepsis?*

Activity 22.2

(Allow a minute)

The most common cause of AKI in sepsis is pre-renal hypotension causing ischemic injury. He seems to have hypertension which is odd given that he has sepsis! Another odd thing is that he has heart failure with hypertension. If this was an acute MI the hypertension can be explained by sympathetic activation but that isn't the case. A better question would be 'what are the causes of heart failure with hypertension?'

P: *Subarachnoid haemorrhage* (increased sympathetic activation), *bilateral renal artery stenosis* (activation of rennin-angiotensin-aldosterone axis), *thyrotoxicosis.*

I like that you are thinking! Most of these conditions cause flash pulmonary oedema (LVF) except perhaps thyrotoxicosis. However, our patient has biventricular failure. Cardio-renal syndrome consists of renal conditions that can affect the heart and vice versa. These include bilateral renal artery stenosis, nephritic syndrome and chronic kidney disease.

Suspecting something was amiss, she asked for a spot urine albumin-creatinine ratio which was $40\,mg\,mmol^{-1}$. She consulted with the on-call Nephrology registrar who suggested a strict input–output chart with fluid restriction, daily U&Es and took over the patient's care.

The repeat Troponin I was 3 and blood cultures grew *Staphylococcus aureus*, sensitive to penicillin. He was diagnosed with post-Staphylococcal glomerulonephritis and required an ACEi to control his hypertension. Once the infection was treated, his creatinine started improving and he was discharged with renal clinic follow-up.

A single piece of the puzzle (hypertension) which was not fitting the picture (sepsis, heart failure, and AKI) necessitated a revision of the diagnosis leading to appropriate management of the patient. One must be aware of these misfits in the data when evaluating patients and revise the hypothesis where necessary.

Example 22.3

A 42 year old man was admitted to A&E with a three day history of sudden onset, non-colicky left flank pain. He had a history of hypertension for which he took amlodipine. There was no history of urinary tract calculi.

J: *SQs- middle aged man + acute left flank pain. Provisional diagnoses – upper UTI, possible pyelonephritis, renal stones will still be in the differential.*

O/E: Pulse 90 bpm, BP 160/90, Saturations 98% on air, Temperature 37.6 °C, BMs 9 mmol l^{-1}, RR 18 per minute. He looked comfortable and the pain was reported as dull. He had left renal angle tenderness and the rest of the examination was normal.

Urine dipstick: blood 2+, protein 1+, leucocyte esterase positive. Abdominal X-ray (AXR): No renal tract calculi.

J: *Severity of illness – ill. Sounds like a UTI.*

Bloods: Hb 120 g l^{-1}, WCC 13 × 10^9 per litre, CRP 60 mg l^{-1}, U&Es normal, with a creatinine of 80 µmol l^{-1}. He was started on trimethoprim for a suspected UTI and urine was sent for MC&S. He was given co-codamol for pain and discharged.

Three days later, he re-presented with ongoing left-flank pain, but was apyrexial. Repeat bloods: Creatinine 120 µmol l^{-1}, CRP 40 mg l^{-1}, and WCC 11 × 10^9 per litre. The urine culture requested previously was negative. Urine sediment did not show any dysmorphic red cells or red cell casts. The admitting registrar ascribed the raised creatinine to trimethoprim, as it blocks tubular epithelial cell secretion of creatinine. However, given the persistence of pain, she requested a CT scan of the renal tract to exclude perinephric abscess.

The CT scan showed polycystic kidneys but no evidence of perinephric abscess or calculi. He was referred to the nephrologists for further management.

Would you have treated him for a UTI with his initial presentation?

Activity 22.3

(Allow a minute)

The answer is yes. UTI seems more likely given the higher prevalence of this condition with this presentation. However, a lack of resolution of symptoms with treatment of the provisional diagnosis should suggest an alternative diagnosis which is what was done in this scenario.

In hindsight, suggestive features for polycystic kidney disease included age, hypertension, and haematuria. One could argue that the hypertension was secondary to pain although the latter was not severe. The mild temperature and inflammatory marker rise did not fit with pyelonephritis. Cyst rupture was the likely cause for pain and haematuria. Polycystic kidney disease commonly presents as hypertension in the fourth decade but other variations of disease presentation include UTI and renal calculi. One must be aware of the variability of disease presentation and pause to think of all the diagnoses that could explain the constellation of signs and symptoms, e.g. symptomatic non-ruptured abdominal aortic aneurysms, acute pancreatitis, and pelvic inflammatory disease in a woman (think of all the anatomical structures in the vicinity of the renal angle).

Reference

Bakris, G.L. and Weir, M.R. (2000). Angiotensin-converting enzyme inhibitor–associated elevations in serum creatinine. *Archives of Internal Medicine* 160 (5): 2413–2446.

23 Haematuria

This chapter tells you how to approach haematuria from a renal perspective

Haematuria can arise from anywhere along the renal tract. Identification of a glomerular source of bleeding warrants a renal work-up as opposed to a urological work-up if it is non-glomerular in origin. Active urinary sediment with dysmorphic red cells, red cell casts, albuminuria, and lipiduria points to a glomerular source.

Example 23.1

> A 26 year old man presents with a two day history of gross haematuria. He has no significant past medical history and is not on any medications. He denies using any recreational drugs.

> P: *SQs – Young man + gross haematuria. Provisional diagnoses – Renal stones, UTI.*

> There was no history of intense exercise preceding the haematuria (thinking of rhabdomyolysis). There were no clots and the urine was brown in colour. He complained of left flank pain but there were no features suggestive of renal colic or history of renal stones. On direct questioning he admitted to an ongoing flu-like illness with sore throat for three days but no cough.

> P: *The flank pain points to either pyelonephritis or nephrolithiasis.*

> O/E: Pulse 90 bpm, BP 150/80, Saturations 96% on air, Temperature 37.8 °C, RR 18 per minute. He had anterior cervical lymphadenopathy but no tonsillar exudates. PA: Left- flank tenderness but no masses felt. The rest of the systemic examination: normal. Urine dipstick: Blood 3+, protein 2+, leucocyte esterase positive, nitrites negative, and pH normal.

> P: *Severity of illness – ill. The examination seems to suggest a UTI with a low grade pyrexia, flank tenderness, and positive urine dipstick.*

> Bloods: WCC 13×10^9 l^{-1}, CRP 120 mg l^{-1}L, Na$^+$ 138 mmol l^{-1}, K$^+$ 4 mmol l^{-1}, Urea 8 mmol l^{-1}, Creatinine 120 μmol l^{-1}, Albumin 35 g l^{-1}, and remaining LFTs: normal. The admitting SHO diagnosed a UTI and treated him with oral trimethoprim.

Activity 23.1

(Allow a minute)

How would you fit the cervical lymphadenopathy and sore throat into this diagnosis?

The Hands-on Guide to Clinical Reasoning in Medicine, First Edition. Mujammil Irfan.
© 2019 John Wiley & Sons Ltd. Published 2019 by John Wiley & Sons Ltd.
Companion website: www.wiley.com/go/irfan/clinicalreasoning

Re-stating the SQs: upper respiratory tract infection (URTI) + active urinary sediment + hypertension. The last two point to nephritic syndrome. Acute haematuria with URTI should raise the possibility of glomerular disease.

The consultant physician noted that the patient had no family history of renal disease and that there were no previous episodes of haematuria. He requested a rapid antigen detection test (RADT) for group A Streptococci (GAS) on a throat swab and treated him with penicillin. The test was positive. The dipstick proteinuria was confirmed with a raised urine ACR of 40 mg mmol⁻¹. Urine microscopy: Dysmorphic red cells and red cell casts. A renal USG did not show any evidence of pyelonephritis or hydronephrosis. He was diagnosed with post-Streptococcal GN.

P: *The high inflammatory markers with a positive GAS test would fit in with Group A Streptococcal pharyngitis. The clinical picture suggests nephritic syndrome with an active urinary sediment and elevated creatinine. However, would you get flank pain with post-Streptococcal GN?*

Any acute GN can cause tissue oedema and stretch the renal capsules causing flank pain.

Given the hypertension and proteinuria, he was started on ramipril 2.5 mg OD. The haematuria persisted with a raised creatinine of 125 μmol l⁻¹, whilst the sore throat settled over a week.

P: *Is the persistently raised creatinine secondary to ramipril?*

I don't think so as the creatinine was already raised prior to its initiation.

A renal consult was skeptical of the diagnosis. They decided to proceed with a renal biopsy owing to the persistent haematuria, proteinuria, and raised creatinine. They postulated that post-Streptococcal GN would have a latent period of one to three weeks rather than the near simultaneous haematuria with pharyngitis in this case.

The renal biopsy confirmed IgA nephropathy, which causes 'synpharyngitic haematuria,' i.e. haematuria with pharyngitis. He was followed up in the renal clinic when his haematuria settled in a few months.

The availability heuristic led the SHO to diagnose a UTI. Although this is more common from a prevalence perspective it is vital to explain all the clinical features with the diagnosis that is being put forward. The inability to explain the pharyngitis with the diagnosis of a UTI should lead one to question the diagnosis.

Example 23.2

A 75 year old lady was admitted with a three day history of cough and green sputum, accompanied by fevers, lethargy, and weight loss over two months. There were no other chest symptoms. She had a history of hypertension for which she took ramipril. This was her third admission for similar complaints over the last two months.

J: *SQs – Elderly lady + acute cough on a background of similar recurrent episodes and hypertension. Provisional diagnoses – acute bronchitis, unresolved CAP, malignancy.*

O/E: Pulse 90 bpm, BP 150/80, Saturations 91% on air, Temperature 37.2 °C, RR 20 per minute. RS: Crepitations in the right lung base and reduced breath sounds with increased vocal resonance. CXR: confirmed right basal consolidation and she was treated with antibiotics. A CT scan was organized given the recurrent presentations to look for underlying lung malignancy.

J: *The hypoxia, clinical findings and CXR fit with CAP however I agree that malignancy needs to be excluded.*

The CT scan showed multiple lung parenchymal opacities, some of which were cavitating. A follow-on CT of abdomen and pelvis did not show any evidence of the primary. Breast examination: normal. The admitting team raised the possibility of TB owing to the prolonged constitutional symptoms and chronic cough.

J: *The differential lies in all the causes of cavitating lung lesions (Gadkowski and Stout 2008).*

Lists of conditions that cause a particular clinical entity are useful as an aide memoire. Checking off exhaustive lists would ensure that no diagnosis is missed but the fallout is that unnecessary tests are requested which can muddy the waters further. For instance, a false positive result can mislead the clinician who does not heed the prior probability of the condition in question. Herein the clinical context dictates who should be your prime suspect. Tests to rule out diseases whose prior probability is greatest should be requested first instead of a blanket screen. Disease prevalence helps, but the clinical context narrows it down. With this in mind, what would your differential be?

Activity 23.2

(Allow two minutes)

....

....

....

....

....

Infections, malignancy, and autoimmune conditions would be on top of the list.

A respiratory consult elicited no personal or family history of TB. In fact, five days into her admission she was feeling well and asymptomatic. There was no significant travel history. Given the cavitating lesions the registrar advised a bronchoscopy to exclude atypical TB and other opportunistic infections. HIV and an autoimmune screen were requested. Bloods: Hb 120 g l^{-1}, WCC 11 × 10^9 l^{-1}, CRP 40 mg l^{-1}, U&Es, and LFTs: Normal. Urine dipstick: blood 2+, protein 1+. Urine microscopy: red cell casts and dysmorphic red cells.

Bronchial washings were negative for atypical TB, other opportunistic organisms and malignancy. PR3-anti-nuclear cytoplasmic antibody (ANCA): positive. HIV: negative. A renal biopsy showed granulomatosis with polyangiitis (GPA) and she was started on immunosuppressants.

Lung lesions with an active urinary sediment and hypertension (the last two pointing to nephritic syndrome) would raise the possibility of pulmonary-renal syndromes like Goodpasture's, GPA and other connective tissue diseases. The creatinine can initially remain normal as we have discovered in the chapter on renal investigations (Figure 21.1).

If bronchial washings had not excluded infections one would be reluctant to give immunosuppressants on the basis of a positive ANCA alone. On the other hand GPA cannot be excluded solely on the basis of a negative ANCA as 10% of patients with GPA can be ANCA negative (Savige et al. 2005). This is where pre-test probability of a disease comes in. If the pre-test probability is high, a negative ANCA should be followed up with a tissue biopsy to confirm or refute GPA.

Example 23.3

An on-call SHO was bleeped by a staff nurse from the ward with a positive urine dipstick: protein 1+, blood 1+, leucocyte esterase and nitrites positive. She requested a review for prescribing antibiotics. The urine dipstick was from an 82 year old man with a history of falls, DM, IHD, MI, and HT. He had a long-term urinary catheter in situ.

P: *SQs – Elderly man + positive urine dipstick + vascular risk factors + catheterised.*
      Provisional diagnoses – Possible UTI.

The urine dipstick was done as the urine smelt strong. On review he denied any abdominal pain. A urine culture on admission a week ago was positive for *Escherichia Coli* sensitive to gentamicin and nitrofurantoin. He was orientated to time and place. O/E: HR 84 bpm, BP 130/80, Temperature 36.6 °C, RR 16 per minute, BMs 14 mmol l⁻¹L, Saturations 95% on air. PA: no suprapubic or costovertebral angle tenderness. Rest of systemic examination: normal.

The SHO started nitrofurantoin and requested the nurse to send the urine specimen for culture and sensitivity.

Would you have started antibiotics?

Activity 23.3

(Allow a minute)

The antibiotics were stopped the next day by the consultant physician as the patient was felt to be asymptomatic. The need for the catheter was reviewed. The catheter had been inserted on a recent hospital admission two months ago for reasons of immobility. A decision was made for a trial without catheter, which was successful and he was discharged when his mobility improved with walking aids and physiotherapy.

This example brings to light the topic of screening tests. An appropriate screening test presupposes intention to treat if it turns out to be positive. Furthermore, treatment should have a mortality/morbidity benefit. Hence screening is utilised in specific populations with risk factors to minimise costs and improve health on a population-wide basis. In addition a good screening test should have low false positive/false negative rate thereby detecting those who have the disease.

Urine dipsticks are often done on admission as a 'routine screening test' but they lack specificity in the context of UTIs. The lack of symptoms (fever, confusion in the elderly, suprapubic or costovertebral pain) or signs of sepsis make it very unlikely that this gentleman has a UTI especially in the setting of a long-term catheter. Long-term catheterisation results in microbial colonisation in a 'biofilm' around the catheter (Nickel et al. 1994) which causes asymptomatic bacteriuria. It also leads to mucosal injury of the bladder causing a false positive 'haematuria.' Asymptomatic bacteriuria is treated only in special circumstances of pregnancy (with risk factors) or prior to urinary tract instrumentation where it has been shown to reduce mortality and morbidity. In short treat symptoms not test results.

References

Gadkowski, L.B. and Stout, J.E. (2008). Cavitary pulmonary disease. *Clinical Microbiology Reviews* 21 (2): 305–333.

Nickel, J.C., Costerton, J.W., McLean, R.J., and Olson, M. (1994). Bacterial biofilms: influence on the pathogenesis, diagnosis and treatment of urinary tract infections. *Journal of Antimicrobial Chemotherapy* 33 (suppl A): 31–41.

Savige, J., Pollock, W., and Trevisin, M. (2005). What do antineutrophil cytoplasmic antibodies (ANCA) tell us? *Best Practice & Research. Clinical Rheumatology* 19 (2): 263–276.

▼

This chapter tells you how to approach oedema from a renal perspective

▲

Oedema in nephrotic syndrome often starts in non-dependent areas with loose subcutaneous tissue, e.g. peri-orbitally and then evolves into abdominal (ascites), peripheral, and generalised oedema (anasarca). Pulmonary oedema is unusual in nephrotic syndrome unless there is co-existent heart disease. In contrast, the salt and water retention causing volume expansion in nephritic syndrome behaves as biventricular failure, i.e. both peripheral and pulmonary oedema. This is distinguished from CCF by hypertension.

Example 24.1

A 65 year old man was referred for exclusion of a right leg DVT. He was being treated for CCF by his GP over the last three weeks. Previous medical history (PMH): hypertension and diabetes mellitus for which he took aspirin, bisoprolol, frusemide, and metformin.

P: *SQs: Middle aged man + (CCF + HT + DM + right leg swelling. Provisional diagnoses – DVT, CCF, local causes of limb oedema.*

O/E: HR 80 bpm, BP 130/70, Saturations 95% on air, Temperature 36.6 °C, RR 18 per minute. He had bilateral pitting pedal oedema with the right leg more swollen than the left up to the knees. No deep vein tenderness. CVS: JVP normal, no added sounds. RS: normal breath sounds. PA: mildly swollen, shifting dullness suggesting free fluid but no masses.

Bloods: Hb 130 g l^{-1}, WCC 14 × 10^9 l^{-1}, CRP 60 mg l^{-1}. LFTs: normal, except albumin 25 g l^{-1}, and protein 60 g l^{-1}. U&Es: normal. The admitting SHO gave him treatment dose enoxaparin and asked him to return for a venous doppler the next day in accordance with the DVT pathway. Whilst filling in his drug chart he noticed a diclofenac prescription for worsening chronic back pain over the last month.

P: *Severity of illness – ill. NSAIDs can cause fluid retention as well as AKI. I suspect this has decompensated the heart failure resulting in worsening oedema.*

The venous doppler was positive for a DVT and he was started on therapeutic anticoagulation. The registrar stopped the NSAIDs and re-visited the history to elicit the risk factors for DVT. There were no risk factors apart from relative immobility over the last three weeks since he started noticing the swollen legs. On further questioning it transpired that he initially noticed swelling around his eyes first thing in the mornings, which later progressed to generalised oedema.

The Hands-on Guide to Clinical Reasoning in Medicine, First Edition. Mujammil Irfan.
© 2019 John Wiley & Sons Ltd. Published 2019 by John Wiley & Sons Ltd.
Companion website: www.wiley.com/go/irfan/clinicalreasoning

Albumin: globulin ratio = albumin/total
protein-albumin
Normal > 1

P: The oedema seems to be of renal aetiology. Can NSAIDs cause nephrotic syndrome?

Yes, they can cause minimal change disease resulting in nephrotic syndrome.

Given the hypoalbuminemia and renal oedema, a urine dipstick, and urine ACR were requested, which showed protein 3+ and ACR 45 g mmol^{-1}, confirming proteinuria. The low albumin/globulin ratio in combination with worsening back pain raised the possibility of myeloma causing nephrotic syndrome. Serum electrophoresis confirmed this diagnosis and a kidney biopsy showed light chain deposition, confirming myeloma kidney.

What factors could have prevented the SHO from getting the full picture?

Activity 24.1

(Allow three minutes)

The admitting SHO was blinkered by the question of DVT that the GP had raised focusing entirely on ruling out DVT in a busy medical admissions unit. We are all guilty of succumbing to such pressures especially when constrained by 'pathways' which further restrict our vision. It is in fact in these pressing situations that one should be alert to the perils of premature closure. The relatively new onset of 'heart failure' which was temporally associated with NSAID use for worsening back pain should have triggered further questioning. Answering the question raised should not be the only focus but should go beyond to explain all the relevant clinical findings.

Example 24.2

A 66 year old dishevelled man with chronic cirrhosis was admitted for worsening ascites and leg oedema over two weeks. He was a regular at the hospital, having paracentesis whenever his ascites worsened. He had ongoing alcohol dependence and chronic hepatitis B (HBV). Drugs included frusemide 40 mg od, spironolactone 50 mg od, and thiamine.

J: SQs – Middle aged man + chronic cirrhosis and ascites + alcohol excess + hepatitis B + worsening oedema. Provisional diagnoses: any failure could cause worsening oedema e.g. decompensated cirrhosis (liver failure) or alcoholic cardiomyopathy (heart failure), AKI from drugs or gastro-intestinal (GI) bleed or sepsis related (renal failure).

This was his fourth admission for paracentesis over the last two months. He denied any recent cardiac sounding chest pains or history of IHD, haematemesis, over the counter drugs, recreational drug use or infective symptoms. The ascites was not associated with any pain (thinking of spontaneous bacterial peritonitis – SBP). His appetite was poor but he had gained weight from the oedema. Current smoker 40 py, alcohol intake 40 units per week.

O/E: Unkempt and strong smelling. HR 90 bpm, BP 130/70, Saturations 90% on air, RR 22 per minute, Temperature 37 °C. PA: soft and non-tender, massive ascites with fluid thrill; bilateral pitting leg oedema until thighs. CVS: JVP normal, no signs of heart failure; RS: chest clear.

J:　*Severity of illness – ill. No features to suggest heart failure, signs point to decompensated cirrhosis.*

Bloods: Hb 120 g l⁻¹, WCC 14 × 10⁹ l⁻¹, platelets 150 × 10⁹ l⁻¹, CRP 40 mg l⁻¹, Na⁺ 130 mmol l⁻¹, K⁺ 3.2 mmol l⁻¹, urea 6 mmol l⁻¹, creatinine 110 μmol l⁻¹, albumin 25 g l⁻¹ L, ALT 20 IU l⁻¹ ALP 120 IU l⁻¹, GGT 80 IU l⁻¹, PT 16s, fibrinogen 2 g l⁻¹, APTT 35s, alpha fetoprotein 10 mcg l⁻¹. CXR: normal. ECG: normal.

J:　*The low albumin, platelets, urea, and ALT is in keeping with advanced cirrhosis.*

He was given IV vitamin K to correct coagulopathy, IV vitamins, lactulose and omeprazole, and fluid restricted to <1 l per day, with daily weights. An ascitic drain was inserted to help with his respiratory compromise. Ascitic fluid: protein 20 g l⁻¹, polymorphonuclear cell count (PMN) <250 cells mm⁻³, serum ascites albumin gradient (SAAG) 10 g l⁻¹.

J:　*Seems to be a transudate with no evidence of SBP.*

What other causes can you think of that present with hypoalbuminemia and oedema?

Activity 24.2

(Allow three minutes)

↓ albumin → ↓ capillary oncotic
Pressure ↝ interstitial oedema

RAAS activation → renal
sodium and water retention →
oedema

Reduced hepatic synthesis of proteins (cirrhosis), protein losses (renal – nephrotic syndrome or gut – protein-losing enteropathy), and reduced protein intake (malnutrition and refeeding oedema) all cause hypoalbuminemia and oedema via reduced capillary oncotic pressures which in turn activates renin-angiotensin-aldosterone system (RAAS) causing renal sodium and water retention.

Five days later repeat creatinine was 130 μmol l⁻¹, urea 12 mmol l⁻¹, and albumin 20 g l⁻¹. Diuretics were witheld as the Na⁺ had also dropped to 126 mmol l⁻¹. The oedema worsened and he developed anasarca. An echo was performed which was normal. The team felt that he had end-stage liver disease and with the ongoing alcohol dependence, liver transplantation was not feasible.

Given the increasing frequency of admissions, the registrar revisited the presentation. He noted the severe hypoalbuminemia and low SAAG, the latter suggesting that this was not due to portal hypertension. This triggered a urine dipstick, showing protein 3+, no blood. Urine ACR was raised. The nephrologists diagnosed membranous nephropathy secondary to hepatitis B causing nephrotic syndrome.

The admitting team was fixated on chronic decompensated alcoholic cirrhosis causing worsening oedema and ascites owing to ongoing alcohol dependence and his dishevelled demeanour. This is called 'attribution error' where a negative stereotype leads us to short cut the reasoning process and we quickly latch on to a single possibility ('anchoring') (Langdridge and Butt 2004). We fall for 'confirmation bias' where we selectively accept or ignore information as long as it confirms our initial impressions. The next time this happens we should pause to think of all other possible alternative explanations for the constellation of signs and symptoms.

Reference

Langdridge, D. and Butt, T. (2004). The fundamental attribution error: a phenomenological critique. *The British Journal of Social Psychology* 43: 357–369.

25 Non-Specific Symptoms

▼

This chapter tells you how to approach non-specific symptoms of renal impairment

▲

Renal impairment can present with non-specific symptoms and get diagnosed on blood tests. When renal dysfunction is eventually picked up it can then be difficult to distinguish AKI from CKD. Clinical features such as new onset oedema, haematuria, oliguria or anuria suggest AKI but are not fail-safe. Investigations are more helpful in distinguishing the two:

- A serial increase in creatinine suggests AKI whilst a stable value points to CKD.
- A renal USG showing small, echo dense kidneys with thin renal cortices suggests CKD although normal sized kidneys do not exclude CKD.
- Renal osteodystrophy (e.g. subperiosteal resorption and loss of bone density of distal third of clavicles on x-rays) suggests CKD.

Example 25.1

A 76 year old man was referred to the medical SHO by A&E with acute confusion.

> J: SQs – Elderly man + acute confusion. Provisional diagnoses: primary neurological conditions like CVA, meningo-encephalitis, and systemic conditions like sepsis, MI.

Bloods: Na^+ 130 mmol l^{-1}, K^+ 7 mmol l^{-1}, urea 30 mmol l^{-1}, creatinine 500 μmol l^{-1}. Cl$^-$ 100 mmol l^{-1}, ALT 70 IU l^{-1}, AST 110 IU l^{-1}, ALP 110 IU l^{-1}, bilirubin 15 μmol l^{-1}, GGT 40 IU l^{-1}, albumin 35 g l^{-1}, protein 70 g l^{-1}, globulin 35 g l^{-1}. Corrected Ca^{2+} 1.7 mmol l^{-1}, PO_4^- 1.8 mmol l^{-1}, glucose 9 mmol l^{-1}, alcohol <17 mmol l^{-1}. Hb 120 g l^{-1}, WCC 15 × 10^9 per litre, platelets 200 × 10^9/l, CRP 40 mg l^{-1}. Paracetamol and salicylate: undetectable. Plasma osmolality 310 mosm kg^{-1}. Clotting profile: normal. No previous blood results available. An ABG was done when renal dysfunction was detected. ABG on air: pH 7.3, $PaCO_2$ 3 kpa, PaO_2 13 kpa, HCO_3^- 11.1 mmol l^{-1}, Saturations 96%, lactate 4 mmol l^{-1}.

How would you interpret these results?

Activity 25.1

(Allow five minutes)

....

....

....

....

....

The Hands-on Guide to Clinical Reasoning in Medicine, First Edition. Mujammil Irfan.
© 2019 John Wiley & Sons Ltd. Published 2019 by John Wiley & Sons Ltd.
Companion website: www.wiley.com/go/irfan/clinicalreasoning

Biochemistry

Ignoring the SQs for a minute, let us start with the U&Es. The raised creatinine with a preserved urea creatinine ratio (in SI units) of <100:1 suggests intrinsic renal disease as opposed to pre-renal failure (Dossetor 1966). Hyponatremia could be secondary to dehydration or the AKI whilst hyperkalemia is secondary to renal dysfunction.

The AST/ALT ratio of 1.5 with a normal GGT makes alcoholic liver disease unlikely. The mild rise in transaminases (assuming it is acute) with the rest of the liver function tests (LFTs) being normal suggests that it is either coming from the liver (viral hepatitis, drug induced) or the muscles (cardiac or skeletal) (Nathwani et al. 2005; Vroon and Israili 1990). The normal clotting profile and albumin mean the synthetic function of the liver is normal, the latter suggesting that the process is acute.

The low Ca^{2+} and high PO_4^- could be due to AKI or part of a wider picture.

Haematology

The mildly raised WCC and CRP implies a stress response although overwhelming sepsis can cause a low WCC and a lag in CRP rise. The clinical context will help in differentiating them.

ABG

↓pH → acidaemia, ↓$PaCO_2$ → not in keeping with acidaemia. Hence, we move on to HCO_3^- which is low → in keeping with acidaemia, therefore has metabolic acidaemia. Now we look at the anion gap (AG) which is elevated at 26. An elevated AG metabolic acidosis has a wide differential illustrated by the mnemonic 'KUSSMAUL.' Plasma ketones, salicylate, and alcohol are all normal. The serum osmolal gap of $3\,mosm\,kg^{-1}$ (normal $<10\,mosm\,kg^{-1}$) rules out other alcohols like methanol and ethylene glycol.

Since urea can move freely across cell membranes it does not exert significant negative charge in the serum which would reduce its contribution to the raised AG. The lactate is mildly elevated which again cannot account for all the AG. We are left with organic acids like sulphates and phosphates that accumulate in renal failure and are contributing to the AG. Rhabdomyolysis can also release sulphates and phosphates from damaged skeletal muscles which then accumulate in AKI. Thus the raised AG seems to be due to a combination of elevated urea, lactate, and unmeasured organic acids such as sulphates and phosphates. Of note, the normal A-a gradient of 3.2 kpa indicates a normal alveolar capillary interface.

Summary

AKI with intrinsic renal disease + elevated AG metabolic acidaemia + mild transaminitis (could be liver, heart, or skeletal muscles). If the source of transaminitis is the liver the differentials would include sepsis or viral hepatitis with glomerulonephritis for starters. Cardiac source could point to MI causing cardiogenic shock and AKI. If the source is skeletal muscles, rhabdomyolysis will be on top of the list given the pattern of electrolyte imbalance (low Ca^{2+}, high K^+ and PO_4^-) and AKI.

He was started on treatment for hyperkalaemia and the history was explored. He was found on the floor at home after a presumed fall and unable to get up. The neighbours had rung 999. There was no prescription, alert bands or Meditags on his person.

O/E: He kept repeating 'I'm a shark and I need to be in water' and appeared drowsy and confused. Looked dry. HR 110 bpm, BP 100/80, Saturations 94% on air, Temperature 38 °C. CNS: no focal neurological deficits, asterixis, tremor, no cerebellar signs or signs of meningeal irritation. No signs of fracture from the fall apart from bruises on the back and legs. Rest of the systemic examination: normal.

CXR: normal. Electrocardiogram (ECG): sinus tachycardia. Urine dipstick: protein 2+, blood 3+, leucocytes, and nitrites positive, urine myoglobin negative. Urine microscopy: no red cells or casts.

J: *Severity of illness – ill. There are no features suggestive of cardiogenic shock but given the pyrexia with haemodynamic instability urinary sepsis would certainly be in. This could explain why he was on the floor. The other possibility would be seizures with post-ictal confusion, e.g. due to alcohol withdrawal or encephalitis. I would treat for sepsis.*

The prolonged immobility on the floor and bruises on the skin suggested rhabdomyolysis despite a negative urine myoglobin, since it has a short half-life and gets cleared by the kidneys unless there is on-going muscle damage. He was given 1 l of normal saline over one hour as he was tachycardic, hypotensive, and appeared dry. He was catheterized to exclude post-renal obstruction and monitor fluid balance and was transferred to ICU for closer monitoring. Antibiotics were started for presumed UTI and cultures confirmed *Escherichia coli* bacteraemia five days later.

CT head excluded structural abnormalities and the lumbar puncture was normal. A serum CK of 20 000 IU l^{-1}, confirmed rhabdomyolysis. Haemofiltration was started for fluid overload and rising hyperkalaemia. USG showed normal sized kidneys. He eventually improved with supportive care and was discharged.

Although we are always taught that history precedes examination and investigations there are exceptions to be made. When there is no history from the patient and collateral history is sketchy we are still expected to make a diagnosis. Often patients are worked up before being referred to relevant specialties from A&E. Scrutinising blood results can help in asking the right questions and in this case looking for the right clues in the clinical examination that will help establish the diagnosis. Being able to process data backwards requires experience but is a useful tool nonetheless and it would bode well to have this in your armamentarium.

Secondly, despite the common adage that we should treat patients and not blood results there are still some results that need to be treated in their own right. Of course, the context is important but the onus should be on action which can be curtailed in light of further information. In this respect the most striking abnormality is the K$^+$ of 7 which needs to be treated before the rest of the results can be analysed.

Finally, we need to ensure that we have explained all the findings with the diagnosis. In this example, the acute confusion can be explained by sepsis and uremic encephalopathy.

Example 25.2

A cardiac arrest call was put out for a 76 year old man who was admitted for gross haematuria, flank pains and clot colic. He was being treated for a UTI and was being investigated for a right-sided renal cell carcinoma. The nurses had found him unresponsive in his bed.

P: *SQs – Elderly man + cardiac arrest call + UTI + Possible renal malignancy. Provisional diagnoses – severe sepsis, PE, MI in short anything causing cardio-respiratory failure. Severity of illness – dying.*

On arrival he was found to have respiratory effort and cardiac output. He was stuporous with HR 80 bpm, BP 100/70, RR 9 per minute, Temperature 37 °C, and Saturations 95% on air.

P: *Revised severity of illness – very ill. He seems to have acceptable vital signs given the scenario of cardiac arrest. I would give him IV fluids, check his bloods, ABG, BMs, and do a quick exam.*

I agree with the approach to which I would add an ECG. It is important to point out that despite his seemingly acceptable observations he is peri-arrest given the neurological obtundation.

Systemic examination: normal apart from the low Glasgow coma scale (GCS) of 7/15 (E 1, M 5, V1). No focal neurological deficits; plantar reflexes: normal (bilaterally upgoing plantars would suggest post-ictal state). The urinary catheter bag contained blood stained urine. He had a history of DM, HT, and chronic back pain. On review of bloods from earlier in the morning: WCC $15 \times 10^9 \, l^{-1}$, Hb $100 \, g \, l^{-1}$, Plt $450 \times 10^9 \, l^{-1}$, CRP $100 \, mg \, l^{-1}$; LFTs: normal except albumin $25 \, g \, l^{-1}$, Ca^{2+} $2.3 \, mmol \, l^{-1}$, PO_4^- $1.8 \, mmol \, l^{-1}$, ALP $200 \, IU \, l^{-1}$, Na^+ $140 \, mmol \, l^{-1}$, K^+ $4 \, mmol \, l^{-1}$, Urea $15 \, mmol \, l^{-1}$, creatinine $200 \, \mu mol \, l^{-1}$ from $110 \, \mu mol \, l^{-1}$ on admission four days ago. ECG: normal sinus rhythm.

P: *He does seem to have an inflammatory marker rise with a ↑WCC suggesting either stress response or sepsis. He has developed an AKI over the last four days perhaps post-renal given the clots. There are no electrolyte imbalances accounting for the low GCS. He does have a low albumin probably in keeping with the malignancy.*

That was a thorough assessment of the blood results. What would you do in this situation?

Activity 25.2

(Allow a minute)

The team considered the possibility of unwitnessed seizures, possibly secondary to brain metastases given his underlying renal cell carcinoma. They organised a CT head with anaesthetic support.

The medical registrar noted the AKI and ran through the drug chart. He noted insulin, gliclazide, atenolol, oxynorm, oxycontin, and anti-thrombotic compression stockings. He quickly requested a capillary glucose – $9 \, mmol \, l^{-1}$ and had a good look at his pupils, which seemed to be equal but small. Given the low RR he administered naloxone 200 mcg IV, which increased his RR and the GCS improved. An ABG confirmed respiratory acidaemia with a pH of 7.28, and $PaCO_2$ of 10 kpa. He was started on a naloxone infusion and titrated to achieve a RR > 12 per minute.

Availability heuristic led the team to suspect cerebral metastases. However, the AKI served as a vital clue which led the registrar to suspect reduced drug clearance. Insulin is normally catabolised and excreted by the kidneys. Gliclazide and opiates are also eliminated by the kidneys. Hypoglycaemia should be the first to be excluded in this scenario which highlights its importance as part of the vital signs to be obtained especially during a 'cardiac arrest' call. Opioid skin patches are another commonly missed entity on clinical examination. Changes in drug pharmacodynamics are common in renal dysfunction and require recognition and dose modification.

References

Dossetor, J.B. (1966). Creatininemia versus uremia. *Annals of Internal Medicine* 65 (6): 1287.
Nathwani, R.A., Pais, S., Reynolds, T.B., and Kaplowitz, N. (2005). Serum alanine aminotransferase in skeletal muscle diseases. *Hepatology* 41 (2): 380–382.
Vroon, D.H. and Israili, Z. (1990). *Aminotransferases.* Butterworths.

PART IV
Endocrinology

▼
**Focussing on relevant aspects of history
from an endocrine perspective**
▲

Nowhere in medicine is clinical acumen more vital than in endocrinology. It is one of those few specialties where clinical features are not restricted to one anatomical site. Indeed it takes a keen eye to look at the person as a whole to diagnose the underlying pathology.

An endocrinopathy can present in different ways as shown below:

- **Non-Specific Symptoms**
  Endocrine problems tend to present to the GP with non-specific symptoms such as weight loss or gain, fatigue, increased thirst, diarrhoea, anxiety, palpitations, amenorrhea, headaches, loss of body hair, or hirsutism. These symptom clusters can be used as SQs and the overall pattern can help point to the diagnosis. For example, a symptom cluster of weight loss, fatigue, increased thirst and appetite signals the possibility of diabetes mellitus.
- **Seemingly isolated organ system involvement getting unified under one endocrinopathy**
  Hospital admissions often tend to be focused on isolated organ systems and an endocrinopathy may come to light by chance. In an era of specialisms, single elements of an endocrinopathy may be treated individually by a specialist before an astute clinician picks up the overarching diagnosis, e.g. depression (psychiatry), renal stones (urology), recurrent admissions with abdominal pains (surgery) before someone picks up hyperparathyroidism (painful bones, abdominal groans, renal stones, and psychic moans).
- **Incidental blood tests revealing an endocrinopathy**
  The proliferation of 'routine' blood tests has resulted in endocrinopathies being increasingly diagnosed in asymptomatic individuals. This throws up the medical/ethical dilemma of whether to treat or not to treat an asymptomatic person. For instance, routine blood tests showing incidental hypercalcaemia may eventually lead to the diagnosis of asymptomatic primary hyperparathyroidism.
- **Finding one endocrinopathy signals the co-existence of another**
  For instance, Schmidt's syndrome (autoimmune polyglandular endocrinopathy type 2) consists of several autoimmune endocrinopathies (hypothyroidism, adrenal insufficiency, type 1 diabetes mellitus) and other autoimmune non-endocrinopathies like myasthenia gravis and vitiligo. Another example is MEN (multiple endocrine neoplasias) syndrome.
- **Symptoms can be shared by several endocrine conditions**
  For example, hyperglycaemia and its osmotic symptoms are commonly ascribed to diabetes mellitus but they can also occur in acromegaly and Cushing's syndrome.

Most presentations in endocrinology are either due to overproduction or underproduction of a specific hormone. Figure 26.1 demonstrates the varied symptom clusters that can occur in major endocrine pathologies. I have started you off with the pathophysiological explanation for the occurrence of these symptoms in each endocrinopathy and I shall leave the rest to you. Any of these symptom clusters should make you explore the possible endocrinopathies with appropriate questions.

The Hands-on Guide to Clinical Reasoning in Medicine, First Edition. Mujammil Irfan.
© 2019 John Wiley & Sons Ltd. Published 2019 by John Wiley & Sons Ltd.
Companion website: www.wiley.com/go/irfan/clinicalreasoning

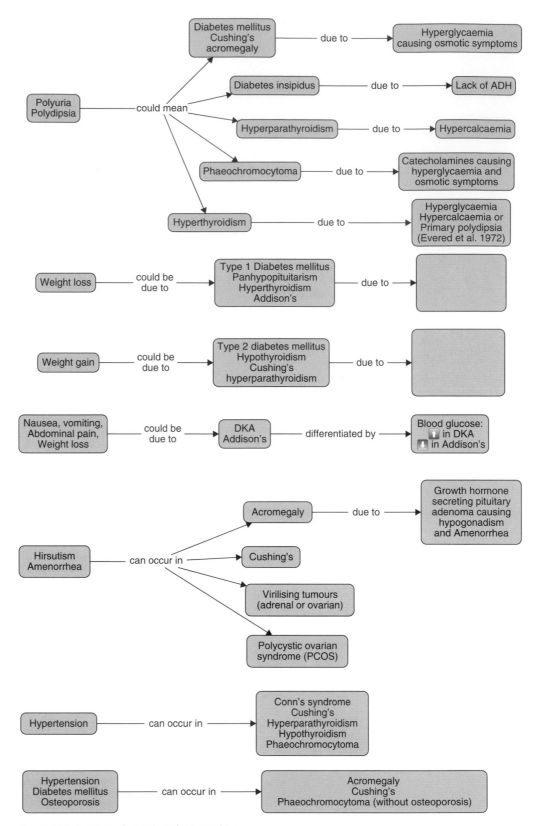

Figure 26.1 Symptom clusters in endocrinopathies

Reference

Evered, D.C., Hayter, C.J., and Surveyor, I. (1972). Primary polydipsia in thyrotoxicosis. *Metabolism* 21 (5): 393–404.

27 Clinical Examination: Looking at the Person as a Whole

▼

Focussing on relevant clinical features and their interpretation from an endocrine perspective

▲

Endocrinological conditions tend to have systemic effects which can only be elicited by a holistic examination. Clinical manifestations of the common under and overactive syndromes have been shown in figures. Each of the figures can be read from the left hand-side starting with the hands, working your way up to the arms, face, neck, chest and abdomen, and finishing with the legs – in keeping with the clinical examination routine. For those who are curious to know the pathophysiological basis of these signs, there is a reference list at the end of the chapter that will give you all the answers.

Once an endocrinological disorder is recognised, examination should proceed to identify the cause, as explained below.

27.1 ACROMEGALY (FIGURE 27.1a)

Clinical manifestations of acromegaly are secondary to excess growth hormone and insulin-like growth factor-1 (IGF-1), which stimulate tissue growth and antagonise insulin activity.

27.2 DIABETES MELLITUS

Clinical examination in DM should focus on assessment of complications of diabetes mellitus and glycaemic control (Figure 27.1b). The former can be divided into macrovascular and microvascular complications, as illustrated in the figure. Rarely, hyperglycaemia diagnosed as 'diabetes mellitus' can be secondary to other endocrine disorders and this is worth bearing in mind.

27.3 THYROID DISORDERS

All aetiologies of hyperthyroidism produce the same clinical manifestations except Grave's disease (Figure 27.2). Grave's disease causes unique autoimmune-mediated infiltrative ophthalmopathy (retro-orbital infiltration) and infiltrative dermopathy (pretibial myxoedema) (Bahn 2010; Burman and McKinley-Grant 2006).

Infiltrative ophthalmopathy causes various eye signs, including proptosis (eyeball visible from above forehead), exophthalmos (sclera visible above lower eyelid), chemosis, keratitis, corneal ulceration, painful diplopia, ophthalmoplegia and loss of colour vision. The last two are indications for surgical intervention.

On the other hand, lid retraction (sclera visible below upper eyelid), stare, and lid lag (white of sclera visible whilst eyeball follows the downward moving finger) can occur in hyperthyroidism of any cause (Bilezikian and Loeb 1983).

Assessment of thyroid status is independent of the presentation, e.g. Grave's ophthalmopathy or pretibial myxoedema does not automatically mean hyperthyroidism. One can still be euthyroid or even hypothyroid with Grave's features, as the physical changes may persist despite treatment. Another example is goitre, where its presence does not equate to hyperthyroidism or hypothyroidism.

The Hands-on Guide to Clinical Reasoning in Medicine, First Edition. Mujammil Irfan.
© 2019 John Wiley & Sons Ltd. Published 2019 by John Wiley & Sons Ltd.
Companion website: www.wiley.com/go/irfan/clinicalreasoning

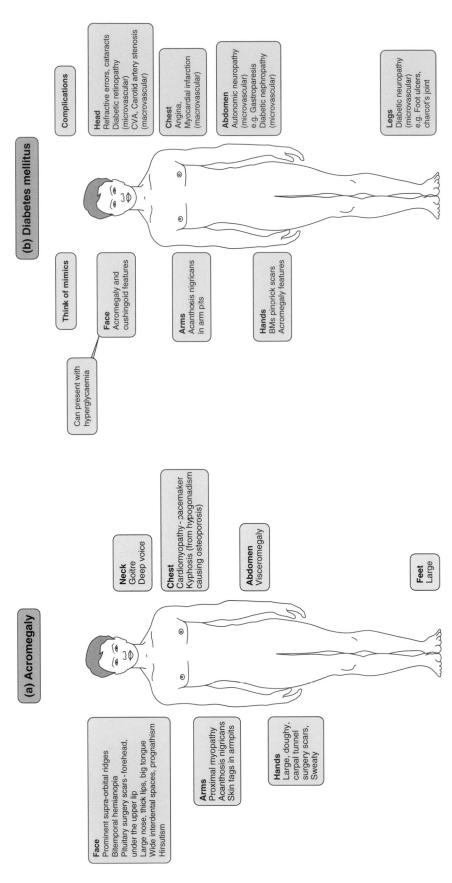

(a) Acromegaly

Face
Prominent supra-orbital ridges
Bitemporal hemianopia
Pituitary surgery scars - forehead, under the upper lip
Large nose, thick lips, big tongue
Wide interdental spaces, prognathism
Hirsutism

Neck
Goitre
Deep voice

Arms
Proximal myopathy
Acanthosis nigricans
Skin tags in armpits

Chest
Cardiomyopathy - pacemaker
Kyphosis (from hypogonadism causing osteoporosis)

Hands
Large, doughy, carpal tunnel surgery scars, Sweaty

Abdomen
Visceromegaly

Feet
Large

(b) Diabetes mellitus

Think of mimics

Can present with hyperglycaemia

Face
Acromegaly and cushingoid features

Arms
Acanthosis nigricans in arm pits

Hands
BMs pinprick scars
Acromegaly features

Complications

Head
Refractive errors, cataracts
Diabetic retinopathy (microvascular)
CVA, Carotid artery stenosis (macrovascular)

Chest
Angina,
Myocardial infarction (macrovascular)

Abdomen
Autonomic neuropathy (microvascular)
e.g. Gastroparesis
Diabetic nephropathy (microvascular)

Legs
Diabetic neuropathy (microvascular)
e.g. Foot ulcers, charcot's joint

Figure 27.1 Clinical examination findings in a) Acromegaly and b) Diabetes mellitus

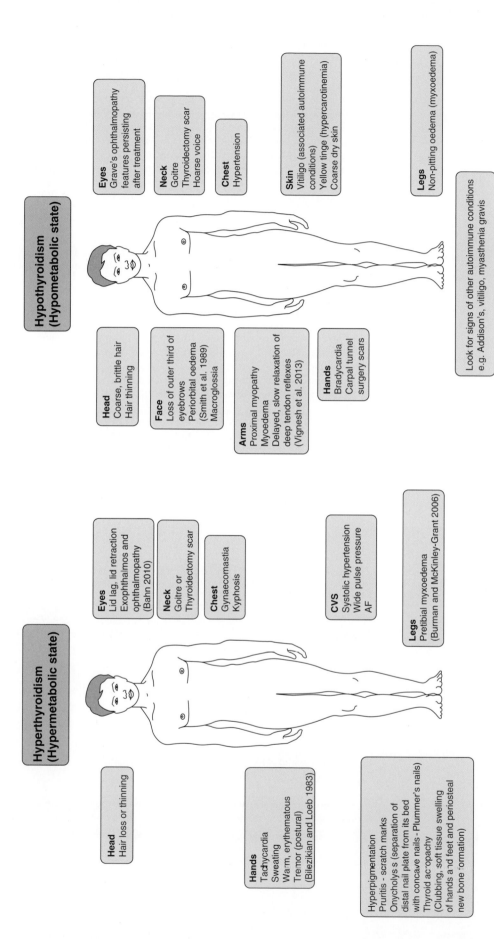

Hyperthyroidism (Hypermetabolic state)

Eyes
Lid lag, lid retraction
Exophthalmos and
ophthalmopathy
(Bahn 2010)

Neck
Goitre or
Thyroidectomy scar

Chest
Gynaecomastia
Kyphosis

CVS
Systolic hypertension
Wide pulse pressure
AF

Legs
Pretibial myxoedema
(Burman and McKinley-Grant 2006)

Head
Hair loss or thinning

Hands
Tachycardia
Sweating
Warm, erythematous
Tremor (postural)
(Bilezikian and Loeb 1983)

Hyperpigmentation
Pruritis - scratch marks
Onycholys s (separation of
distal nail plate from its bed
with concave nails - Plummer's nails)
Thyroid acropathy
(Clubbing, soft tissue swelling
of hands and feet and periosteal
new bone formation)

Hypothyroidism (Hypometabolic state)

Eyes
Grave's ophthalmopathy
features persisting
after treatment

Neck
Goitre
Thyroidectomy scar
Hoarse voice

Chest
Hypertension

Skin
Vitiligo (associated autoimmune
conditions)
Yellow tinge (hypercarotinemia)
Coarse dry skin

Legs
Non-pitting oedema (myxoedema)

Head
Coarse, brittle hair
Hair thinning

Face
Loss of outer third of
eyebrows
Periorbital oedema
(Smith et al. 1989)
Macroglossia

Arms
Proximal myopathy
Myoedema
Delayed, slow relaxation of
deep tendon reflexes
(Vignesh et al. 2013)

Hands
Bradycardia
Carpal tunnel
surgery scars

Look for signs of other autoimmune conditions
e.g. Addison's, vitiligo, myasthenia gravis

Figure 27.2 Clinical examination findings in a) Hyperthyroidism and b) Hypothyroidism

Lack of features suggestive of hyperthyroidism (signs of sympathetic overactivity – tachycardia, eye signs, sweating) or hypothyroidism (myxoedema, bradycardia, hypothyroid myopathy causing delayed relaxation of deep tendon reflexes), would be in keeping with euthyroid status.

Examination of a goitre involves assessing the thyroid gland and the thyroid status. The thyroid gland is examined as follows. Inspection: midline swelling in the neck which moves on deglutition, confirms that it is the thyroid gland. Palpation from behind: Look for features of diffuse enlargement (e.g. physiological, Graves), multinodular goitre (multiple nodules of variable size), or a solitary nodule. Look for associated lymphadenopathy (e.g. thyroid carcinoma). Tenderness suggests viral thyroiditis (De Quervain's) or radiation thyroiditis. Percussion: Retrosternal dullness confirms inferior extension of goitre. Auscultation: for bruit over the goitre (e.g. Graves).

Upon encountering a solitary thyroid nodule, 5 differentials must be considered – benign adenoma, toxic adenoma, thyroid carcinoma, single palpable nodule of multinodular goitre and thyroid cyst.

27.4 CUSHING'S SYNDROME (FIGURE 27.3a)

- Cushing's syndrome should be considered in the following circumstances – Simultaneous development of epidemiologically prevalent conditions such as hypertension, obesity and glucose intolerance.
- The presence of skin bruising, hypertension, and proximal myopathy is highly predictive of Cushing's syndrome (Ross and Linch 1982).

It is vital to look for the aetiology of Cushing's when examining. Concurrent steroid responsive diseases like rheumatoid arthritis and COPD should bring iatrogenic Cushing's to mind. Adrenal mass, hirsutism, and virilisation in females should raise suspicion of adrenal carcinoma. Hyperpigmentation and visual field defects should suggest pituitary adenoma causing Cushing's disease. Hyperpigmentation with bilateral adrenalectomy scar suggests Nelson's syndrome, where the adrenalectomy was done for Cushing's disease. Some of these patients then show a corticotroph progression i.e. an enlarging pituitary adenoma secreting adrenocorticotropin hormone (ACTH). This causes hyperpigmentation via stimulation of melanocyte stimulating hormone receptors in the dermis.

27.5 ADRENAL INSUFFICIENCY (FIGURE 27.3b)

ACTH stimulates the zona fasciculata (glucocorticoid synthesis) and zona reticularis (androgen synthesis). The zona glomerulosa (mineralocorticoid synthesis) is regulated by plasma volume and potassium. Hence, primary adrenal insufficiency results in a deficiency of all the above hormones plus the epinephrine from the medulla, whereas secondary or tertiary adrenal insufficiency (ACTH deficiency) spares the mineralocorticoid and epinephrine production.

Hyperpigmentation and a lack of mineralocorticoid activity (postural hypotension) point to primary adrenal insufficiency (Addison's). The opposite suggests secondary or tertiary adrenal failure.

Autoimmune polyglandular endocrinopathy as an aetiology of adrenal insufficiency can be identified by the presence of other autoimmune features, such as vitiligo, hyper- or hypo-thyroidism, type 1 DM, myasthenia gravis, etc.

An improved glycaemic control with reduced insulin requirements in type 1 DM, should suggest the co-existence of Addison's (Armstrong and Bell 1996). This is due to lack of gluconeogenesis by cortisol deficiency and hypoglycaemia due to epinephrine deficiency.

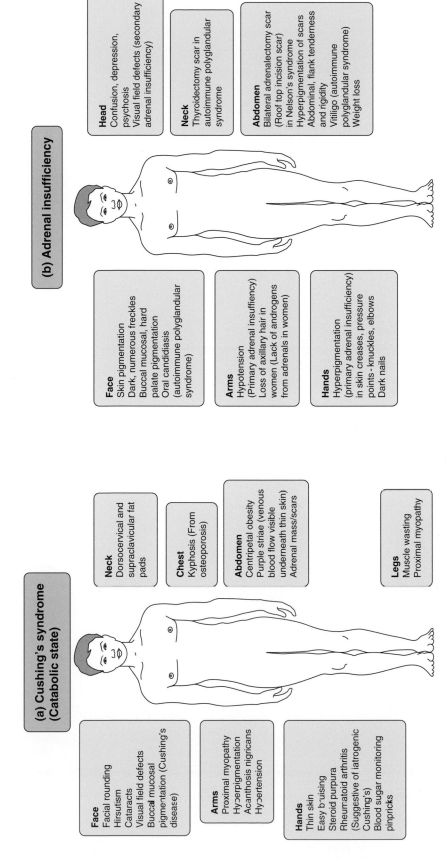

(a) Cushing's syndrome (Catabolic state)

Neck
Dorsocervical and supraclavicular fat pads

Chest
Kyphosis (From osteoporosis)

Abdomen
Centripetal obesity
Purple striae (venous blood flow visible underneath thin skin)
Adrenal mass/scars

Legs
Muscle wasting
Proximal myopathy

Face
Facial rounding
Hirsutism
Cataracts
Visual field defects
Buccal mucosal pigmentation (Cushing's disease)

Arms
Proximal myopathy
Hyperpigmentation
Acanthosis nigricans
Hypertension

Hands
Thin skin
Easy bruising
Steroid purpura
Rheumatoid arthritis (Suggestive of iatrogenic Cushing's)
Blood sugar monitoring pinpricks

(b) Adrenal insufficiency

Head
Confusion, depression, psychosis
Visual field defects (secondary adrenal insufficiency)

Neck
Thyroidectomy scar in autoimmune polyglandular syndrome

Abdomen
Bilateral adrenalectomy scar (Roof top incision scar) in Nelson's syndrome
Hyperpigmentation of scars
Abdominal, flank tenderness and rigidity
Vitiligo (autoimmune polyglandular syndrome)
Weight loss

Face
Skin pigmentation
Dark, numerous freckles
Buccal mucosal, hard palate pigmentation
Oral candidiasis (autoimmune polyglandular syndrome)

Arms
Hypotension (Primary adrenal insufficiency)
Loss of axillary hair in women (Lack of androgens from adrenals in women)

Hands
Hyperpigmentation (primary adrenal insufficiency) in skin creases, pressure points - knuckles, elbows
Dark nails

Figure 27.3 Clinical examination findings in a) Cushing's syndrome and b) Adrenal insufficiency

References

Armstrong, L. and Bell, P.M. (1996). Addison's disease presenting as reduced insulin requirement in insulin dependent diabetes. *BMJ (Clinical Research Eduation)* 312 (7046): 1601–1602.

Bahn, R.S. (2010). Graves' ophthalmopathy. *The New England Journal of Medicine* 362 (8): 726–738.

Bilezikian, J.P. and Loeb, J.N. (1983). The influence of hyperthyroidism and hypothyroidism on alpha- and beta-adrenergic receptor systems and adrenergic responsiveness. *Endocrine Reviews* 4 (4): 378–388.

Burman, K.D. and McKinley-Grant, L. (2006). Dermatologic aspects of thyroid disease. *Clinics in Dermatology* 24 (4): 247–255.

Ross, E.J. and Linch, D.C. (1982). Cushing's syndrome–killing disease: discriminatory value of signs and symptoms aiding early diagnosis. *Lancet (London, England)* 2 (8299): 646–649.

▼
Focussing on an overview of screening tests in endocrinology
▲

General principles:

- *Most hormones are released in a pulsatile fashion*
  Exceptions include thyroxine and parathormone, which tend to have relatively constant blood levels and are therefore reliably measured.
- *Hormones display physiological variation with time and age*
  Static tests mislead the clinician if not used in the right context. For example, a 'static' single random blood sugar gives a snapshot view of the glycaemic status and cannot be used to diagnose diabetes mellitus unless there are symptoms consistent with diabetes. An oral glucose tolerance test on the other hand is a dynamic test which consists of a stimulus (glucose challenge) and measures the response (plasma glucose levels over a two hour period). In this case, the response is an indirect measure of insulin secretion and the overall test is a better physiological reflection of glycaemic control.
- *Indirect ways of measuring hormone production*
  A stable co-factor that is secreted along with the active hormone can be a surrogate measure, e.g. C-peptide levels in suspected insulinoma. Twenty-four hour urine collection for a specific hormone or its metabolic end-products can also be a surrogate measure, e.g. 24 hour urinary free cortisol (protein-bound portion is not excreted) and catecholamines.
- In general, *stimulatory tests* are used in underactive endocrine conditions, whilst *suppressive tests* are used in overactive conditions, e.g. short synacthen test in Addison's disease and dexamethasone suppression test in Cushing's syndrome.
- *Testing the integrity of endocrine axes*
  Loss of feedback control is an important mechanism of disease. Measuring end-products (hormones) of these axes helps in localising the site of the disorder, e.g. a low thyrotropin releasing hormone and high thyroid stimulating hormone (TSH) with a high free T4 (FT4), suggests a pituitary problem, possibly a thyrotroph adenoma.

It is so easy to get overwhelmed by the many investigations available, that it would serve us well to focus on suitable screening tests in our capacity as general physicians. Further confirmation and management can then be left to specialist endocrinologists. With this in mind here is a list of screening tests for the major endocrinological disorders.

28.1 PITUITARY ADENOMAS

The anterior pituitary gland consists of thyrotrophs (TSH), somatotrophs (growth hormone), lactotrophs (prolactin), gonadotrophs (gonadotropins), and corticotrophs (ACTH). Most endocrinological adenomas are true benign (monoclonal) neoplasms rather than malignant and this applies to pituitary adenomas (Herman et al. 1990). They should be differentiated from hyperplasias arising secondary to stimulation factors, which are polyclonal in origin, e.g. TRH causing thyrotroph hyperplasia.

Some adenomas are functional, producing excess hormones, whilst others are non-functional. Both however, can compress surrounding tissues as they expand and cause symptoms, e.g. somatotroph pituitary adenoma can cause acromegaly, visual field defects, and decreased secretion of other hormones like ACTH, TSH by compression of the optic chiasma and normal pituitary tissue respectively.

The Hands-on Guide to Clinical Reasoning in Medicine, First Edition. Mujammil Irfan.
© 2019 John Wiley & Sons Ltd. Published 2019 by John Wiley & Sons Ltd.
Companion website: www.wiley.com/go/irfan/clinicalreasoning

Pituitary adenomas <1 cm are called microadenomas, whilst those >1 cm are called macroadenomas. Incidental pituitary adenomas on MRI are called incidentalomas. Hormonal hypersecretion should be measured in all macroadenomas to identify the cause, i.e. thyrotroph (TSH, FT4), somatotroph (IGF-1), lactotroph (prolactin), gonadotroph (gonadotropins, TRH stimulated gonadotropin concentrations), and corticotroph (ACTH, 24 hour free urinary cortisol levels) hypersecretion. Measuring hyposecretion identifies hormones needing replacement. The best cost-effective investigation of a microadenoma, is a serum prolactin level.

28.2 PROLACTINOMAS

Any pituitary adenoma can enlarge and compress the pituitary stalk, causing loss of dopaminergic tonic inhibitory control by the hypothalamus on the lactotrophs – resulting in mild increases in prolactin levels (up to $200 \, \text{ng} \, \text{ml}^{-1}$). A true lactotroph macro-adenoma (>1 cm) produces levels of $5000–10\,000 \, \text{ng} \, \text{ml}^{-1}$, whilst a micro-adenoma (<1 cm) produces up to $5000 \, \text{ng} \, \text{ml}^{-1}$, which should be distinguished from stalk compression.

28.3 ACROMEGALY

Screening test - Serum IGF-1 levels. IGF-1 is normally produced by the liver. Examples of false negatives are poorly controlled type 1 diabetes mellitus, malnutrition, renal, and liver failure. In this case, use an oral glucose tolerance test where a 75 g glucose load normally suppresses the two hour GH levels to $<1 \, \text{ng} \, \text{l}^{-1}$. If $>1 \, \text{ng} \, \text{l}^{-1}$ we should look for acromegaly.

28.4 DIABETES INSIPIDUS (DI)

Screening test – Serum sodium, plasma, and urine osmolality. Polyuria + urine osmolality $<200 \, \text{mosmol} \, \text{kg}^{-1}$ or raised serum sodium with urine osmolality < plasma osmolality points to DI (Makaryus and McFarlane 2006).

Water deprivation test: Lack of anti-diuretic hormone (ADH) → loss of renal concentrating ability. Poor fluid intake → concentrated plasma, but instead of concentrating the urine, the kidneys continue excreting dilute urine. This causes Na^+ to be $>145 \, \text{meq} \, \text{l}^{-1}$ and urine osmolality to be < plasma osmolality. At the end of the test, administration of desmopressin corrects the urine osmolality in central DI, but not in nephrogenic DI.

Copeptin, a co-peptide secreted with ADH can be used as a surrogate marker to diagnose DI. A baseline level $>21.4 \, \text{pmol} \, \text{l}^{-1}$ discriminates nephrogenic DI from the rest, obviating the need for water deprivation test (Timper et al. 2015).

28.5 THYROID DISORDERS

The most important test in thyroid disorders is TSH ($0.4–5 \, \text{mU} \, \text{l}^{-1}$), since minor fluctuations in T4 levels cause major changes in TSH. Third generation TSH assays are highly sensitive and levels $<0.1 \, \text{mU} \, \text{l}^{-1}$ are reliable in diagnosing hyperthyroidism.

A low TSH implies hyperthyroidism and a high TSH implies hypothyroidism. Free T4 is only useful in secondary and tertiary thyroid disorders. For instance, a high TSH despite high T4 implies a loss of feedback inhibition, localising the site of disease to the pituitary (secondary) or hypothalamus (tertiary). Measurement of TRH will help discriminate the two.

Adequate thyroxine replacement in hypothyroidism is assessed by measuring TSH, not T4. If the TSH is adequately suppressed by a given dose of thyroxine, it is the right dose. On the other hand, free T4 and T3 should be monitored during the treatment of hyperthyroidism as the TSH can remain suppressed for weeks to months during early treatment (Ehrmann and Sarne 1989).

28.6 PARATHYROID GLAND

Hyperparathyroidism is suspected when a frankly elevated or a seemingly 'normal' PTH is detected in the face of hypercalcaemia. The normal response to $\uparrow Ca^{2+}$ is $\downarrow$PTH – often $<10 \, \text{pg} \, \text{ml}^{-1}$ (normal range $10–60 \, \text{pg} \, \text{ml}^{-1}$). Hence, finding a normal PTH with $\uparrow Ca^{2+}$ is inappropriate and points to primary hyperparathyroidism.

Incidental hypocalcaemia accompanied by hyperphosphatemia is investigated with serum creatinine, magnesium, and PTH levels. An inappropriately low or normal PTH is in keeping with hypoparathyroidism.

28.7 DIABETES MELLITUS

Diagnostic criteria for diabetes mellitus include:

- Fasting plasma glucose (FPG) (≥ 8 hours) ≥ 7 mmol l^{-1}
- Two hours post-prandial plasma glucose (PPG) during oral glucose tolerance test (OGTT) ≥ 11.1 mmol l^{-1}
- Glycosylated haemoglobin (HbA1C) $\geq 6.5\%$ or 48 mmol mol^{-1}

These readings will have to be repeated subsequently to make a diagnosis of diabetes mellitus, however symptomatic patients do not need a second test to confirm the diagnosis. These cut-offs were stipulated, as values higher than these were associated with an increased incidence of diabetic retinopathy, a surrogate marker of diabetic microvascular complications.

Diagnostic criteria in symptomatic patients (osmotic symptoms and weight loss):

$$random plasma glucose (RPG) \geq 11.1 \, mmol \, l^{-1}$$

FPG, PPG, and HbA1C test three different physiologic processes. Hepatic insulin resistance and defective early phase insulin secretion results in fasting hyperglycaemia seen in impaired fasting glucose (IFG). In contrast, skeletal muscle insulin resistance, some hepatic insulin resistance and defective delayed insulin secretion underlies the prolonged hyperglycaemia into the postprandial phase (up to two hours later) seen in IGT (Nathan et al. 2007). HbA1C is a non-enzymatically glycosylated product of HbA over the 120 day lifespan of a red blood cell (Ludwig 2002). Hence, it gives an average measure of glycaemic control over the last three months.

28.8 CUSHING'S SYNDROME

Broadly speaking there are two types of hypercortisolism – physiological (pseudo-Cushing's) and pathological (true Cushing's syndrome). Pseudo-Cushing's, is defined as physiological hypercortisolism $\pm$ some clinical features of true Cushing's syndrome + resolution of hypercortisolism when the primary disorder remits, e.g. severe depression, chronic alcoholism. It goes without saying, that all exogenous steroids should be stopped before Cushing's is considered.

Tests with high sensitivity are used to detect Cushing's at the expense of specificity, with the true negatives excluded by more specific tests (Lacroix et al. 2015).

Patients with a low pre-test probability need a single screening test, whilst those with a high pre-test probability need two.

- Late night salivary cortisol:
  Takes advantage of cortisol's diurnal variability (two measurements)
- Twenty-four hour urinary free cortisol (UFC):
  Assesses the physiologically – active free cortisol and is more likely to correlate with cushingoid features (two measurements)
- Low dose (1 mg overnight or 2 mg over two days) dexamethasone suppression test:
  Dexamethasone suppresses corticotropin releasing hormone (CRH) and ACTH production by the hypothalamus and pituitary respectively. It does not interfere with serum, urinary or salivary cortisol as the antibody assays do not interact with dexamethasone.

In order to maximise sensitivity, upper limit of normal for salivary cortisol and 24 hour UFC and a serum cortisol of <50 nmol l^{-1} for the dexamethasone test have been recommended as cut offs.

28.9 ADRENAL INSUFFICIENCY

Short synacthen (synthetic ACTH) test.

28.9.1 Primary Adrenal Insufficiency

For chronic adrenal insufficiency, high dose (250 mcg) short ACTH test is the best. In this scenario, the adrenal is non-functional and therefore unable to produce cortisol when stimulated. If iatrogenic HPA axis suppression is suspected, ensure that dexamethasone is substituted for any other long term steroid that the patient is on, since serum cortisol assays will not react with dexamethasone.

28.9.2 Secondary Adrenal Insufficiency

If new or recent onset ACTH deficiency is suspected, treatment is initiated with hydrocortisone to allow adrenal atrophy. A short synacthen test is then done after four to six weeks. If secondary adrenal insufficiency is suspected to be of a longer duration, the long synacthen test is performed to distinguish from primary adrenal insufficiency.

28.10 PHEOCHROMOCYTOMA

Catecholamines include dopamine, epinephrine, and norepinephrine. The adrenal medulla secretes norepinephrine and epinephrine in a 1:4 ratio, whereas paragangliomas predominantly secrete norepinephrine. In pheochromocytoma, these catecholamines are metabolised within the tumour and excreted into the urine as metanephrine, normetanephrine and vanillylmandelic acid.

One can measure these products in either the urine or the plasma. Twenty-four hour urinary fractionated metanephrines and catecholamines have a 98% sensitivity and specificity (Sawka et al. 2003), making it a useful screening test for pheochromocytoma.

Plasma fractionated metanephrines have a high sensitivity but low specificity, making them more useful in diagnosing familial syndromes that can present with pheochromocytoma. This group tends to have small tumours, which secrete low levels of catecholamines that can be picked up with a highly sensitive test. Moreover, this is more convenient to the patient than a 24 hour urine collection.

Many drugs like tricyclic antidepressants and Levodopa can interfere with measurement of these products and where possible should be stopped prior to testing.

28.11 PRIMARY HYPERALDOSTERONISM OR CONN SYNDROME

Adrenal aldosterone production is under the control of the renin-angiotensin-aldosterone axis and not ACTH. The primary stimulus for renin secretion is hypovolemia. Primary hyperaldosteronism is characterised by excessive aldosterone secretion, which occurs independent of the plasma renin levels. Hyperaldosteronism causes sodium and water retention → hypervolemia → ↓ renin levels. Accompanying renal potassium losses result in hypokalemia and metabolic alkalosis.

Biochemical evaluation of suspected Conn's follows this simple physiological explanation – A high plasma aldosterone/plasma renin activity ratio with a raised plasma aldosterone concentration is the hallmark of Conn's syndrome (Blumenfeld et al. 1994). If the plasma renin activity is also found to be high this is likely to be secondary hyperaldosteronism.

References

Blumenfeld, J.D., Sealey, J.E., Schlussel, Y. et al. (1994). Diagnosis and treatment of primary hyperaldosteronism. *Annals of Internal Medicine* 121 (11): 877–885.

Ehrmann, D.A. and Sarne, D.H. (1989). Serum thyrotropin and the assessment of thyroid status. *Annals of Internal Medicine* 110 (3): 179–181.

Herman, V., Fagin, J., Gonsky., R. et al. (1990). Clonal origin of pituitary adenomas. *The Journal of Clinical Endocrinology and Metabolism* 71 (6): 1427–1433.

Lacroix, A., Feelders, R.A., Stratakis, C.A., and Nieman, L.K. (2015). Cushing's syndrome. *Lancet (London England)* 386 (9996): 913–927.

Ludwig, D.S. (2002). The glycemic index: physiological mechanisms relating to obesity, diabetes, and cardiovascular disease. *Journal of the American Medical Association* 287 (18): 2414–2423.

Makaryus, A.N. and McFarlane, S.I. (2006). Diabetes insipidus: diagnosis and treatment of a complex disease. *Cleveland Clinic Journal of Medicine* 73 (1): 65–71.

Nathan, D.M., Davidson, M.B., DeFronzo, R.A. et al. (2007). Impaired fasting glucose and impaired glucose tolerance: implications for care. *Diabetes Care* 30 (3): 753–759.

Sawka, A.M., Jaeschke, R., Singh, R.J., and Young, W.F. Jr. (2003). A comparison of biochemical tests for pheochromocytoma: measurement of fractionated plasma metanephrines compared with the combination of 24-hour urinary metanephrines and catecholamines. *The Journal of Clinical Endocrinology and Metabolism* 88 (2): 553–558.

Timper, K., Fenske, W., Kühn, F. et al. (2015). Diagnostic accuracy of Copeptin in the differential diagnosis of the polyuria-polydipsia syndrome: a prospective Multicenter study. *The Journal of Clinical Endocrinology and Metabolism* 100 (6): 2268–2274.

29 Weight Gain

Obesity is a world-wide phenomenon of epidemic proportions. Patients often seek an underlying endocrinological cause although this is very unlikely in the vast majority (Tsai and Wadden 2013). It should however be considered in the differential as obesity is an important risk factor for cardiovascular disease. Furthermore some untreated endocrinological disorders increase cardiovascular mortality in their own right.

Example 29.1

A 42 year old man was referred by the GP with hyperglycaemia and suspected diabetic ketoacidosis (DKA). PMH: HIV, hypertension, asthma, and DM. Medications – Truvada (tenofovir/emtricitabine) and kaletra (lopinavir/ritonavir) for HIV, ramipril, seretide 500 accuhaler, salbutamol inhaler, rosuvastatin, and gliclazide. He was a current smoker of 40 py.

P: *SQs – middle aged man + raised BMs + HIV +*
   vascular risk factors + asthma. Provisional diagnoses – possible DKA, underlying infection – chest, urine, missed medications.

He denied missing any medications. Blood glucose levels had become difficult to control despite an increased dose of gliclazide although previous glycaemic control was good. He had dramatically put on weight over the last month with an increased appetite. There were no infective symptoms.

O/E: pulse 94 bpm, BP 150/90, saturations 96% on air, RR 12 per minute, Temperature 37.2 °C, BMs 17 mmol l^{-1}. Well hydrated with an elevated BMI. RS: bilateral scattered wheeze, rest of the systemic examination normal. Urine: ketones 1+, glucose 2+, protein 1+.

Serum ketones, arterial pH and HCO$_3^-$ were normal thereby excluding DKA. CXR and ECG: normal. Bloods: WCC 18 g l^{-1}, neutrophil 15 × 10^9 per litre, eosinophil 1 × 10^9 per litre, CRP 30 mg l^{-1}, glucose 18 mmol l^{-1}, Na 134$^+$ mmol l^{-1}, urea 4 mmol l^{-1}, plasma osmolality 290 mosm kg^{-1} and rest normal.

P: *Severity of illness – relatively well. He seems to have hyperglycaemia but no clinical*
   features of DKA/hyperosmolar hyperglycaemic state (HHS) although urine ketones are
   positive. Could it still be DKA?

   Ketonuria does not imply DKA as it is non-specific. However, ketonemia is characteristic
   of DKA in the right context. In summary he appears to have poor glycaemic control
   over the last one month which seems to be the clue. There is a mild neutrophilia with a
   mildly raised CRP but the lack of focal infective symptoms or signs makes it non-specific.
   The eosinophilia could be secondary to atopy as he has asthma.

He was discharged on additional metformin, advised to exercise regularly and referred to the diabetes clinic. During his clinic visit it came to light that he had been started on seretide accuhaler two months ago for poor asthma control. The ritonavir in his antiretroviral therapy was a strong CYP3A4 inhibitor which resulted in an accumulation of fluticasone (seretide) causing iatrogenic Cushing's (Samaras et al. 2005). This was confirmed with low 24 hour urinary free cortisol levels and low ACTH levels. The seretide was switched to fostair (beclometasone/formoterol) and he was followed up.

What was the reason for the diagnosis to be missed in the first instance?

Activity 29.1

(Allow a minute)

The heuristic 'common things are common' was inappropriately applied in this situation whilst ignoring important clues. This was compounded by a lack of awareness of variations of disease presentation as described below.

Abrupt onset of poor glycaemic control and weight gain were the clues that suggested an underlying endocrine disorder. Endocrine mimics of 'diabetes mellitus' should always be considered consciously in such presentations. Other causes include poor compliance, drugs, intercurrent illness, worsening insulin resistance, erratic absorption of insulin due to lipoatrophy and in type 2 DM, development of latent autoimmune diabetes in adults (LADA).

Iatrogenic Cushing's differs from spontaneous Cushing's syndrome in the abrupt onset of symptoms including rapid weight gain, higher incidence of osteoporosis, avascular necrosis, psychiatric manifestations, pancreatitis, and benign intracranial hypertension (Raveendran 2014). It also results in suppression of the HPA axis, with patients requiring maintenance steroids once they are off the culprit synthetic glucocorticoid.

Beclometasone and ciclesonide are not metabolised by CYP3A4 and hence are preferred in HIV patients who are on protease inhibitor boosters like ritonavir and cobicistat. In hindsight the neutrophilia was likely secondary to the demargination of neutrophils seen in patients who are on exogenous steroids.

Example 29.2

A 56 year old current smoker of 40 py was admitted to medical admissions unit (MAU) for worsening right leg cellulitis. PMH: obesity, hypertension. Medications: bendroflumethiazide, perindopril. She had noticed increasing swelling and erythema in the right leg over three days when her GP had started PO flucloxacillin.

J: *SQs – middle aged woman + unilateral leg swelling + obesity + HT. Provisional diagnoses – DVT, cellulitis, lymphedema.*

There were no risk factors for VTE except relative immobility due to obesity. There were no red flag symptoms or features to suggest unilateral venous or lymphatic compression (enlarged lymph nodes, abdominal malignancy, pelvic tumours compressing veins and lymphatics).

O/E: Dehydrated. Pulse 110 bpm, BP 150/90, Saturations 97% on air, Temperature 38.6 °C, RR 16 per minute, and BMs 12 mmol l⁻¹. Right leg: swollen, tender with an erythematous well demarcated area in keeping with cellulitis. No deep vein tenderness, rest of the systemic examination: normal.

Just before the house officer left the room she reported increasing lethargy and puffiness around her eyes over six months. She persistently questioned the possibility of hypothyroidism since it would also account for the weight gain and hypertension as she had read on the Internet. The house officer sent bloods along with TFTs.

J: *Severity of illness – ill. I would treat for cellulitis and send blood cultures along with routine blood tests.*

However, you will still have to give her an explanation for not doing the TFTs. The correct way of dealing with this would be to clinically assess the thyroid status as TFTs in a sick patient are very tricky to interpret. Unless there is a good clinical reason for doing the test, e.g. new atrial fibrillation, TFTs are best left for out-patient assessment. Even in this group pre-test probability should be assessed by an evaluation of thyroid status. Clear-cut results, i.e. TSH < 0.01 or > 20 mU l⁻¹ are better indicators of thyroid dysfunction than ambiguous results, in order to have an impact on patient management.

Bloods: Hb 130 g l⁻¹, WCC 15 × 10⁹ l⁻¹, Platelets 400 × 10⁹ l⁻¹, CRP 120 mg l⁻¹, Na⁺ 136 mmol l⁻¹, K⁺ 4 mmol l⁻¹, urea 14 mmol l⁻¹, creatinine 150 mmol l⁻¹, RBS 12 mmol l⁻¹, LFTs in particular albumin, normal, TSH 6 mU l⁻¹ and FT4 10 pmol l⁻¹. Urine dipstick: normal. CXR: normal.

She was given IV fluids and IV antibiotics. The consultant questioned the rationale behind doing TFTs as the TSH was mildly elevated and FT4 low normal. She assessed the thyroid status of the patient and felt she was euthyroid (Attia et al. 1999). In retrospect the periorbital puffiness was episodic and secondary to ACEi. She switched the perindopril to bisoprolol and counselled the patient that the TFTs were not indicated to start with. She suggested repeating them in the out-patients six weeks post-discharge. Repeat TFTs in clinic were normal but a fasting plasma glucose was raised at 11 mmol l⁻¹. She was diagnosed with type 2 DM and started on treatment.

What do you think prompted the house officer to request the TFTs?

Activity 29.2

(Allow a minute)

This example shows commission bias in action. We are all guilty of succumbing to this where we are expected to 'do something' either by the patient, the situation, our colleagues or by ourselves (Croskerry 2002). This was made worse by the house officer cutting corners and not assessing the thyroid status. He instead took the easy way out by requesting tests.

It has been hypothesised that hospitalised sick patients tend to have relative central hypothyroidism (↓TSH, ↓FT3, and FT4) as the low catabolic rate is protective. During recovery the TSH can ↑ whilst the FT4 normalises (Koulouri et al. 2013). Obesity can complicate matters by causing ↑TSH and ↑FT3 due to ↑ leptin levels secreted by adipose tissue (Biondi 2010). The message is: as in every aspect of medicine, assess the pre-test probability of disease (thyroid dysfunction) which is low in this patient and interpret the results with post-test probability based on the sensitivity/specificity of the test in question.

Lastly, stress hyperglycaemia is common in sick patients secondary to ↑insulin antagonists (cortisol, catecholamines, growth hormone, etc.). However, severe stress hyperglycaemia (>11 mmol l⁻¹) has a higher likelihood of developing DM (up to 47%) in the long run (Macintyre et al. 2012).

▼

Think of endocrine mimics of diabetes mellitus in patients with poor glycaemic control.

Consciously consider variations in disease presentation.

Remember commission bias; never be coerced into making management decisions for the sake of it.

▲

References

Attia, J., Margetts, P., and Guyatt, G. (1999). Diagnosis of thyroid disease in hospitalized patients a systematic review. *Archives of Internal Medicine* 159: 658–665.

Biondi, B. (2010). Thyroid and obesity: an intriguing relationship. *Journal of Clinical Endocrinology and Metabolism* 95 (8): 3614–3617.

Croskerry, P. (2002). Achieving quality in clinical decision making: cognitive strategies and detection of bias. *Academic Emergency Medicine: Official Journal of the Society for Academic Emergency Medicine* 9 (11): 1184–1204.

Koulouri, O., Moran C., , Halsall, D., et al. 2013. Pitfalls in the measurement and interpretation of thyroid function tests.' *Best Practice & Research. Clinical Endocrinology & Metabolism* 27(6), pp. 745–62.

Macintyre, E.J., Majumdar, S.R., Gamble, J.M. et al. (2012). Stress hyperglycemia and newly diagnosed diabetes in 2124 patients hospitalized with pneumonia. *The American Journal of Medicine* 125: 1036.e17–1036.e23.

Raveendran, A.V. (2014). Inhalational steroids and iatrogenic Cushing's syndrome. *The Open Respiratory Medicine Journal* 8: 74–84.

Samaras, K., Pett, S., Gowers, A. et al. (2005). Iatrogenic Cushing's syndrome with osteoporosis and secondary adrenal failure in human immunodeficiency virus-infected patients receiving inhaled corticosteroids and ritonavir-boosted protease inhibitors: six cases. *The Journal of Clinical Endocrinology and Metabolism* 90 (7): 4394–4398.

Tsai, A.G. and Wadden, T.A. (2013). In the clinic: obesity. *Annals of Internal Medicine* 159 (5): ITC3-1-ITC3-15; quiz ITC3-16.

30 Palpitations

▼

This chapter tells you how to approach palpitations from an endocrinological perspective

▲

Endocrinological causes of palpitations are often found in small print. Symptoms can often overlap with psychiatric conditions such as panic attacks or generalised anxiety disorder which expectedly are a diagnosis of exclusion.

Example 30.1

> As part of a work-up for new onset AF, TFTs were done on a 42 year old man with no PMH. Medications – nil. He was a non-smoker and a teetotaller. TFTs: TSH < 0.5 µl⁻¹, FT4 10 pmol l⁻¹.

J: *SQs – middle aged man + new onset AF + hyperthyroidism. Provisional diagnoses – AF secondary to hyperthyroidism.*

His FT4 is normal with a low TSH. Would you say he has hyperthyroidism?

J: *I'd like to assess him clinically for hyperthyroidism.*

He had no other clinical features to support hyperthyroidism.

J: *Then I'd just repeat the TFTs in a few weeks.*

I don't think you have interpreted the tests correctly. A ↓TSH with normal FT4, assuming a normal FT3 too is biochemically subclinical hyperthyroidism. A ↓TSH with ↑FT3 and FT4 is biochemically hyperthyroidism. Since he has presented with AF would you treat the subclinical hyperthyroidism?

Activity 30.1

(Allow a minute)

J: *But he has no clinical features to support hyperthyroidism.*

Partly right, but AF is a symptom of hyperthyroidism and subclinical hyperthyroidism carries a threefold increased risk of AF (Sawin et al. 1994). Moreover, it can also progress to overt hyperthyroidism and cause hypertension, tachycardia, and ↓bone mineral density/osteoporosis (Klein and Danzi 2007).

The Hands-on Guide to Clinical Reasoning in Medicine, First Edition. Mujammil Irfan.
© 2019 John Wiley & Sons Ltd. Published 2019 by John Wiley & Sons Ltd.
Companion website: www.wiley.com/go/irfan/clinicalreasoning

J: *In that case I would treat.*

The AF was managed with bisoprolol and rivaroxaban as per guidelines. A radio-active iodine uptake scan and thyroid ultrasound identified a toxic adenoma and he was given a choice of surgery, radio-iodine or long term thionamides. He opted for radio-iodine. Once he was hypothyroid (look for ↓FT4, not TSH as TSH can remain low for months) he was started on replacement thyroxine and titrated. The AF reverted to sinus rhythm (happens in up to 75% of patients). The bisoprolol and rivaroxaban were stopped six months later.

Our practice population determines the pre-test probability of disease and the context certainly influences this. Test results then modify this by increasing or decreasing this probability. They do not provide a binary yes/no answer. Interpretation of test results also rests on sound knowledge which plays a central role in clinical reasoning. In line with the adage, 'what the eye does not know, the mind cannot see,' knowledge deficits are common. They can be personal deficits or limitations in current knowledge. Incorrect interpretation of test results can be partly avoided by recognising personal lack of knowledge. Unfortunately, there can be a genuine lack of insight into our shortcomings. Indeed, research has shown that overconfidence leads to diagnostic errors (Berner et al. 2008). Awareness of knowledge gaps, personal or otherwise must stem from the humility to accept that we cannot know it all.

Example 30.2

A 53 year old lady was admitted with acute chest discomfort, breathlessness, sweating, and palpitations. She was unable to pinpoint the initial symptom. Three similar episodes over the last six months had been ascribed to panic attacks. Current smoker 50 py. PMH: Type 2 diabetes mellitus, hypertension. Medications: gliclazide, sitagliptin, lantus insulin, aspirin, simvastatin, and ramipril.

P: *SQs – middle aged lady + chest discomfort, breathlessness, sweating, and palpitations + vascular risk factors. Provisional diagnoses – ACS, PE, CAP, panic attacks.*

Previous episodes would settle with fizzy drinks which she attributed to their 'burping action.' This episode was worse than previous occurrences but symptoms subsided with another fizzy drink and oxygen in the ambulance. No triggering factors.

O/E: pulse 120 bpm, BP 160/70, saturations 94% on air, Temperature 37.4 °C, RR 26 per minute, BMs 8. Systemic examination: normal. ECG: sinus tachycardia, CXR: normal. ABG: FiO_2 0.21, pH 7.46, PaO_2 12 kpa, $PaCO_2$ 3 kpa, HCO_3^- 24 mmol l^{-1}. The registrar calculated the Well's score as 4.5 (intermediate probability) and started enoxaparin.

P: *Severity of illness – ill. There is tachycardia, but the A-a gradient is only mildly elevated at 4.2 kpa. Respiratory alkalosis points to hyperventilation which can be seen in PE but is non-specific. I'm not entirely convinced of a PE.*

Bloods: normal. D dimer positive (false-positive). CPTA showed no PE but an incidental left adrenal mass. 24 hour urine was sent for fractionated metanephrines and catecholamines. She was referred to the endocrinologists for possible pheochromocytoma given the episodic symptoms.

The next day she had a similar episode. A keen-eyed nurse checked her BMs which were 3.2 mmol l^{-1}. Oral glucose gel improved her symptoms immediately. The 24 hour urinary tests were positive but they were felt to be an appropriate secondary response to the hypoglycaemic episode (Figure 30.1). The recently started insulin regime was modified and the hypoglycaemic episodes settled. The adrenal incidentaloma was followed up by the endocrinologists. She remained well, five years later.

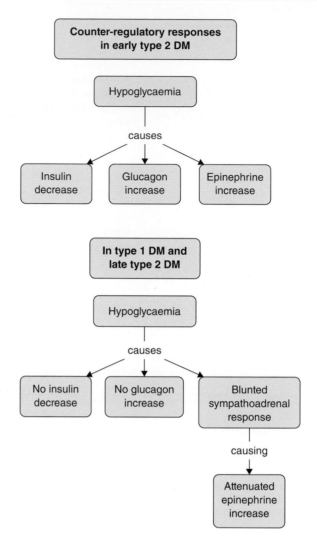

Figure 30.1 Counter-regulatory responses to hypoglycaemia in diabetes mellitus

How would you approach incidental findings?

Activity 30.2

(Allow a minute)

Incidental findings are being increasingly reported given the proliferation of high fidelity imaging studies (Lumbreras et al. 2010). Although guidelines to deal with adrenal incidentalomas have been drawn up recently, they often involve increasingly invasive and intensive investigations and treatments (Fassnacht et al. 2016). These interventions result in both cost and emotional burden on the patient concerned, especially since, incidental findings are often found in asymptomatic patients who may be wary of initiating treatments. Unsurprisingly, the responsibilities of a clinician upon encountering such findings are mired in ethical and legal controversies. Some authors have therefore even advocated counselling patients regarding the possibility of incidental findings before the investigation is requested.

Incidental findings, on a blood test or imaging study, should be interpreted in light of the context. Before embarking on invasive investigations, the pros and cons of the investigations will have to be balanced against the cons of missing a diagnosis which may or may not be treatable. For example, finding an incidental malignancy on a CT scan in a patient with severe co-morbidities does not immediately warrant a tissue biopsy to confirm the diagnosis if no treatment can be offered. An opposing view is that some patients would rather have a diagnosis even if it is untreatable, than live a life in fear. Hence these decisions should be taken in concurrence with patients and their philosophy of life.

As you can see there is no right or wrong answer, but it is worth thinking from all these angles. A hypoglycaemic episode coinciding with her symptoms enabled causal reasoning based on sound pathophysiology of counter-regulatory responses to hypoglycaemia (Cryer 2004). This fortuitous event saved our patient from a series of what may have been increasingly invasive investigations perhaps culminating in a surgical resection of the adrenal gland.

▼

Endocrinological causes of palpitations include hypoglycaemia, hyperthyroidism, and rarely pheochromocytoma.

Knowledge is an important pre-requisite in sound clinical reasoning.

Management of incidental findings should be based on the context and four pillars of ethical decision making.

▲

References

Berner, E.S. and Graber, M.L. (2008). Overconfidence as a cause of diagnostic error in medicine. *The American Journal of Medicine* 121 (5): S2–S23.

Cryer, P.E. (2004). Diverse causes of hypoglycemia-associated autonomic failure in diabetes. *The New England Journal of Medicine* 350 (22): 2272–2279.

Fassnacht, M., Arlt, W., and Bancos, I. (2016). Management of adrenal incidentalomas: European Society of Endocrinology Clinical Practice Guideline in collaboration with the European Network for the Study of Adrenal Tumors. *European Journal of Endocrinology* 175 (2): G1–G34.

Klein, I. and Danzi, S. (2007). Thyroid disease and the heart. *Circulation* 116 (15): 1725–1735.

Lumbreras, B., Donat, L., and Hernández-Aguado, I. (2010). Incidental findings in imaging diagnostic tests: a systematic review. *The British Journal of Radiology* 83 (988): 276–289.

Sawin, C.T., Geller, A., Wolf, P.A. et al. (1994). Low serum thyrotropin concentrations as a risk factor for atrial fibrillation in older persons. *The New England Journal of Medicine* 331 (19): 1249–1252.

31 Weight Loss

▼

This chapter tells you how to approach weight loss from an endocrinological perspective

▲

Unintentional weight loss of >5% from baseline over 6–12 months is considered to be significant (Gaddey and Holder 2014). It often results from ↑ energy expenditure (e.g. fever, hyperthyroidism) or ↓ food intake, the latter being most common. Malignancy, non-malignant gastrointestinal conditions (e.g. peptic ulcer disease, inflammatory bowel disease), and psychiatric conditions (e.g. depression) account for the bulk of unintentional weight loss (Vanderschueren et al. 2005). Weight loss + ↑ appetite → think of malabsorption syndromes and endocrinopathies (hyperthyroidism, diabetes mellitus, pheochromocytoma) although Addison's is an exception. If a clear cause is not apparent on initial assessment, close follow-up is better than escalating, invasive investigations (commission bias). The fear of missing occult malignancy fuels this search, but this is a very rare cause of unintentional weight loss if the initial investigations are negative (Marton et al. 1981).

Example 31.1

A 24 year old woman was admitted under the surgeons with a one day history of abdominal pain. There were six previous admissions over the last three months for drug overdoses and recurrent UTIs. PMH: alcohol excess, intravenous drug abuse, and groin abscesses. She was unemployed and not on medications. On shift changeover, she was highlighted by the nursing staff as a 'frequent flyer.'

J: SQs: *Young woman + acute abdominal pain + recurrent UTIs + alcohol and substance abuse + groin abscesses. Provisional diagnoses: surgical causes of abdominal pain, ectopic pregnancy, pyelonephritis, pancreatitis secondary to alcohol, and since we are on endocrinology placement Addison's, hyperparathyroidism or DKA.*

She reported non-colicky, non-radiating, diffuse abdominal pain, with persistent dysuria and vulvovaginal irritation despite two courses of antibiotics. She denied missing any antibiotic doses. Previous urine cultures grew *Escherichia coli* on one occasion and candida on another. She admitted to injecting herself with heroin and drinking alcohol the previous day.

O/E: Dehydrated, emaciated, unkempt, covered in tattoos, and IV injection marks over the arms and groins. Pulse 112 bpm, BP 110/70, saturations 95% on air, RR 18 per minute, Temperature 38 °C. Oral candidiasis. PA: Diffuse abdominal tenderness with no signs of peritonism. No renal angle tenderness. Rest of the examination: normal. Urine dipstick: nitrites +, protein 1+, glucose 2+, ketones 2+, βhcg negative.

The Hands-on Guide to Clinical Reasoning in Medicine, First Edition. Mujammil Irfan.
© 2019 John Wiley & Sons Ltd. Published 2019 by John Wiley & Sons Ltd.
Companion website: www.wiley.com/go/irfan/clinicalreasoning

J: *Severity of illness: ill. She appears to have a UTI. I would treat her with fluids and antibiotics that she was sensitive to on her previous cultures. I think she has DKA given the glucosuria.*

Urine and blood cultures were sent. Bloods: Hb 110 g l⁻¹, WCC 16 × 10⁹ l⁻¹, platelets 200 × 10⁹ l⁻¹, CRP 120 mg l⁻¹; U&Es, and LFTs: normal, except ALT 70 IU l⁻¹ and amylase 150 U l⁻¹. CXR: normal, no air under the diaphragm. AXR: normal. She was treated with IV antibiotics and fluids. The SHO sent an HIV and hepatitis screen.

J: *There is an inflammatory marker rise with mildly raised amylase (non-specific) and mild transaminitis. The last could be due to alcohol excess. I would request a serum lipase and ABG to exclude pancreatitis and metabolic acidosis.*

The registrar noted the glucosuria and asked for BMs which were 22 mmol l⁻¹. This was confirmed with plasma glucose levels. She was referred to the medical registrar who re-visited the history and noticed she had lost 10 kg in weight over the last four months with classic symptoms of polyuria and polydipsia. The serum ketones were 3.5 mmol l⁻¹ and the ABG confirmed metabolic acidosis. She diagnosed DKA and initiated sliding scale of insulin. Urine and blood cultures, HIV, and hepatitis screen were negative on day 5. She was found to have vulvovaginal candidiasis and was treated appropriately.

Why do you think the diagnosis was delayed over several months?

Activity 31.1

(Allow a minute)

There seem to be several factors accounting for the delay:

1. Attribution error – the patient fitting a negative stereotype (alcohol and substance abuse) and therefore likely to have HIV/hepatitis as well as compliance issues. Although their likelihood is increased, this should not deter the physician from looking at alternatives. Diabetes mellitus has a higher prevalence in the general population than HIV and is also known to cause immunosuppression.
2. Ascertainment bias – the label 'frequent flyer' did not help matters as this immediately elicited a negative reaction downplaying any strong pertinent data that appeared later. The clues of oral candidiasis, recurrent UTIs, and glucosuria were initially side lined. We can only presume that these were wrongly attributed to HIV and 'stress hyperglycaemia' secondary to sepsis respectively.
3. The 'unpacking principle' is also well illustrated in this example where the presence of glucosuria triggered the hypothesis of diabetes mellitus leading to the uncovering of other symptoms. The failure to do so by the admitting SHO upon encountering recurrent UTIs, candidiasis, and glucosuria cannot be justified. One should always strive to 'unpack' all the information and not make decisions based on what is visible. Some patients are unable to verbalise their symptoms or disregard them by playing them down as unimportant. It is up to the physician to dig deeper and ascertain all the facts before making a diagnosis.

4. Lastly, the current admission brings contextual factors into focus where a surgical admission resulted in fixation on surgical causes of acute abdomen. Similarly, the inclusion of this example in the endocrinology section triggered the generation of various endocrinopathies in Jenny's (and your) mind. We seem to be heavily inclined to assess patients based on where we find them – medical or surgical ward or accident and emergency unit (A&E), rather than assessing them as individual presentations bereft of their environment. In the burgeoning world of specialisms, it is imperative that we maintain a broad approach to clinical evaluation, otherwise we risk missing the diagnosis altogether.

Example 31.2

A 72 year old lady was referred to the medical registrar on nights to exclude a medical cause for hypotension. She had been admitted under the orthopaedics in A&E for a right hip fracture. She had risen quickly from her chair, lost balance, and fallen. PMH: depression on mirtazapine.

P: *SQs – elderly lady + hypotension + right hip fracture + depression. Provisional diagnoses – bleeding from hip fracture, underlying sepsis, arrhythmia causing hypotension.*

The registrar bemoaned that the obvious cause of hypotension was bleeding from the hip fracture but grudgingly reviewed the patient. She had been recently investigated for significant weight loss of 10 kg over six months. She had received extensive non-diagnostic investigations including blood tests, oesophagogastroduodenoscopy (OGD), colonoscopy, CT thorax, abdomen and pelvis, and serum tumour markers. Interferon gamma release assay (IGRA)-negative for latent TB. HIV and coeliac screen negative.

P: *Severity of illness – ill. Revised provisional diagnoses – underlying malignancy +/– osteoporosis but no new pointers to hypotension.*

O/E: emaciated, dehydrated. Pulse 82 bpm, BP 86/60, Saturations 96% on air, RR 17 per minute, BMs 4 mmol l^{-1}, Temperature 38 °C. Systemic and per rectal examination: normal, except external rotation and shortening of right leg. ECG: sinus rhythm, CXR: normal. Urine dipstick: negative.

Bloods: Hb 120 g l^{-1}, WCC 10 × 10^9 l^{-1}, platelets 250 × 10^9 l^{-1}; LFTs normal; Na$^+$ 126 mmol l^{-1}, K$^+$ 3.6 mmol l^{-1}, urea 12 mmol l^{-1}, creatinine 120 μmol l^{-1}, CRP 50 mg l^{-1}.

Given the new information of chronic weight loss, hypotension, and hyponatremia the registrar felt this could be Addison's as he had recently seen a similar presentation. Baseline serum cortisol, ACTH, plasma renin activity, and aldosterone levels were sent. She was then given IV hydrocortisone, normal saline, and empiric antibiotics to cover the possibility of underlying sepsis.

What other possible alternatives can you think of, that can account for these findings?

Activity 31.2

(Allow a minute)

P: *All causes of shock need to be considered. If the hyponatremia is ascribed to dehydration*
     or sepsis (syndrome of inappropriate ADH secretion SIADH), the obvious ones include
     hypovolemic and septic shock.

Distributive shock due to myxoedema coma (depression, hyponatremia) is another possibility. However, the lack of bradycardia and hypothermia argue against it.

> Later her husband mentioned incidentally that he had noticed his wife turn darker over the last few months. The bloods and a short synacthen test confirmed Addison's. TFTs were normal. She improved quickly over the next two weeks post hip replacement and was discharged to the rehabilitation ward with endocrinology input.

The initial heuristic of 'common things are common' led to the bias of 'anchoring' (hypotension is obviously due to hypovolemia from hip fracture). Fortunately, when more information was available (weight loss and hyponatremia) other possibilities were considered. The recency of a similar presentation (availability heuristic) helped the registrar to make the right – albeit a rare diagnosis.

This example has been deliberately included to show that heuristics (mental shortcuts) are not inherently bad. Heuristics are efficient, time-saving, and accurate in the majority of cases. They are especially helpful when information is sketchy and an urgent working diagnosis is essential to initiate treatment. Otherwise we would all be snowed under by the volume of data to the point of exhaustion (Eva and Norman 2005). Equally, knowing when to use them and when not to, is important. The intention of exercise 31.2 was to illustrate how new information should trigger a switch from non-analytic reasoning processes (heuristics) to analytic reasoning (e.g. causal reasoning – other causes of hypotension).

▼
Every presentation should be assessed with a clean slate bereft of the setting in which it takes place.

Heuristics are useful but one needs to know when to use them and when not to.
▲

References

Eva, K.W. and Norman, G.R. (2005). 'Heuristics and biases – a biased perspective on clinical reasoning. *Medical Education* 39 (9): 870–872.

Gaddey, H.L. and Holder, K. (2014). Unintentional weight loss in older adults. *American Family Physician* 89 (9): 718–722.

Marton, K.I., Sox, H.C. Jr., and Krupp, J.R. (1981). Involuntary weight loss: diagnostic and prognostic significance. *Annals of Internal Medicine* 95 (5): 568–574.

Vanderschueren, S., Geens, E., Knockaert, D., and Bobbaers, H. (2005). The diagnostic spectrum of unintentional weight loss. *European Journal of Internal Medicine* 16 (3): 160–164.

32 Thirsty and Confused

The Hands-on Guide to Clinical Reasoning in Medicine, First Edition. Mujammil Irfan.
© 2019 John Wiley & Sons Ltd. Published 2019 by John Wiley & Sons Ltd.
Companion website: www.wiley.com/go/irfan/clinicalreasoning

▼

This chapter tells you how to approach confusion from an endocrinological perspective

▲

Example 32.1

An 82 year old psychiatry in-patient was referred to the Geriatric Medicine registrar as she was found to have primary hyperparathyroidism. PMH: Alzheimer's disease with behavioural issues, HT, IHD, glaucoma, and stroke with partial recovery of left hemiparesis.

P: *SQ – Elderly lady + primary hyperparathyroidism + Alzheimer's + vascular risk factors. She already has a diagnosis. I would look for the clinical features that support this diagnosis.*

She was frail, bed-bound, needing a hoist for transfer, and completely dependent for all her activities of daily living. She lacked capacity to make decisions with regards to her diagnosis or therapy. The hypercalcaemia (2.9 mmol l⁻¹) was incidentally discovered on 'routine blood tests.' The creatinine was 100 μmol l⁻¹ and PTH was 50 pg ml⁻¹. No other reason for hypercalcaemia was found on subsequent work-up. There were no risk factors for fragility fracture.

P: *The normal PTH in the face of hypercalcaemia suggests primary hyperparathyroidism. Although, she does not fit with the well known description of painful bones, abdominal groans, psychic moans, and renal stones does hypercalcaemia make this symptomatic?*

Primary hyperparathyroidism manifests itself with symptoms related to both excess parathormone and hypercalcaemia. It is difficult to assess these symptoms in someone with severe dementia as they are unable to communicate. It is worth exploring her neuropsychiatric symptoms to elicit if there are any subtle features of hyperparathyroidism. An abdominal kidney-ureter-bladder (KUB) X-ray would be a minimum to identify renal stones indicative of progression of primary hyperparathyroidism. The dementia would once again make it difficult to appreciate thirst (polydipsia). Of note there is no renal impairment. Surgery would be off the table in this scenario in view of her co-morbidities and frailty regardless of whether she has symptoms or not.

Assuming she is asymptomatic, what factors would you consider in making treatment decisions?

Activity 32.1

(Allow three minutes)

....

....

....

....

....

159

This example illustrates situations where treatment decisions have to be made despite a poor evidence base. Uncertainty is all pervasive in clinical practice. To paraphrase Renee Fox, there are three types of uncertainty, the first stems from a personal lack of knowledge (no one can know everything), the second from limitations in current level of understanding of a disease process and the third, from a personal inability to discriminate between the two aforementioned (Fox 1980). Ideally one must communicate this uncertainty to patients before embarking on treatments which will also temper patient expectations.

Individualising treatment and utilising the four principles of ethical decision-making will help. Remember this is an asymptomatic patient – a situation commonly encountered in conditions identified on screening like hypertension, diabetes mellitus, etc. Risks vs benefits of treatment should be weighed against a strategy of observation in terms of complication rates, patient discomfort, and economic burden. Patient views should also be considered.

Medical management of asymptomatic hyperparathyroidism has not been conclusively shown to reduce complications except in certain specific circumstances (Marcocci et al. 2014). Furthermore, studies have prospectively looked at asymptomatic patients over a 10 year period to ascertain clinical risk (Silverberg et al. 1999). In this context, life-expectancy of the individual patient needs to be taken into consideration before treatment decisions are made. Immobility is a well-known risk factor for losing bone mass which worsens with the high bone turnover in hyperparathyroidism, so patients can be at risk of fragility fractures even with routine nursing and turning in bed. If the expected benefits outweigh the potential risks, the least disruptive treatment should be considered which does not worsen the quality of life.

Her significant co-morbidities precluded her from surgery and it was felt that further investigations would not be in her best interests. She was started on annual intravenous bisphosphonates in consultation with her next of kin. The serum calcium levels were monitored at regular intervals with a view to starting cinacalcet for severe hypercalcaemia or symptomatic hypercalcaemia.

Example 32.2

A 45 year old man presented with increasing confusion over three days. PMH: bipolar disorder, hypertension. Medications: lithium, amlodipine.

P: *SQs – middle aged man + psychiatric disorder + hypertension. Provisional diagnoses – encephalitis, stroke, epilepsy, alcohol intoxication, DKA (first presentation), recreational drugs.*

All causes of cerebral hypoperfusion and toxic/metabolic derangements can cause confusion.

No collateral history. O/E: Confused, agitated, dehydrated. Pulse 100 bpm, BP 140/90, saturations 96% on air, temperature 37.3 °C, RR 18 per minute, BMs 9 mmol l^{-1}. CNS: AMT 6/10, no signs of meningeal irritation or cerebellar signs. Pupils normal and reactive, fundi normal. Limbs – Hypertonic, hyper-reflexic, clonus with myoclonic jerks, plantars down-going. Power – normal. Rest of systemic examination normal. ECG, CXR normal, urine dipstick: specific gravity 1.003, trace protein.

Bloods: FBC, LFTs, Glucose, ABG normal. CRP 30 mg l^{-1}, Na 148 mmol l^{-1}, K 3.8 mmol l^{-1}, Urea 15 mmol l^{-1}, Creatinine 145 μmol l^{-1}, calcium 2.9 mmol l^{-1}, phosphate, and ALP normal, Alcohol normal.

P: *Severity of illness – ill. I'm not sure what this is!*

What possible hypotheses can be ruled out based on the available clinical information?

Activity 32.2

(Allow three minutes)

....
....
....
....
....

All we do is cross-check the data against the provisional diagnoses:

Signs	Reduces chances of
No lateralizing signs	stroke, intracranial space-occupying lesions
Normal pupils and ABG	Recreational drugs
Down-going plantars	Seizures (post-ictal state – plantars up-going)
Normal BMs	DKA (although not impossible)
Normal temperature, CRP mildly elevated	Encephalitis

We have someone taking lithium for a psychiatric disorder who presents acutely with neurological signs, electrolyte imbalance, and AKI. It is worth exploring their temporal association and attempting to explain these findings using first principles of pathophysiology.

Physiology: The low specific gravity of urine indicates a dilute urine despite hypernatremia. This provides a clue to diabetes insipidus commonly seen with chronic lithium usage.

Pharmacology: The kidneys handle lithium similarly to sodium. Hence lithium toxicity can be precipitated by volume depletion or renal impairment, both of which reduce its excretion. Patients with psychiatric disorders can have polydipsia or sometimes stop drinking water. The latter causes hypovolemia precipitating lithium re-absorption by the proximal tubules in parallel with sodium re-absorption. The higher lithium levels interfere with aquaporin-2 water channels and induce ADH resistance in the principal cells of the collecting tubule. This results in dilute urine worsening the hypovolemia and setting up a vicious cycle.

Lithium toxicity causes neuromuscular excitability resulting in hypertonia, hyper-reflexia and clonus. It also increases the threshold of calcium sensing receptors in the parathyroid glands causing uninhibited PTH secretion. This results in hypercalcemia which worsens the nephrogenic diabetes insipidus. Lastly, lithium, hypercalcemia, and hypernatremia contribute to the confusion.

The registrar requested urgent lithium levels which were $6\,mmol\,l^{-1}$. IV fluids and haemodialysis were initiated since he was symptomatic. Upon recovery it transpired he had stopped drinking water a few days prior to admission precipitating lithium toxicity.

This example illustrates causal reasoning whereby a seemingly non-related constellation of signs and symptoms are explained very easily by their temporal associations and patho-physiologic reasoning. It is easy to see that causal reasoning rests on a sound knowledge of patho-physiologic processes – a feat not many of us can boast of given the ever expanding field of medicine. Nevertheless, this provides a good example where engaging an analytic model of reasoning by reverting to first principles helps solve clinical dilemmas.

▼

Endocrinological causes of confusion include diabetic emergencies (DKA, hyperosmolar hyperglycaemic state (HHS), hypoglycaemia), and hyper or hypo function of the pituitary, thyroid, parathyroid, and adrenal gland.

Uncertainty, especially in rare diseases should be communicated to patients and personal knowledge gaps should be addressed.

Causal reasoning needs a good grasp of pathophysiology.

▲

References

Fox, R.C. (1980). The evolution of medical uncertainty. *The Milbank Memorial Fund Quarterly. Health and Society* 58 (1): 1–49.

Marcocci, C., Bollerslev, J., Khan, A.A., and Shoback, D.M. (2014). Medical management of primary hyperparathyroidism: Proceedings of the Fourth International Workshop on the Management of Asymptomatic Primary Hyperparathyroidism. *The Journal of Clinical Endocrinology and Metabolism* 99 (10): 3607–3618.

Silverberg, S.J., Shane, E., Jacobs, T.P. et al. (1999). A 10-year prospective study of primary hyperparathyroidism with or without parathyroid surgery. *New England Journal of Medicine* 341 (17): 1249–1255.

33 History Taking: What a Headache

▼
This chapter tells you how to approach relevant aspects of history from a neuro-logical perspective
▲

In neurology, one can often place the pathological process in an anatomical location provided a good history has been obtained and the examination findings are correctly interpreted. A comprehensive neurological history and examination is beyond the scope of this book, but I will certainly give you a road map to develop your skills further.

There are five pathological processes that can occur in neural tissue which point to the aetiology:

- Vascular
- Neoplastic
- Inflammatory
- Degenerative/demyelination
- Infection

It is useful to envisage history taking along these lines. Vascular events (e.g. stroke, subarachnoid haemorrhage) are sudden in onset, infections and inflammatory conditions can be sub-acute; whilst neoplastic and degenerative conditions are chronic.

General principles

- *Negative symptoms carry greater significance in neurology*. For instance, loss of sensa-tion is more significant than positive symptoms like pins and needles or tingling.
- *Pattern recognition* is a useful technique for novices. Neurology has five different but integrated systems: Cortical (e.g. pyramidal), subcortical (e.g. extra-pyramidal) cerebellar, autonomic nervous system (ANS), and peripheral nervous system (PNS) consisting of motor and sensory systems. Different combinations of these fit into a pattern which provides clues to the diagnosis. For example, extra-pyramidal features + ANS = multi-system atrophy.
- *Dominant hemisphere*. All right-handed and 70% of left-handed people have a dominant left hemisphere. Lesions of dominant frontal and parieto-temporal lobes result in speech disorders. Lesions in dominant parietal lobe lead to left-right disorientation, acalculia, agraphia, and finger agnosia (ALFA). By derivation, these are all cortical signs.
- *Bilateral cortical representation*. Upper facial muscles upper motor neurone (UMN of facial nerve), articulation of speech, and swallowing have bilateral cortical representa-tion. This is a fail-safe mechanism to protect basic human functions, e.g. swallowing is usually affected in the initial stages following stroke. It often returns back to normal over a variable period of time provided there is no extensive bilateral brain damage.
- *Drugs*. Never forget to review medications and recreational drugs since they are a common cause of neurological deficits.

33.1 HEADACHE

In the general population, tension-type headache, and migraines are the most common. However, in the emergency department headache evokes the possibility of life-threatening diagnoses. Often, it is the story of headache, its context, accompanying symptoms, age and gender that direct us to the cause (Figure 33.1).

The Hands-on Guide to Clinical Reasoning in Medicine, First Edition. Mujammil Irfan.
© 2019 John Wiley & Sons Ltd. Published 2019 by John Wiley & Sons Ltd.
Companion website: www.wiley.com/go/irfan/clinicalreasoning

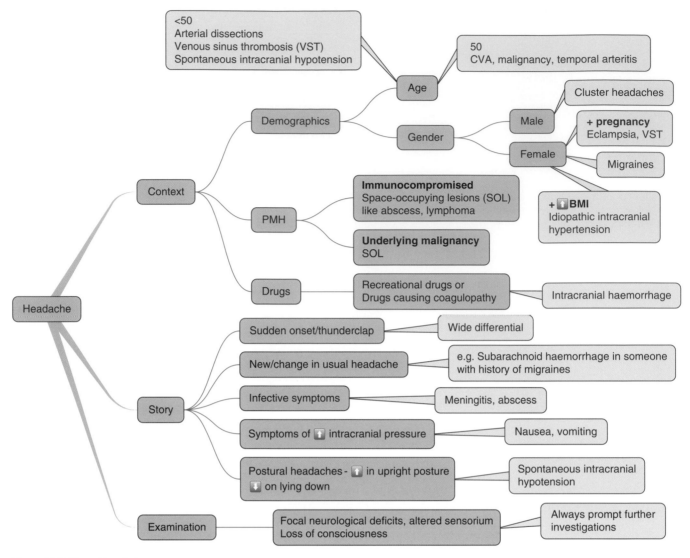

Figure 33.1 Story of headache

Vexatiously, headache can also be very non-specific e.g. it can accompany any febrile illness hence blurring the margins further.

33.2 SPEECH DISORDERS

From a neurological perspective, a speech disorder strictly refers to dysphasia and dysarthria. Conditions like deafness, dementia, and delirium especially in the elderly can impact speech and confound assessment hence the 5 Ds of speech disorder. The context as always helps in deciphering the problem e.g. a UTI with acute confusion points to delirium; a gradual decline in cognitive function implies dementia; a concurrent hemiparesis implies dysphasia. An abbreviated mental test (AMT), confusion assessment method (CAM) screen, and a quick check of hearing aids would help in weeding out the confounding variables (Inouye et al. 1990).

History taking often reveals the presence of a speech disorder even before a formal assessment is undertaken. Again, onset of symptoms (sudden or gradual) gives clue to the aetiology of dysphasia or dysarthria.

33.3 DYSPHASIA (LANGUAGE DISORDERS)

There are six components of language assessment (Table 33.1).

Table 33.1 Components of language assessment

		Receptive/sensory/Wernicke's/ (temporo-parietal) dysphasia	Expressive/motor/Broca's/ (frontal lobe) dysphasia
Fluency	Inferred from history/describe your house/ job, etc.	++ (neologisms – made-up words, paraphrasia – half right words)	–
Comprehension	Simple task: lift your left arm up Complex task: lift your left arm up and touch your right ear	–	+
Repetition	'No ifs ands or buts' or 'British constitution'	–/+ (preserved in transcortical sensory aphasia)	+ (preserved in transcortical motor aphasia)/–
Naming objects (isolated defect in nominal dysphasia)	Point to your watch, pen, and ask them to name it	–	–
Reading[a]	Dyslexia – unable to read a written passage	–	+/–
Writing[a]	Dysgraphia – incoherent writing	+	+/–

[a]Illiteracy can affect reading and writing.

33.4 DYSARTHRIA (DISORDERS OF ARTICULATION): LANGUAGE IS INTACT

Speech originates in the cortex and travels down the corticobulbar pathways to the brainstem nuclei of lower cranial nerves which innervate the tongue, pharyngeal, and laryngeal muscles where speech is articulated. The impulses in corticobulbar pathways are modulated by the cerebellum and extra-pyramidal system that affects the flow of speech. Therefore, dysarthria occurs from problems in:

Cortex, corticobulbar pathways – spastic dysarthria/cortico-bulbar palsy – strained speech. Tongue is slow.

Cerebellum – disjointed speech – slow + abnormal separation of syllables

Extra-pyramidal system (EPS) – monotonous fast speech

Lower cranial nerve nuclei and nerves – flaccid dysarthria/bulbar palsy – labial (p), lingual (t), and guttural (ga) consonants affected. Hot potato speech. Tongue is flaccid ± 'bag of worms' fasciculations.

Neuromuscular junction – fatiguability – myasthenia

Some patients have functional disorders presenting as speech abnormality e.g. unable to phonate. A normal cough reduces the probability of organic disease.

33.5 DIZZINESS

Patients are often unclear about what they mean by dizziness. Dizziness encompasses vertigo, presyncope (near fainting), disequilibrium, psychiatric disorder, or non-specific dizziness.

The description of vertigo was traditionally taught as the discriminating feature that indicated vestibular disorders. However, it has been shown that this is flawed (Kerber and Baloh 2011). Just as we elicit onset, duration, precipitating, and relieving factors for any other symptom in medicine so should we focus on these features in dizziness.

Points to note:

• Dizziness that does not worsen with head movement is not vertigo.
• Dizziness that worsens with turning in bed eliminates orthostatic hypotension as a cause since the blood pressure remains constant.

Recurrent episodes of vertigo (~1 minute) representing benign paroxysmal positional vertigo can be detected by the Dix-Hallpike manoeuvre with high sensitivity (88%).

Acute onset of dizziness lasting ≥24 hours, worsened by head movement, accompanied by nausea, vomiting, gait unsteadiness, and nystagmus is defined as acute vestibular syndrome which can be peripheral (e.g. vestibular neuritis – dizziness; labyrinthitis – dizziness + hearing loss or tinnitus) or central (e.g. posterior circulation strokes, multiple sclerosis) (Venhovens et al. 2016).

The HINTS (Head Impulse test, Nystagmus, Test of Skew deviation) exam differentiates peripheral from central vestibular dysfunction (videos demonstrating this test are easily accessible on the Internet).

- Head impulse test – look for the catch-up saccade (a corrective eye movement to re-fixate on the object e.g. your nose) when the head is moved briskly to the centre in a vertical plane. A vestibular nerve problem will result in the catch-up saccade whilst the absence of it implies normal or central vestibular lesion.
- Nystagmus – assess in primary gaze and lateral gaze. Unidirectional nystagmus implies peripheral whilst bidirectional indicates central causes.
- Vertical skew deviation – cover/uncover test. Look for torsional nystagmus (rotatory) in a vertical plane when the eye is uncovered whilst asking the patient to look straight ahead.

Peripheral. Catch-up saccade on head impulse test, unidirectional nystagmus, and no vertical skew deviation. Central: No catch-up saccade, bi/multi-directional nystagmus with vertical skew deviation.

Another red flag for central vestibular dysfunction in acute settings is associated acute hearing loss. This results from vascular disorders affecting the internal auditory branch of anterior inferior cerebellar artery (AICA) which is an end-artery supplying the inner ear. AICA syndrome results in hearing loss and acute vestibular syndrome.

33.6 TRANSIENT LOSS OF CONSCIOUSNESS (TLOC)

Metabolic, electrical disturbances, and global cerebral hypoperfusion of any cause (e.g. arrhythmias, low-flow states) will result in TLOC (see Table 10.1). Posterior circulation transient ischemic attacks (TIAs) can rarely cause TLOC by reduced perfusion to the ascending reticular activating system (ARAS). This is a diffuse collection of nuclei in the brainstem which acts as the sleep-awake switch.

33.7 MOTOR AND SENSORY DEFICITS

Onset of symptoms, pattern of muscles involved and associated symptoms help in establishing the diagnosis. Sensory deficits can be central or peripheral. Once again, the onset, diffuse or differential sensory loss (specific modalities affected e.g. pain and temperature only), associated symptoms, and in the case of spinal cord lesions a clear sensory level will help in establishing the diagnosis – all dealt with in the next chapter.

References

Inouye, S.K., van Dyck, C.H., Alessi, C.A. et al. (1990). Clarifying confusion: the confusion assessment method. A new method for detection of delirium. *Annals of Internal Medicine* 113 (12): 941–948.

Kerber, K.A. and Baloh, R.W. (2011). 'The evaluation of a patient with dizziness. *Neurology: Clinical Practice* 1 (1): 24–33.

Venhovens, J., Meulstee, J., and Verhagen, W.I. (2016). Acute vestibular syndrome: a critical review and diagnostic algorithm concerning the clinical differentiation of peripheral versus central aetiologies in the emergency department. *Journal of Neurology* 263 (11): 2151–2157.

34 Clinical Examination: Walking Straight

▼

This chapter tells you how to synthesise examination findings from a neurological perspective

▲

This chapter is not a detailed discourse on 'how to examine' instead, the focus is on explanation of signs, and their synthesis to help you arrive at a diagnosis which is often missing in most books. As elsewhere, the diagnosis should begin to take form as soon as the examination commences. The right combination of words should be used to clearly instruct the patient in order to avoid confusion. Sometimes it is worth mirroring the action expected of the patient whilst standing next to them. I suggest that you develop your own routine that you will be comfortable with.

34.1 LIMB EXAMINATION

Figure 34.1 shows the line of thinking that is needed when you examine the limbs. Imagine the motor pathway as a vertical motorway with various exits/entry points corresponding to the horizontal levels at which the lesion is found (Figure 34.3). Your task is to:

1. Locate the lesion on the vertical line in the upper motor neuron (UMN) or lower motor neuron (LMN) segment using examination findings from Figure 34.1.
2. Find accessory signs that help localise the lesion further. For example, if UMN signs are detected, the lesion could be anywhere between the motor cortex, and the lateral corticospinal tract (brain – spinal cord). Sensory examination can be used to elicit signs that localise the lesion within this segment in a horizontal plane. In other words, the specific sensory signs behave as sign posts on the motorway pointing to the exit.

   For instance:
   Cortical sensory signs → places the lesion in the cortex.
   Sensory level at L1 → lesion in spinal cord around L1.

34.1.1 Upper Limbs (UL)
Look around the patient for cervical collar, hand therapy ball, walking aids, etc. which give a clue to the diagnosis or the functional impact of neurological disability.

Inspection: Note the pattern of wasting (muscle groups involved), asymmetry, fasciculations, contractures (uni-/bilateral), surgical scar over cervical spine. Of note, spontaneous fasciculations carry greater significance than those induced by tapping.

Arms out-stretched with palms facing up and eyes closed:

- Pronator drift → UMN lesion since supinators are weaker than pronators.
- Pseudo-athetosis (wandering fingers/hands) → loss of proprioception (Romberg's equivalent in UL).
- Rebound phenomenon when displaced → hypotonia in cerebellar lesions.

Tone: Spasticity is velocity dependent. Look for 'supinator catch.' After passively moving the wrist in supination/pronation a couple of times to help the patient relax, one *quickly* supinates the wrist which catches mid-way. If the wrist is supinated *slowly* there is no catch. This differentiates it from rigidity where supination done quickly or slowly has a feel of stiffness throughout the range of movement (Bhimani and Anderson 2014). Spasticity is often associated with clonus – look for it in the wrist (Biotti and Vighetto 2013).

The Hands-on Guide to Clinical Reasoning in Medicine, First Edition. Mujammil Irfan.
© 2019 John Wiley & Sons Ltd. Published 2019 by John Wiley & Sons Ltd.
Companion website: www.wiley.com/go/irfan/clinicalreasoning

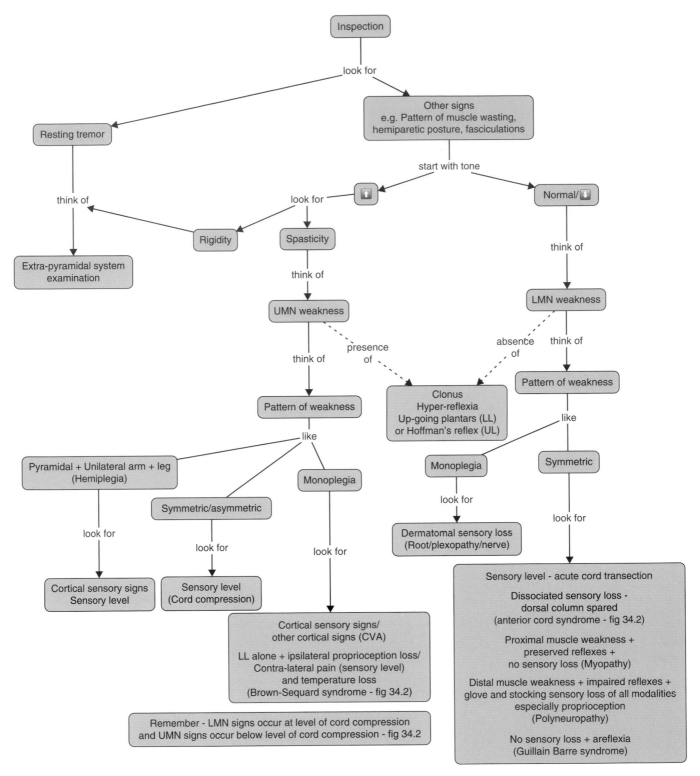

Figure 34.1 Concept map showing how to think when doing a neurological examination

Power: Spasticity → UMN lesion. It commonly results in the pyramidal pattern of
weakness (hemiparetic posture) i.e. arm held in flexion (extensors weaker than flexors)
and leg in extension (flexors weaker than extensors). The inability of the leg to flex
causes the circumduction (the foot tracing a semicircle to avoid catching the toes) seen
in the hemiparetic gait.

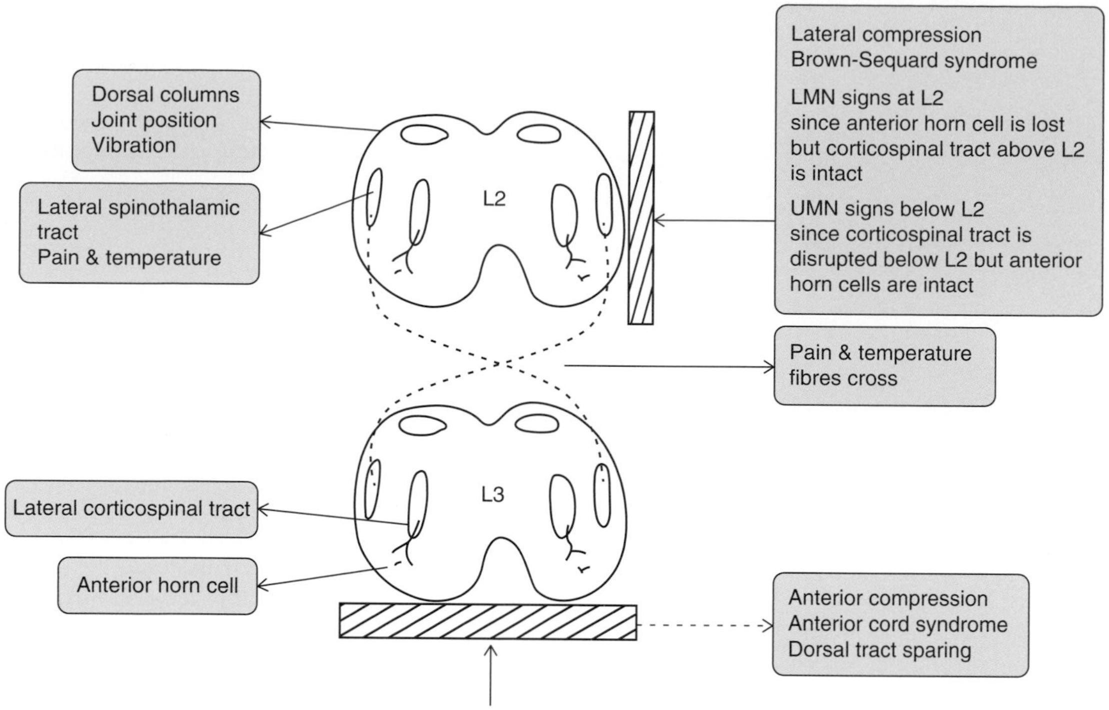

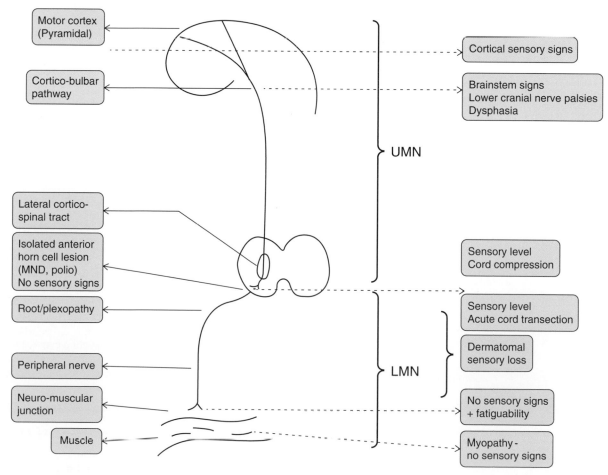

Dorsal columns
Joint position
Vibration

Lateral spinothalamic
tract
Pain & temperature

Lateral compression
Brown-Sequard syndrome

LMN signs at L2
since anterior horn cell is lost
but corticospinal tract above L2
is intact

UMN signs below L2
since corticospinal tract is
disrupted below L2 but anterior
horn cells are intact

Pain & temperature
fibres cross

Lateral corticospinal tract

Anterior horn cell

Anterior compression
Anterior cord syndrome
Dorsal tract sparing

Figure 34.2 Anatomy of anterior and lateral cord compression

Motor cortex
(Pyramidal)

Cortico-bulbar
pathway

Cortical sensory signs

Brainstem signs
Lower cranial nerve palsies
Dysphasia

UMN

Lateral cortico-
spinal tract

Isolated anterior
horn cell lesion
(MND, polio)
No sensory signs

Root/plexopathy

Peripheral nerve

Neuro-muscular
junction

Muscle

Sensory level
Cord compression

Sensory level
Acute cord transection

Dermatomal
sensory loss

No sensory signs
+ fatiguability

Myopathy -
no sensory signs

LMN

Figure 34.3 Motorway and exits of neuroanatomy helping in interpretation of examination findings and localising the lesion

Normal/↓ tone + muscle wasting/weakness + fasciculation → LMN pattern of weakness.

- Look for muscle weakness following spinal root/peripheral nerve distribution e.g. wrist drop in radial nerve palsy – extensor muscle weakness.
- Distal muscle weakness → peripheral neuropathy (reflexes absent/↓).
- Proximal muscle weakness → myopathy (reflexes present).

Co-ordination: If power is normal check co-ordination and other cerebellar signs. Conversely, muscle weakness will interfere with co-ordination making its assessment impractical.

Reflexes: Spasticity, clonus, hyper-reflexia, and extensor plantars (UMN) all go together. Reflexes may be diminished/absent in LMN lesion. Assess with reinforcement and if still absent report them as such. Learn to grade them.

Sensory examination: Sensory examination is directed by preceding motor examination findings.

- UMN monoplegia → look for cortical sensory signs (sensory inattention/extinction, 2-point discrimination, astereognosis, graphesthesia) in affected UL and sensory level on the opposite side if lower limb (LL) also involved (Figure 34.3).
- Symmetrical/asymmetrical UMN weakness (possible cord compression) → look for sensory level with pin-prick (most discriminatory).
- Unilateral LMN weakness → root/plexopathy/nerve → dermatomal examination.
- Symmetric LMN weakness (distal muscle) → polyneuropathy → glove and stocking distribution of sensory loss in all modalities (joint position, vibration lost first).

34.1.2 Lower Limbs (LL)

Look around the patient for wheelchair, callipers, special shoes with soles, stick, etc. as in UL examination.

Assess gait, tandem walking and Romberg's if the patient is able to stand. Romberg's: stand with heels together. If the patient is unsteady with eyes open and worse with eyes closed → cerebellar ataxia. If they are unsteady only with eyes closed → sensory ataxia – Romberg's positive (peripheral neuropathy/polyneuropathy).

Inspection: Similar to UL.

Tone: Once the patient is relaxed (use distraction if needed), roll the leg longitudinally on the bed holding it with your hands above and below the knee. Check if the foot moves en-bloc with the leg (hypertonia) or flops around independently (normal tone). Proceed to hold the knee with two hands and *suddenly* (velocity dependent) lift the knee from underneath so as to flex it. Pay close attention to the heel of the foot and check if it scrapes the bed (normal tone) or gets lifted off the bed ('knee catch' – spasticity). If there is hypertonia, look for knee and ankle clonus.

Power, co-ordination, reflexes, and sensory examination are similar to the UL. The following points are explained for emphasis.

Cerebellar signs in LL – foot tapping, heel-shin test.

Physiologic causes of extensor plantars: sleep, first nine months of infancy, post-ictal (the last is not strictly physiological).

Pin-prick sensation: Start by showing the patient how the neurological pin feels on the chest or the forehead (in cases of suspected high cervical lesions). Then test the limbs and each time ask them if it feels similar to the 'sharp' sensation they felt on the chest or forehead (reference point) with a 'yes' or 'no' rather than dull or sharp. This eliminates all the confusion with 'adjectives.'

Traditional teaching emphasises comparing pinprick sensation between the two limbs as expected in OSCEs. This is useful in unilateral dermatomal loss of sensation. However, other lesions (e.g. sensory level, glove, and stocking) are much easily detected when pinprick is compared to the chest/forehead as the reference.

34.2 EXAMINATION OF THE SENSORY SYSTEM

This should include, assessment of loss of sensation in all the five modalities in a dermatomal distribution (root/plexus/nerve), glove and stocking distribution (circumferential loss in polyneuropathy), looking for a sensory level (cord lesion), and cortical sensory signs (cortical lesion). Deep tendon reflexes (DTR) comprise of a

Table 34.1 Patterns of weakness in LL with sensory signs. Fill in the missing information to make it your own

Unilateral UMN weakness/monoplegia + sensory level	Brown-Sequard syndrome: pain and temperature loss on opposite side; proprioception loss on same side (lateral cord compression)
Unilateral UMN weakness/monoplegia + cortical sensory signs	
Asymmetric UMN weakness + sensory level	
Symmetric UMN weakness + sensory level	
Unilateral LMN weakness + dermatomal sensory loss	
Symmetric LMN weakness + sensory level	Acute (traumatic) cord transection/ flaccid paralysis. Other features: priapism in males, urinary retention, and faecal incontinence
Symmetric LMN weakness + dissociated sensory loss (preserved dorsal column sensation)	Anterior cord syndrome e.g. anterior spinal artery occlusion
Symmetric LMN weakness + no sensory loss + areflexia	
Symmetric LMN weakness with distal muscle involvement + glove and stocking distribution sensory loss	
Symmetric UMN signs (hypertonia, hyper-reflexia, clonus) + *normal power* + sensory level	Hereditary spastic paraparesis
	Cauda equina

sensory (afferent) neuron too. Hence sensory examination is incomplete without assessing DTRs. For example, a predominantly sensory polyneuropathy can still be accompanied by a loss of reflexes despite muscle power being normal.

Table 34.1 gives various combinations of patterns of muscle weakness with different sensory signs in the lower limbs. Work out the diagnosis (and pattern for the last one) using what you have learnt so far.

34.3 GENERAL PRINCIPLES OF CRANIAL NERVE EXAMINATION

- Cranial nerve nuclei can be placed in groups of four in the brain stem except the first two: III–IV (mid-brain), V–VIII (pons), and IX–XII (medulla). Therefore, they act as exits on the motorway pointing to the horizontal level at which the lesion can be placed.
- All cranial nerve nuclei are controlled by higher cortical centres which often have bilateral cortical representation (e.g. VII). Lesions in these pathways cause UMN cranial nerve palsies whereas lesions at the level of the nucleus or below cause LMN palsies (like everywhere else in peripheral nervous system).
- It can't be stressed enough that anatomy helps in understanding the signs elicited e.g. III, IV, V_1, V_2, VI, and sympathetic nerve plexus travel in the cavernous sinus and a lesion here can cause multiple cranial nerve palsies.

34.4 EYE EXAMINATION – A PHYSICIAN'S PERSPECTIVE

This involves assessing the integrity of the visual pathway (visual acuity/visual fields/pupils/ colour vision/fundoscopy), ocular movements (cranial nerves III, IV and VI/nystagmus, and fatiguability), and cortical signs of visual inattention (a form of sensory inattention).

Glasses are a big clue: Check if they are concave/convex (visual acuity). Fresnel glasses/ prismatic lenses have vertical or horizontal lines on them (diplopia/homonymous hemianopia) and a patch on one eye could point to severe diplopia or enucleation. A glass eye does not move with the other eye.

Strabismus: e.g. divergent squint at neutral position. Cover test – ask the patient to look at you. Cover the left eye – the right eye does not move; Cover the right eye – the left eye moves to look at you. Diagnosis: Divergent strabismus with right dominant eye. If no accompanying diplopia – congenital, if not – acquired.

34.4.1 Visual Field Defects
Visual field assessment must be performed one eye at a time whereas visual inattention is assessed with both eyes open (Figure 34.4).

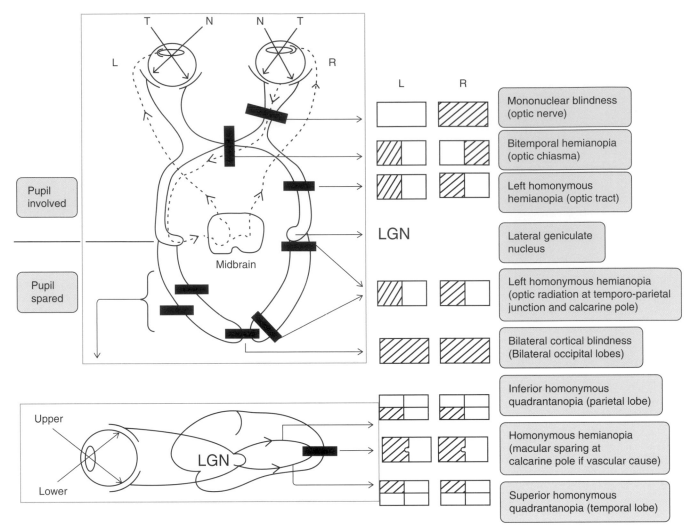

Figure 34.4 Visual field defects explained using anatomy

Points of interest:

- Temporal fibres of optic nerve look at the nasal field of vision whilst the nasal fibres look at the temporal field of vision since the lens flips the image (left-right and upside-down).
- The nasal fibres crossing over at the optic chiasma carry temporal fields of vision. Hence the bitemporal hemianopia from a lesion here.
- Pupillary nerve fibres also cross over at the chiasma, but each innervates both Edinger-Westphal nuclei in the mid-brain (hence the consensual light reflex).
- Pupil is involved in any lesion anterior to the lateral geniculate nucleus and spared in lesions posterior to it.
- The parietal fibres of optic radiation carry lower field of vision whilst the temporal fibres carry upper field of vision (caused by the lens again).
- Macular sparing occurs with a vascular lesion at the calcarine pole owing to dual blood supply.

34.4.2 Ocular Movements

Look at the eyes in their primary position of gaze (looking straight ahead) and check if they already have diplopia.

- Eye is down and out (i.e. upward, inward movements are impaired) with an associated ptosis and non-reactive dilated pupil → Compressive III nerve palsy. Any combination of these components with pupillary sparing → ischemic III nerve palsy.
- Head tilt – one eye above the other + Fresnel glasses → IV nerve palsy (inability of affected eye to look down in adduction – i.e. looking towards the tip of the nose).

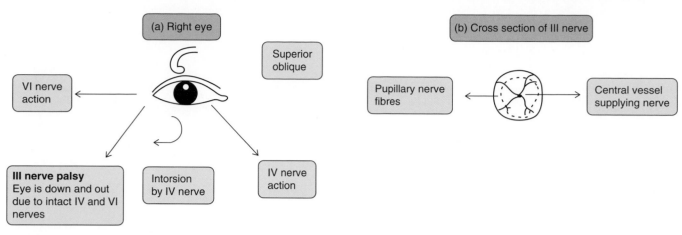

Figure 34.5 Third nerve palsy

- None of the above → ask them to look to one side in both horizontal planes e.g. cross eyed + diplopia on looking to right side in the horizontal plane → right VI nerve palsy.

Figure 34.5a shows the primary action of IV and VI and illustrates why the eye is down and out in III nerve palsy. Ischemic infarct of the III nerve (vascular supply from the centre) spares the superficial pupillary nerve fibres whereas the latter get compressed from the outside in compressive lesions (Figure 34.5b)

Trace an imaginary 'H' (nine cardinal positions of gaze) in front of the patient whilst getting them to follow your finger. Ask them to let you know if they see any double vision. If they do report double vision mentally record the quadrant in which it was seen. For example, if they report diplopia on looking right, upward and outward, hold your finger in that position and identify the eye which has not moved into that quadrant. Sometimes following a conjunctival vessel and ascertaining that it is not moving will help identify subtle nerve palsies.

Ideally one should use a red filter in front of each eye to identify the abnormal side with the cranial nerve palsy. In this scenario you can apply the oft quoted 'which image disappears on closing the eye' which is what most books recommend. Short of that, it can be very confusing to use this approach without a filter!

A combination of impaired ocular movements not following a particular cranial nerve palsy implies complex ophthalmoplegia e.g. Grave's ophthalmopathy, myasthenia gravis, etc.

34.4.3 V Cranial Nerve
Sensory examination of ophthalmic, maxillary and mandibular divisions must be combined with a search for dissociated sensory loss of pain and temperature (pin-prick) in an onion-skin pattern (Figure 34.6). An ascending brain-stem syrinx (as in syringobulbia) will spare the central target area until the last.

34.4.4 VII Nerve
Figure 34.7 shows accessory signs that help localise the VII nerve lesion along its anatomical pathway for LMN (nuclear/infranuclear) facial nerve palsy. For example, Bell's palsy spares lacrimation (but the eye is dry from a lack of eyelid closure) but is associated with loss of taste and hyperacusis since the lesion is in the facial canal. UMN palsy occurs from a lesion in the contralateral cortex resulting in facial paralysis of the lower half of the face. The upper half of the face has bilateral cortical representation and is therefore spared.

34.4.5 Cerebello-pontine (CP) Angle Lesion
Anatomically, this results in V_1 (earliest sign is loss of corneal reflex), VII, and VIII nerve palsies (Figure 34.7).

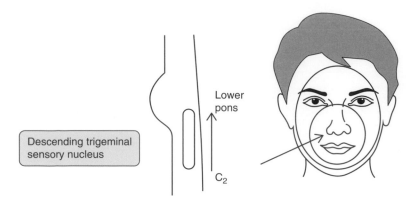

Figure 34.6 Sensory examination of pain and temperature in fifth nerve palsy

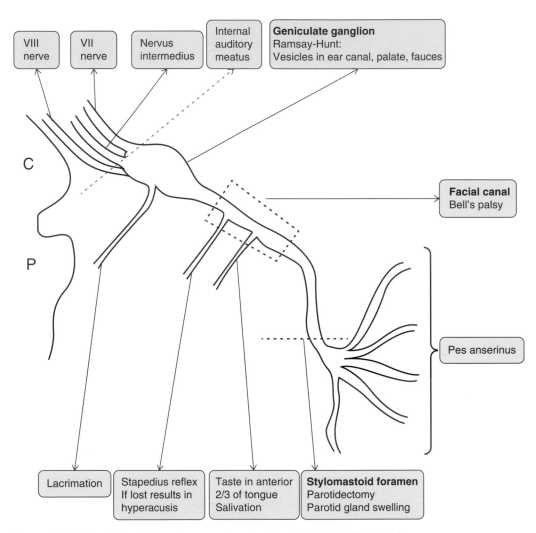

Figure 34.7 Anatomical correlation of accessory signs localising the lesion in 7th nerve palsy

34.4.6 Lower Cranial Nerve Palsies

Swallowing has bilateral cortical representation and is therefore likely to recover post stroke. Unilateral vagus (X) nerve palsy causes difficulty in swallowing (nasal regurgitation), phonation (hoarseness), and coughing. Hypoglossal nerve (XII) is usually affected in combination with other lower cranial nerves i.e. glossopharyngeal (IX) and X. Bilateral lesions of these nerves together, cause corticobulbar (UMN), and bulbar palsy (LMN).

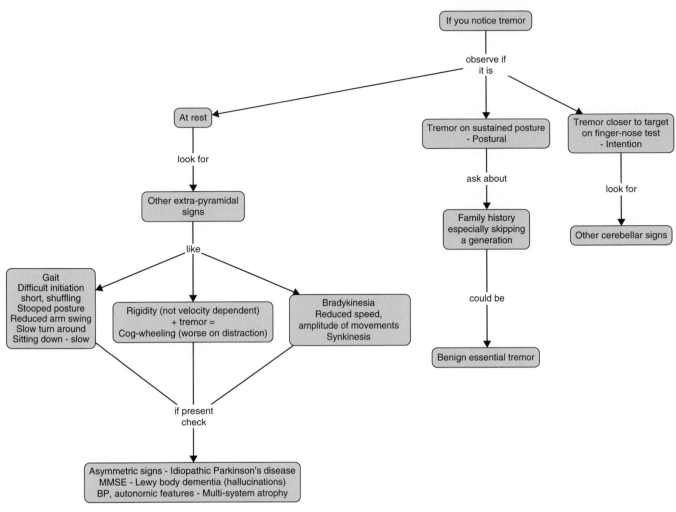

Figure 34.8 Concept map showing examination of tremor

34.4.7 Cerebellar Signs
Acronym: 'DANISH' – Ipsilateral signs of

*D*ysdiadochokinesia
*A*taxia
*N*ystagmus
*I*ntention tremor
*S*taccato speech
*H*ypotonia

34.4.8 Meningeal Signs of Irritation
Nuchal rigidity/neck stiffness – inability to touch chin to chest either passively or actively.

Brudzinski sign – the hips and knees flex on passively flexing the neck in supine position.

Kernig's sign – in the supine position the hip and knee is flexed at 90° and the knee is then passively extended. The test is positive if the opposite knee flexes or there is resistance to knee extension > 135°/pain in lower back or back of thigh.

All signs have poor sensitivity but the last two have a high specificity.

34.4.9 Tremor and Extra-Pyramidal System Examination
Figure 34.8 shows a concept map to explain this symptom.

References
Bhimani, R. and Anderson, L. (2014). Clinical understanding of spasticity: implications for practice. *Rehabilitation Research and Practice* 2014: 279175.
Biotti, D. and Vighetto, A. (2013). Upper limb clonus. *New England Journal of Medicine* 369 (10): e12.

35 Investigations: The Light Bulb

▼
This chapter tells you how to interpret CT head scans and CSF results
▲

As always investigations should be interpreted in their clinical context. Perron et al. (1998) used the mnemonic '*Blood can be very bad*' to ensure vital signs are not missed on emergency CTs which would do well to serve our purpose (Figure 35.1).

Association of each word in the mnemonic Blood Can Be Very Bad with corresponding emergency.

Blood Can Be Very Bad

- **Blood:** Acute blood is bright white on CT. Types include:
  EDH (lens-shaped)
  SDH (sickle-shaped)
  Intraparenchymal (especially basal ganglia)
  Intraventricular (watch for hydrocephalus)
  SAH (blood in cisterns)
- **Cisterns (Can):** CSF collections jacketing the brain. Look for blood in cisterns (SAH), and effacement (increased ICP), 4 key cisterns:
  Circummesencephalic (ring around midbrain)
  Suprasellar (star-shaped) Circle of Willis
  Quadrigeminal (W-shaped)
  Sylvian (between temporal and frontal lobes)
- **Brain (Be):** Look for:
  Symmetry
  Gray-white differentiation
  Shift
  Hyper/hypodensity
  Pneumocephalus
- **Ventricles (Very):** CSF produced in lateral ventricles (back-to-back commas) → III ventricle (slit-shaped) → aqueduct of Sylvius → IV ventricle (helmet-shaped). Approximately 20 mL/h. Look for:
  Effacement
  Shift
  Blood
- **Bone (Bad):** Note soft tissue swelling. Look for blood in sinuses/mastoid air cells, widened sutures.

EDS, Epidural hematoma; **SDH,** subdural hemorrhage; **SAH,** subarachnoid hemorrhage; **CSF,** cerebrospinal fluid; **ICP,** intracranial pressure.

Figure 35.1 Source: Perron et al. 1998. Reproduced with permission of Elsevier

General principles
- Cerebrospinal fluid (CSF) physiology shows that the ventricles, subarachnoid space, central canal of the spinal cord, and the cisterns all communicate with each other (Figure 35.2). Problems in one area of this system will affect the rest. For example, blood from sub-arachnoid haemorrhage (SAH) can show up in the cisterns, ventricles, or subarachnoid space.
- Grey-white matter differentiation in the brain – counter-intuitively, white matter is located centrally, appearing blacker on CT whilst the grey coloured grey matter is on

The Hands-on Guide to Clinical Reasoning in Medicine, First Edition. Mujammil Irfan.
© 2019 John Wiley & Sons Ltd. Published 2019 by John Wiley & Sons Ltd.
Companion website: www.wiley.com/go/irfan/clinicalreasoning

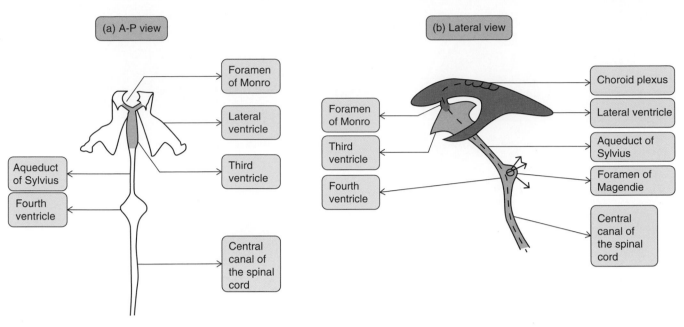

Figure 35.2 Anatomy of CSF production and flow

the outside. This is because the myelin in the axons comprising white matter is fatty thus appearing darker on CT.

- The skull is a rigid compartment with not much extra space. Therefore, anything extra like oedema, space occupying lesion (SOL), or blood in one hemisphere results in the loss of sulci as they get squashed against the skull (sulcal effacement) ipsilaterally and the midline shifts to the opposite side.

Blood – Fresh blood appears white on CT turning grey (isodense with grey matter – outer cortex) to black (isodense with CSF) as the clot resolves (Figure 35.3c). Extra-axial haemorrhage is of three types:

Extradural haematoma (EDH) – lens shaped, limited by sutures in skull +/− skull fractures (Figure 35.3a).
Subdural haematoma (SDH) – crescent/sickle shaped, blood does not enter sulci (Figure 35.3b).
SAH – see under 'cisterns'.

- *Cisterns* – These are pools of CSF collections that occur naturally in the subarachnoid space owing to separation of arachnoid mater from pia mater where the pia mater dips in to line the brain parenchyma e.g. in sulci. Major vessels like the circle of Willis lie in these cisterns which can rupture causing blood to accumulate in them. Of note, lumbar cistern (L2–S2) is where the lumbar puncture is performed (Figure 35.4).

SAH – aneurysmal bleeding in this space results in blood collecting in cisterns/ ventricles since they are all continuous with each other and blood clots cause obstructive hydrocephalus (Figure 35.5). Traumatic SAH can be accompanied by EDH, SDH, ICH, or skull fractures.

- *Brain* – cell death in brain parenchyma appears as a hypodensity (e.g. ischemia/infarction) whereas parenchymal blood appears as hyperdensity (e.g. ICH) (Figure 35.7). Points of interest:

i. A wedge-shaped lesion involving both grey and white matter with loss of differentiation is likely to be vascular (stroke).
ii. Presence of a lesion in grey or white matter alone with surrounding oedema is likely to be a SOL like tumour (Figure 35.7c).
iii. Underlying parenchymal lesions can cause early sulcal effacement, best appreciated by comparing right with left.
iv. Insular ribbon sign and dense middle cerebral artery (MCA) sign are early signs of ischemic infarct involving the MCA which can be seen on 0.625 thin CT cuts (Figures 35.6 and 35.7a).

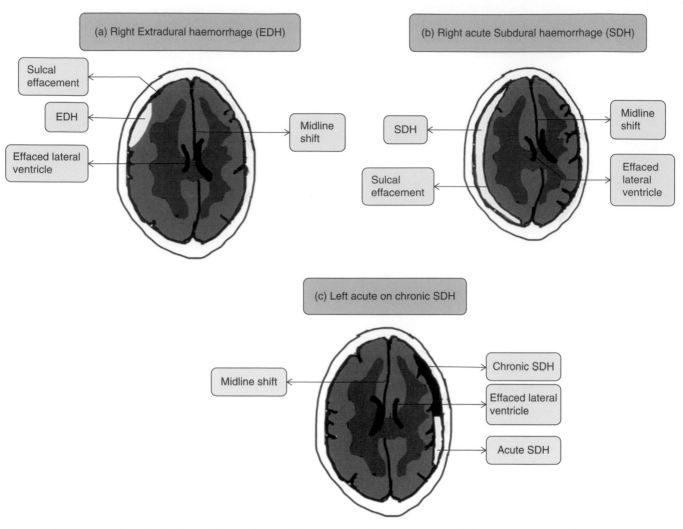

Figure 35.3 CT head showing a) right extradural haemorrhage b) right acute subdural haemorrhage and c) left acute on chronic subdural haemorrhage

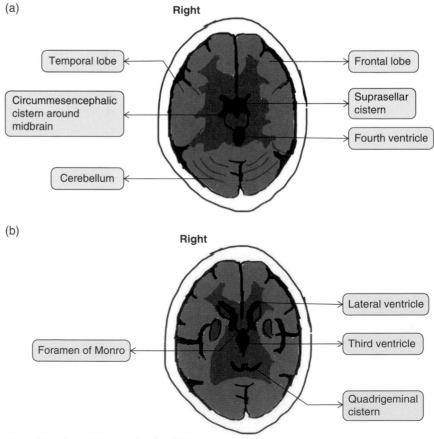

Figure 35.4 Normal CT head showing CSF cisterns

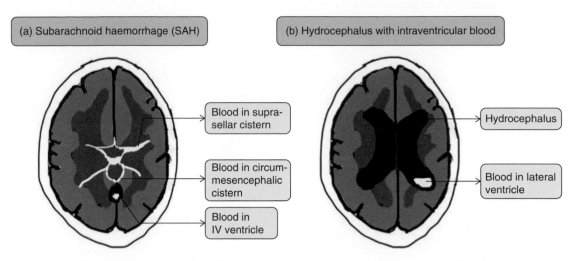

Figure 35.5 CT head showing a) sub-arachnoid haemorrhage and b) hydrocephalus with intraventricular blood

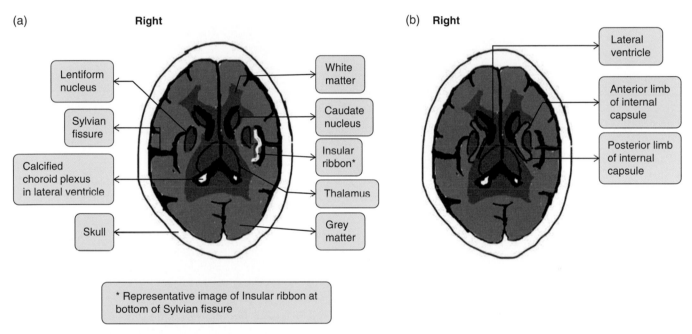

Figure 35.6 Normal CT head anatomy from a stroke perspective

Ventricles – Blood in the ventricles appears white and clot formation can obstruct the outflow of CSF resulting in hydrocephalus. This is anatomically illustrated by enlarged ventricles and physiologically by raised intracranial pressure (ICP). Normal pressure hydrocephalus as the name suggests is an exception.

Bone – (Switch to bone window on CT) look for fractures with subcutaneous oedema +/− blood, air/fluid levels in sinuses.
Common errors: IV contrast that is used to detect SOL, arteriovenous malformation (AVM), and aneurysms can mimic blood. It is often restricted to vessels.
Calcification in basal ganglia, pineal body, and choroid plexus in ventricles can mimic blood on CT.

35.1 CEREBROSPINAL FLUID (CSF) ANALYSIS

Figure 35.8 shows the various components of CSF analysis in various combinations. I have got you started with a few diagnoses. Fill in the empty boxes with the information given below and add more diagnoses to make it your own.

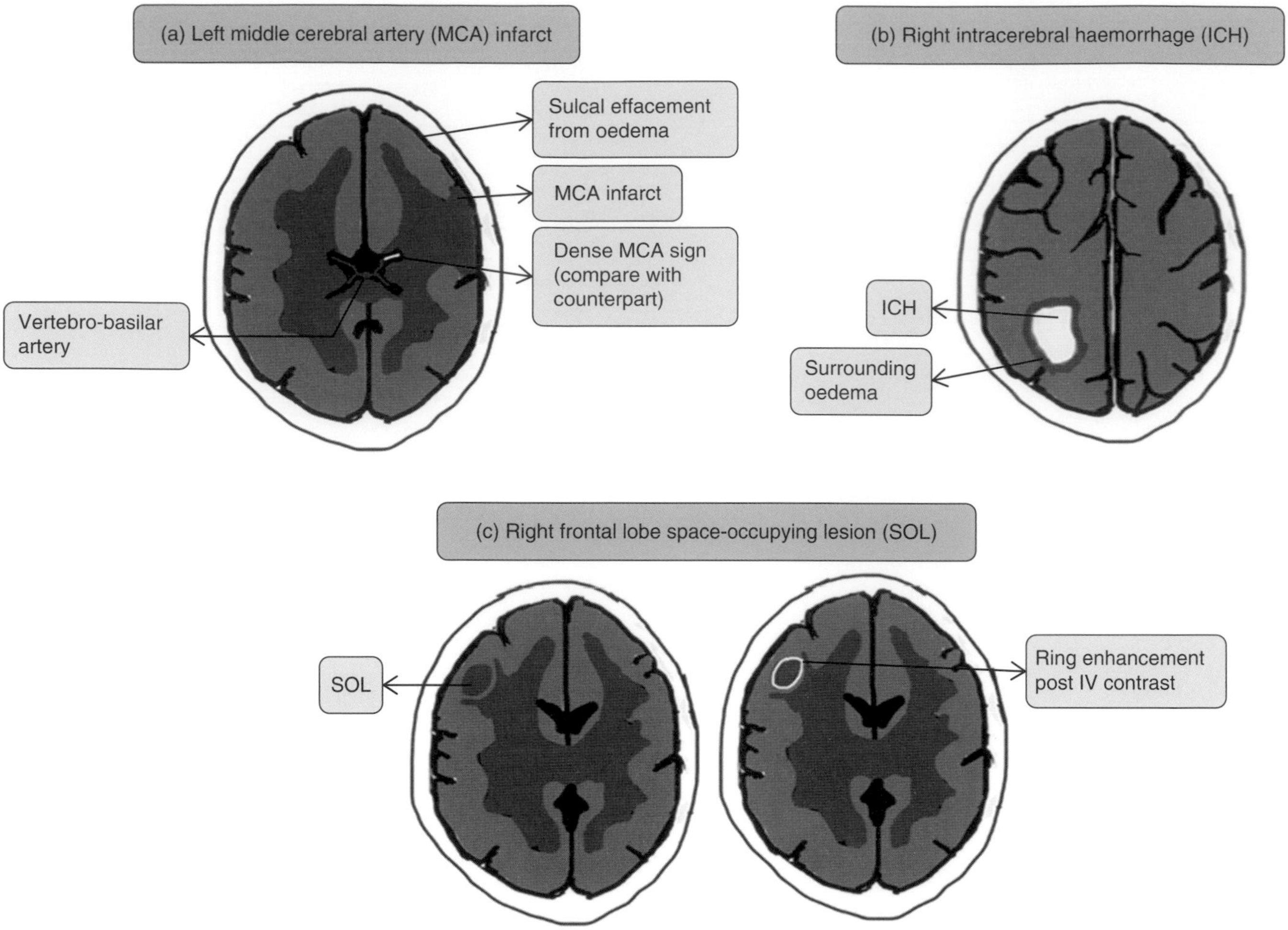

Figure 35.7 CT head showing a) Left MCA infarct b) Right intracerebral haemorrhage and c) Right frontal lobe space occupying lesion

Opening pressure (OP) in lateral decubitus position with the legs extended is 6–20 cm of H_2O. Low OP occurs with iatrogenic or traumatic CSF leak and Froin's syndrome (Dancel and Shaban 2016). Figure 35.8 shows the causes of high OP.

Xanthochromia is a fancy word for pink or yellow tint:
  Red cell haemolysis in the CSF results in breakdown of haemoglobin (red) → oxyhaemoglobin (pink) → methaemoglobin → bilirubin (yellow). This process takes two to four hours. Hence CSF analysed within two hours from collection will theoretically eliminate the possibility of traumatic tap. Additionally, bilirubin can only be produced in the CSF (since it needs heme oxygenase which is found in macrophages, arachnoid mater, and choroid plexus) but not in a test tube whereas oxyhaemoglobin can be produced in either. Therefore, finding bilirubin in the CSF by spectrophotometry is the most reliable way of establishing the diagnosis of SAH (Vermeulen et al. 1989). Bilirubin can be falsely high if CSF protein is ≥ 150 mg dl^{-1} or serum bilirubin is > 170 μmol l^{-1}. Hence a corresponding serum sample should be taken for bilirubin, protein, and glucose (UK National External Quality Assessment Scheme for Immunochemistry Working Group 2003).

Points to note in SAH:

- The sensitivity of CT approaches 100% in the first 6–12 hours from ictus. This drops to 83% in one day and 58% in five days (Sames et al. 1996; Perry et al. 2011).
- A lumbar puncture (LP) should be performed 12 hours from ictus since xanthochromia is at its peak in 95% of patients with SAH. This drops to 70% in three weeks and 40% in four weeks (Vermeulen et al. 1989). Hence recording the timing of the sample relative to the suspected ictus is essential.
- It follows that a delayed presentation will often need an angiography.

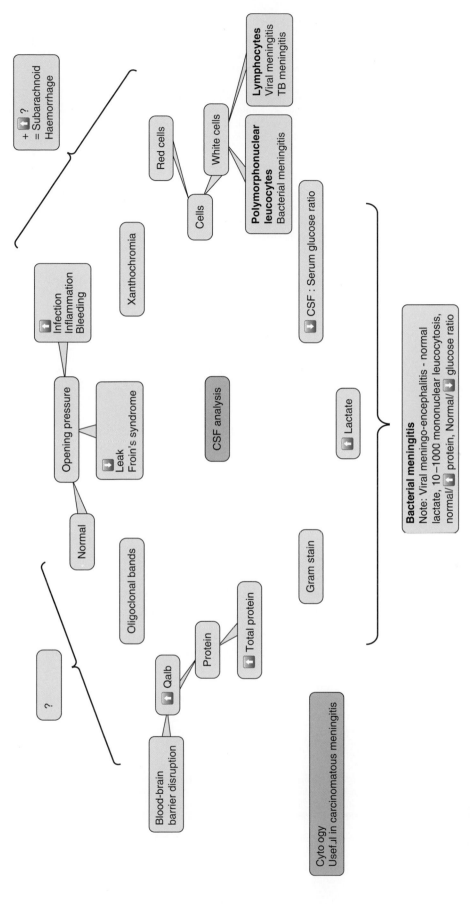

Figure 35.8 Interpretation of CSF analysis

35.2 CELLS

Red cells (normal 5/µl): Traumatic tap, SAH (see above), and in the appropriate setting – herpes simplex virus (HSV)-1 encephalitis (since it causes a necrotizing haemorrhagic encephalitis).

White cells (normal 5/µl): Initial polymorphonuclear cell predominance changes to lymphocyte predominance in 12–24 hours in bacterial meningitis. Mononuclear (lymphocyte) predominance is seen in viral meningo-encephalitis and TB meningitis. WCC > 1000 is seen in acute bacterial meningitis.

35.3 PROTEIN (NORMAL < 0.45 G L⁻¹)

CSF is normally bereft of protein. Total protein includes immunoglobulins which passively move across blood brain barrier (BBB) + intrathecal immunoglobulin synthesis + pathological Q_{alb} (CSF: serum albumin concentration gradient). It follows that infections can increase protein content owing to movement of immunoglobulins into CSF. A high Q_{alb} implies disruption of BBB as in infection, inflammation, bleeding, and leptomeningeal metastases.

Albuminocytologic dissociation (high total protein but normal cell count) – acute inflammatory demyelinating polyneuropathy (AIDP) (i.e. Guillain-Barre syndrome) and chronic inflammatory demyelinating polyneuropathy (CIDP).

35.4 *CSF*: SERUM GLUCOSE RATIO < 0.4 IS ABNORMAL

Glucose is actively transported across BBB. Therefore, conditions like infection, inflammation, leptomeningeal metastases, and bleeding that alter this can cause a low ratio. Viral infections cause a lesser degree of low glucose levels.

35.5 LACTATE (NORMAL 2.8–3.5 MMOL L⁻¹)

This is independent of serum lactate.
Lactate can be helpful in discriminating bacterial (high) from viral (normal) meningitis.

35.6 OLIGOCLONAL BANDS (OCBs)

Intrathecal immunoglobulin synthesis is increased (often IgG) in conditions like multiple sclerosis (MS), subacute sclerosing pan-encephalitis (SSPE), and neurosyphilis. If a sample of the CSF is applied on a gel and an electric voltage is applied to it, similarly charged immunoglobulins will clump together to form visible bands which can be single, >2 (oligoclonal) or multiple (polyclonal). These are compared against serum electrophoresis to identify any congruent bands. MS will often have OCBs that are not seen in the serum.

Gram stain and polymerase chain reaction (PCR) are techniques used to identify bacteria, viruses in the CSF. India ink preparation is used to identify cryptococcus.

References

Dancel, R. and Shaban, M. (2016). Froin's syndrome. *New England Journal of Medicine* 374 (11): 1076–1076.

Perron, A.D., Huff, J.S., Ullrich, C.G. et al. (1998). A multicenter study to improve emergency medicine residents' recognition of intracranial emergencies on computed tomography. *Annals of Emergency Medicine* 32 (5): 554–562.

Perry, J.J., Stiell, I.G., M.L.A., S. et al. (2011). Sensitivity of computed tomography performed within six hours of onset of headache for diagnosis of subarachnoid haemorrhage: prospective cohort study. *BMJ* 343: d4277–d4277.

Sames, T.A., Storrow, A.B., Finkelstein, J.A. et al. (1996). Sensitivity of new-generation computed tomography in subarachnoid hemorrhage. *Academic Emergency Medicine: Official Journal of the Society for Academic Emergency Medicine* 3 (1): 16–20.

UK National External Quality Assessment Scheme for Immunochemistry Working Group (2003). National guidelines for analysis of cerebrospinal fluid for bilirubin in suspected subarachnoid haemorrhage. *Annals of Clinical Biochemistry* 40 (5): 481–488.

Vermeulen, M., Hasan, M.D., Blijenberg, B.G. et al. (1989). 'Xanthochromia after subarachnoid haemorrhage needs no revisitation. *Journal of Neurology, Neurosurgery, and Psychiatry* 52 (7): 826–828.

36 Headache

▼
This chapter tells you how to approach headache from a neurological perspective
▲

Thunderclap headache always conjures up images of life-threatening subarachnoid haemorrhage but there are several other causes of the same and it is important to keep an open mind to other possibilities (Ducros and Bousser 2013).

Example 36.1

A 32 year old woman presented with a one day history of severe headache. She was having breakfast when she developed a generalised headache. She denied any focal neurological symptoms. PMH: nil, medications: oral contraceptive (OC) pill.

P: *Semantic qualifiers (SQs) – Young woman + severe headache + contraceptive pill.*
    Provisional diagnoses: wide differential. I would need some more information.

What questions would you ask her?

Activity 36.1

(Allow few seconds!)

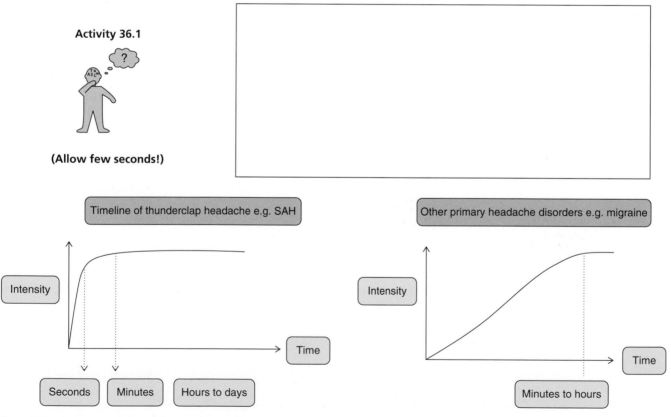

Figure 36.1 Discriminatory features of thunderclap headache

The Hands-on Guide to Clinical Reasoning in Medicine, First Edition. Mujammil Irfan.
© 2019 John Wiley & Sons Ltd. Published 2019 by John Wiley & Sons Ltd.
Companion website: www.wiley.com/go/irfan/clinicalreasoning

The primary question is whether this was a thunderclap headache. The speed of onset and time to reach its maximal intensity will be important (Figure 36.1). As you can see the intensity (severity) of the headache does not discriminate one from the other. A moderate headache can still represent SAH whilst a very 'severe' headache can still be migraine. Secondly, the context of the headache has to be elicited (Figure 33.1).

She reported a sudden onset headache that reached maximal intensity within a minute and was associated with vomiting. She was treated for sinusitis a week ago and denied any confusion, seizures or headache free interval. No family history of aneurysmal rupture.

P: *Provisional diagnoses – cerebral sinus thrombosis* (OC pill), *SAH* (thunderclap headache), *cerebral abscess or meningitis* (sinusitis), *migraine* (OC pill).

Primary headache disorders like tension headache and migraines cannot be diagnosed with a single episode hence that would be a diagnosis of exclusion. SAH, meningitis, and cerebral sinus thrombosis can present as thunderclap headache.

O/E: Temperature 38 °C, pulse 94 bpm, BP 150/70, RR 18 per minute, BMs 9 mmol l^{-1}, Saturations 98% on air. Systemic examination: normal, including neurological examination. In particular, there were no signs of meningeal irritation or altered sensorium. Bloods: Hb 140 g l^{-1}, WCC 12 × 10^9 l^{-1}, platelets 300 × 10^9 l^{-1}, CRP 50 mg l^{-1}, rest normal.

Hypertension (HT) often occurs in neurological conditions secondary to one/more of:

- Endothelial dysfunction following disruption in blood brain barrier e.g. stroke
- Sympathetic discharge
- Pain i.e. headache as in SAH

P: *Severity of illness – ill. Pyrexia points to an infective pathology (meningitis or cerebral abscess). The low grade inflammatory response, lack of signs of meningeal irritation or rash argues against it. The HT could be due to pain.*

Signs of meningeal irritation cement the diagnosis of meningitis (specific) but they lack sensitivity, therefore their absence does not exclude meningitis. Cerebral abscess does not cause meningism unless it has ruptured into the ventricles. Meningeal irritation can also occur with blood (SAH) and pyrexia can occur with SAH and venous sinus thrombosis. Palpable maculopapular rash is a sign of meningococcal septicaemia, where the patient would be very unwell with septic shock. Given this information, would you treat her for meningitis? What factors would you base your decision on?

Activity 36.2

(Allow three minutes)

....

....

....

....

Blood cultures were drawn, and analgesia and ceftriaxone were given. A non-contrasted computerised tomography (CT) scan of the head was normal with no evidence of focal lesions, bleed, or abscess.

P: *Would you proceed with an LP?*

I would keep an open mind with regards to the possibilities including SAH (xanthochromia) and cerebral venous sinus thrombosis (↑opening pressure). An LP would certainly be discriminatory since the headache has been > 12 hours. Given the CT scan was non-contrasted, cerebral abscess would be difficult to diagnose although this and meningitis seem unlikely.

LP: CSF opening pressure 24 cm of H_2O, protein $0.6\,g\,l^{-1}$, serum: CSF glucose ratio 0.7, xanthochromia was positive for bilirubin. She was diagnosed with SAH and referred to the neurosurgeons. A magnetic resonance angiogram (MRA) showed a right middle cerebral artery aneurysm which was coiled and she was discharged.

Prognostic model for meningitis uses: hypotension, seizures, and altered mental status.

0 – low risk
1 – intermediate risk
2–3 – high risk

This example illustrates hypothesis generation very succinctly. By establishing that this was thunderclap headache in an ill patient (severity of illness) the differentials were narrowed down to a few suspects.

Treatment decisions (IV antibiotics in this case) should be viewed through the prism of benefits vs risks. Mortality of untreated bacterial meningitis reaches 100% but rests on the certainty of the diagnosis. Meningitis can be excluded by the absence of all three features: fever > 38 °C, neck stiffness and altered mental status (Attia et al. 1999). The recent sinusitis plus fever raises the possibility of meningitis. Low grade inflammatory response mitigates it but does not exclude it! Assuming she has meningitis, a prognostic model would put her at low risk of mortality and neurological deficits (Aronin et al. 1998). Treatment risks include allergic reactions, selection of resistant micro-organisms, opportunistic infections e.g. Clostridium and risk of over-treatment. Ultimately clinical judgement will have to be exercised in deciding to treat but it is worth considering the basis for the decision.

Example 36.2

A 42 year old man presented with a three day history of worsening generalised headache, neck pain, and flashes of light in the eyes. He had had similar episodes over the last three months with increasing severity which would previously respond to ibuprofen. The recent episode was unresponsive to analgesia prompting the admission.

J: *SQs – middle aged man + acute on chronic headaches + neck pain + visual symptoms. Provisional diagnoses – migraines, tension headache but visual symptoms go against it, cluster headache* (no autonomic features), *new headache* (worse) *could be a new diagnosis e.g. SAH, meningitis, SOL.*

I would add the possibility of analgesic rebound headache.

The headache was gradual in onset with associated nausea. PMH: Hidradenitis suppurativa. Medications: doxycycline. Smoker of 30 py. Alcohol: occasional.

O/E: pulse 90 bpm, BP 150/90, Temperature 37.6 °C, RR 14 per minute, BMs $11\,mmol\,l^{-1}$. Elevated BMI. CNS: no focal neurological deficits except neck stiffness but Kernig's and Brudzinski's signs were negative. Co-Codamol was given for the headache. Non-contrasted CT head scan: normal. Bloods: normal. An LP was planned to exclude SAH.

J: *Severity of illness – ill. Since bloods are normal, meningitis is unlikely but not off the list. Can you do an LP three days after a suspected SAH?*

An LP can be done up to two weeks post ictus. What differentials would you have in this context in an order of decreasing probability?

Activity 36.3

(Allow two minutes)

....

....

....

....

....

J: SAH, migraines, or analgesic rebound headache. Meningitis is highly unlikely given the story and normal bloods.

It is important to note that we are in the territory of chronic headaches. If we focus on this context we would come up with further differentials like cerebral venous thrombosis and idiopathic IIH.

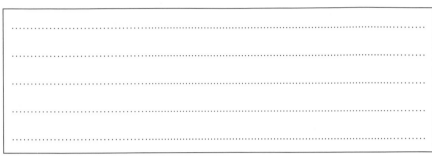

Eye examination and fundoscopy in headache

- Terson's syndrome (sub hyaloid or vitreous haemorrhage), diplopia, dilated pupil – SAH
- Papilloedema – cerebral venous sinus thrombosis, intracranial hypertension (IIH), SOL
- Retinal haemorrhages – hypertensive crisis
- Horner's syndrome – cervical artery dissection
- Acutely painful red eye – acute angle closure glaucoma
- Visual field defects and diplopia – pituitary apoplexy

He was transferred to a different ward from the admissions unit where he was reviewed by another team. An astute clinician noted the doxycycline on his drug chart and confirmed that he had been on it for nearly six months. The episodic headaches had been qualitatively similar over three months but the intensity had worsened. With his elevated BMI, they surmised that he might have IIH and a fundoscopy confirmed bilateral papilloedema (Frisén 1982).

The neurologist concurred with this diagnosis which was confirmed by an opening pressure of 30 cm of H_2O on LP and an MR venogram showing flattened posterior sclera and no cerebral venous thrombosis. Doxycycline was stopped, and he was followed up in the clinic with no recurrence of headaches.

This example demonstrates how a single clue (doxycycline) in the presentation can reveal new hypotheses provided we do not succumb to 'diagnosis momentum' (of SAH) from the previous team (Groopman 2007). The importance of a complete physical examination (fundoscopy) cannot be overemphasised as this could have also drawn the clinician's attention to the right diagnosis (see opposite).

Activity 36.3 illustrates the importance of not closing the loop despite a proposed working diagnosis of SAH by the admitting team. This would be the suggested solution to counter 'diagnosis momentum' in clinical practice.

▼

The speed of onset and time to reach its maximal intensity is the most discriminating aspect of thunderclap headache.

A single discrepant clue can reveal a new hypothesis that stops diagnosis momentum in its tracks.

▲

References

Aronin, S.I., Peduzzi, P., and Quagliarello, V.J. (1998). Community-acquired bacterial meningitis: risk stratification for adverse clinical outcome and effect of antibiotic timing. *Annals of Internal Medicine* 129 (11): 862–869.

Attia, J., Hatala, R., Cook, D.J., and Wong, J.G. (1999). The rational clinical examination. Does this adult patient have acute meningitis?'. *Journal of the American Medical Association* 282 (2): 175–181.

Ducros, A. and Bousser, M.-G. (2013). Thunderclap headache. *BMJ* 346 (15): e8557–e8557.

Frisén, L. (1982). Swelling of the optic nerve head: a staging scheme. *Journal of Neurology, Neurosurgery, and Psychiatry* 45 (1): 13–18.

Groopman, J.E. (2007). *How Doctors Think*. New York: Houghton Mifflin.

▼

This chapter tells you how to approach cranial nerve palsies using diplopia as an example

▲

Diplopia can be monocular (with one eye open) or binocular (both eyes open). The former is due to local eye problems e.g. refractive errors which is an ophthalmological issue whilst the latter is a neurological problem. Cranial nerve palsies can be localised to a point anywhere along the supranuclear (higher cortical centres) pathways → level of the nucleus → cranial nerve pathway, neuromuscular junction (NMJ), and the muscle itself. However, they often present with other neurological deficits and help localise the 'exit on the motorway' as discussed in Chapter 34. Listing the five pathological processes in relation to onset (acute or chronic) will help in identifying the aetiology.

Example 37.1

A 79 year old gentleman presented with a two week history of double vision. PMH: HT, previous DVT, osteoarthritis (OA). Medications: telmisartan and hydrochlorothiazide, paracetamol, and aspirin.

P: *SQs – elderly man + short history of diplopia + HT, previous DVT and OA. Provisional diagnoses – diplopia with a history of HT would point to a vascular cause but the differential is wide.*

Two weeks ago he developed sudden onset severe occipital headache radiating to the back associated with sickness. He was left with a dull headache when he noticed a right-sided droopy eyelid and blurry vision. Over the next two weeks the droopy eyelid improved but the diplopia persisted. He saw his GP who referred him to the hospital. Of note his baseline ET was 10–20 yards secondary to SOB and pain in his knees.

P: *Revised provisional diagnoses – Thunderclap headache and its differentials.*

O/E: Elevated BMI. Temperature 37 °C, pulse 80 bpm, BP 160/90, Saturations 97% on air, RR 14 per minute, BMs 10 mmol l^{-1}. CNS: Right eye ptosis with a dilated, non-reactive pupil, and the eye was resting down and out. No other focal neurological deficits or signs of meningeal irritation. Fundoscopy: normal. Bloods: fibrinogen 3 g l^{-1}, CRP 40 mg l^{-1}, WCC 12 × 10^9 l^{-1}, Platelets 450 × 10^9 l^{-1}; U&Es and LFTs: normal.

The Hands-on Guide to Clinical Reasoning in Medicine, First Edition. Mujammil Irfan.
© 2019 John Wiley & Sons Ltd. Published 2019 by John Wiley & Sons Ltd.
Companion website: www.wiley.com/go/irfan/clinicalreasoning

Using the principles of anatomy and physiology and the time course of events what would be your differentials?

Activity 37.1

(Allow three minutes)

P: *The resting position of the eye and the dilated pupil points to a compressive right third nerve palsy. Given the short history, vascular (e.g. aneurysmal SAH, cerebral venous thrombosis), and infective (e.g. meningitis) causes would be in the differential.*

Figure 37.1 schematically shows the anatomical regions where an aneurysm can compress the third nerve. Meningitis and cavernous sinus thrombosis would cause multiple cranial nerve palsies rather than an isolated palsy. These facts lessen their probability but do not eliminate them just as yet.

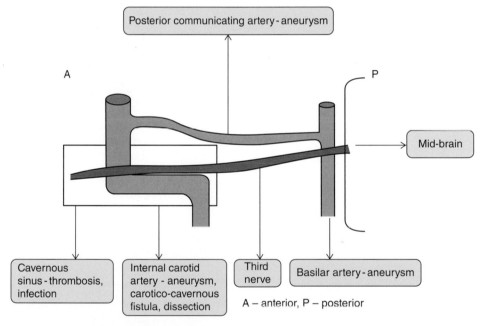

Figure 37.1 Potential sites of aneurysms along third cranial nerve pathway

An urgent MRA did not show any evidence of intracranial aneurysm or mass lesions. An LP was normal and the diplopia resolved in four days.

Activity 37.1

(Allow few seconds!)

Would you have done an LP?

P: *Since the symptoms are resolving, aneurysmal SAH is unlikely. Moreover, LP loses its
     sensitivity to detect SAH two weeks post ictus. The normal MRA is reassuring in excluding
     an aneurysm. I wouldn't do an LP but refer him to the neurosurgeons for further
     evaluation.*

He was discharged from the hospital with a diagnosis of ischemic third nerve palsy.
He re-presented in three weeks with similar symptoms. An urgent Computed
tomography angiogram showed a SAH from a right posterior communicating artery
aneurysm which was coiled. He was discharged to a care home.

There are several issues at hand here.

Causal reasoning: This example beautifully illustrates causal reasoning utilising basic
sciences to arrive at a differential. This is a good strategy especially in neurology where
precise localization is very important to request the right imaging study.

Variability in disease presentation: Pain is not a useful discriminator between the
causes of a third nerve palsy. Ischemic third nerve palsy can be just as painful as an
aneurysmal SAH. Likewise, resolution of symptoms does not reduce the likelihood
of aneurysmal SAH (Foroozan et al. 2002). A normal imaging study should always
be followed by an LP which can be done up to four weeks although with reduced
sensitivity. Moreover, the LP is useful in ruling out other conditions like meningitis
and inflammatory disorders.

Recognising the limitations of the tests we use especially with delayed clinical presentations.
A conscious evaluation of the sensitivity/specificity of the test at hand helps in its judicious
application.

How far would you investigate the first presentation? This can only be answered once a
holistic assessment of the patient has been undertaken. This includes their functional status
(frailty), co-morbidities, and their informed choices. Counselling the patient regarding the
risks of further tests (digital subtraction angiography) vs expectant management (with the
risk of rupture of an unidentified aneurysm) and its accompanying mortality/morbidity
would be the way forward. The final decision will have to rhyme with their philosophy
of life.

Example 37.2

A 65 year old lady presented with a three day history of worsening diplopia. PMH:
HT, type 1 DM, pernicious anaemia. Medications: bisoprolol, aspirin, gliclazide,
insulin, monthly vitamin B12 injections.

J: *SQs – middle aged woman + acute diplopia + vascular risk factors + pernicious anaemia.
     Provisional diagnoses – acute diplopia + vascular risk factors imply vascular aetiology but
     the differential remains wide.*

She reported previous self-resolving episodes of intermittent blurred vision. She
denied any headache or other neurological symptoms including red flag symptoms.

O/E: Pulse 84 bpm, BP 140/86, temperature 37.3 °C, RR 12 per minute, BMs
12 mmol l⁻¹, saturations 95% on air. She had right sided ptosis with binocular
diplopia in the quadrants shown in Figure 37.2a. The eye that failed to move into
that quadrant is marked with an X. The pupil was normal and reactive and fundoscopy was normal. The rest of the systemic and neurological examination was normal.
CXR and bloods: normal.

(a)

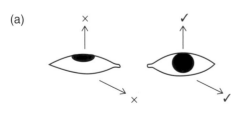

(b)

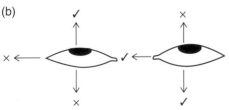

Figure 37.2 Eye examination findings

How would you interpret these findings?

Activity 37.2

(Allow three minutes)

....
....
....
....
....

J: *Severity of illness – ill. Ptosis points to right sided third nerve palsy or Horner's but I can't seem to interpret the diplopia.*

An urgent CT scan of the head performed to exclude aneurysmal SAH or SOL was normal. LP: CSF protein $0.4\,g\,l^{-1}$, CSF serum glucose ratio 0.7, no oligoclonal bands, WCC<5 and red cells<5 and xanthochromia was negative.

J: *Compressive third nerve palsy seems unlikely. It could be ischemic, given the vascular risk factors.*

On day 3 of admission, she reported difficulty in washing her face. The house officer noted bilateral ptosis with persistent diplopia in the quadrants shown in Figure 37.2b.

			Upper limbs			Lower limbs	
			Right	Left		Right	Left
Tone			Normal	Normal		Normal	Normal
Power	Shoulder	F	3/5	4/5	Hip	5/5	5/5
		E	3/5	4/5			
	Elbow	F	4+/5	4+/5	Knee	5/5	5/5
		E	4+/5	4+/5			
	Wrist	F	5/5	5/5	Ankle	5/5	5/5
		E	5/5	5/5			
Reflexes	Biceps		+	+	Knee	+	+
	Triceps		+	+	Ankle	+	+
	Supinator		+	+	Plantar	↓	↓
Sensation			Normal in all four limbs				

No cerebellar signs/signs of meningeal irritation.
F – flexion, E – extension, DF – dorsi-flexion, PF – plantar flexion.

J: *I'm confused!*

Let's look at the pattern. There are eye signs with predominantly proximal myopathy (preserved reflexes). Think of all the diseases that can present with this pattern – generalised muscle/NMJ problems are the prime suspects e.g. myasthenia gravis, botulism (starts with face → descending paralysis from arms to legs), mitochondrial cytopathies like Kearns-Sayre syndrome (chronic presentation), Miller Fisher variant of Guillain-Barre syndrome (GBS) (ascending paralysis from legs to arms).

The initial eye examination represented 'complex ophthalmoplegia' wherein the ophthalmoplegia does not correspond to a particular cranial nerve problem. The normal sized pupil in the ptotic eye was another clue that this was a neuromuscular problem. Ptosis is best approached in three steps:

1. Is the ptotic eye normal or abnormal? Normally the upper eyelid covers 1 mm of the superior aspect of cornea. Ensure that there is no lid retraction or proptosis of the opposite eye. Once this is excluded, the ptotic eye is the abnormal eye.

Complex ophthalmoplegia

Thyroid eye disease
Myasthenia gravis
Mitochondrial cytopathies
Oculopharyngeal dystrophy

2. Look at the pupil – miosis implies Horner's and mydriasis implies third nerve palsy. Normal pupil could mean this is the normal eye, incomplete third nerve palsy or a muscular problem causing the ptosis.
3. The muscular problem can then be localised to the NMJ or the muscle itself (myopathy or muscle restriction e.g. thyroid eye disease).

Fatiguability and curtaining can be used to look for NMJ disorders whilst painful eye movements imply myopathy (Averbuch-Heller et al. 1995). It is likely that she initially had asymmetric ptosis which could have been unravelled with these tests. Hence it is useful to incorporate these tests into routine eye examination.

> An edrophonium test was positive and she was started on low dose prednisolone (as high dose steroids can worsen myasthenia) + pyridostigmine. Stool and serum botulinum toxin was negative and an electromyography (EMG) confirmed the diagnosis of myasthenia gravis.

Pattern recognition is a useful technique in neurology for novices. Breaking down the findings to nerve problem (sensory/motor/mixed neuropathy – reflexes absent), NMJ or muscle problem (myopathy – preserved reflexes), proximal or distal findings, symmetric or asymmetric involvement, associated cortical/subcortical/autonomic/cerebellar findings, and summarising them together on paper will help one to see the patterns emerge. Differential diagnoses that fit the pattern can be tested with clinical findings and/or investigations.

In our patient the variability in the pattern of ophthalmoplegia pointed to myasthenia gravis which declared itself with proximal myopathy of the arms. Misinterpretation of clinical findings invoked the wrong context (SAH/SOL) resulting in a delayed diagnosis.

Hypothesis generation is a fluid state of affairs where the importance of follow-up examination cannot be overemphasised (Schiff 2008). Re-stating the SQs with new data generates new hypotheses especially since some conditions may evolve in the fullness of time and declare themselves.

▼
Pain and resolution of symptoms do not discriminate aneurysmal from ischaemic third nerve palsy.

Pattern recognition is a useful technique in Neurology.
▲

References

Averbuch-Heller, L., Poonyathalang, A., von Maydell, R.D., and Remler, B.F. (1995). Hering's law for eyelids: still valid. *Neurology* 45 (9): 1781–1783.

Foroozan, R., Slamovits, T.L., Ksiazek, S.M., and Zak, R. (2002). Spontaneous resolution of aneurysmal third nerve palsy. *Journal of Neuro-Ophthalmology: The Official Journal of the North American Neuro-Ophthalmology Society* 22 (3): 211–214.

Schiff, G.D. (2008). Minimizing diagnostic error: the importance of follow-up and feedback. *The American Journal of Medicine* 121 (5 Suppl): S38–S42.

▼

This chapter tells you how to approach leg weakness from a neurological perspective

▲

Example 38.1

A 46 year old woman presented with a three day history of worsening breathlessness and productive cough. She had been treated for recurrent chest infections with three courses of antibiotics over the last month. PMH: HT, DM, IHD, asthma, current smoker 35 py, and occasional alcohol. Medications: aspirin, atenolol, ramipril, simvastatin, isosorbide mononitrate, symbicort and ventolin inhalers, metformin, and lantus insulin.

P: *SQs – middle aged lady + acute SOB and cough + recurrent chest infections + asthma + vascular risk factors. Provisional diagnoses – all causes of non-resolving pneumonia.*

There were no red flag symptoms other than reduced appetite and a five pound weight loss over the last week.

O/E: Temperature 38 °C, pulse 90 bpm, BP 110/70, saturations 91% on air, BMs 12 mmol l^{-1}, RR 22 per minute. RS: Reduced breath sounds on the right with increased vocal resonance and dull percussion note. Rest of the systemic examination: normal. CNS: grossly intact, not formally examined.

P: *Severity of illness – ill. Working diagnosis – CAP perhaps atypical. DD: malignancy (smoker).*

Bloods: Hb 100 g l^{-1}, WCC 15 × 10^9 l^{-1}, platelets 400 × 10^9 l^{-1}, MCV 90 fl, CRP 120 mg l^{-1}; U&Es and LFTs: normal, except albumin 29 g l^{-1}. CXR: right upper lobe extensive consolidation. Following blood cultures, she was started on levofloxacin and IV fluids as per local guidelines. The nurses reported to the admitting doctor that she was unable to mobilise to the commode. It came to light that she hadn't been able to get out of bed for the last two days with right leg weakness. The patient was handed over to the night team for review as the junior doctor was finishing his shift.

P: *I'm thinking of cord compression given the suspicion of malignancy.*

The registrar prioritised her review owing to suspected cord compression. There were no bowel/bladder disturbances, back pain, or other focal neurological symptoms. Per-rectal (PR) examination: normal anal tone with no saddle anaesthesia.

The Hands-on Guide to Clinical Reasoning in Medicine, First Edition. Mujammil Irfan.
© 2019 John Wiley & Sons Ltd. Published 2019 by John Wiley & Sons Ltd.
Companion website: www.wiley.com/go/irfan/clinicalreasoning

CNS – cranial nerves normal, no cerebellar, or meningeal signs.

			Upper limbs				Lower limbs	
			Right	Left			Right	Left
Tone			Normal	Normal			Normal	Normal
Power	Shoulder	F	5/5	5/5	Hip	F	5/5	5/5
		E	5/5	5/5		E	5/5	5/5
	Elbow	F	5/5	5/5	Knee	F	5/5	5/5
		E	5/5	5/5		E	5/5	5/5
	Wrist	F	5/5	5/5	Ankle	DF	1/5	5/5
		E	5/5	5/5		PF	4+/5	5/5
Reflexes	Biceps		+	+	Knee		+	+
	Triceps		+	+	Ankle		−	−
	Supinator		+	+	Plantar		↓	↓
Sensation			Normal in all four limbs except dermatomal loss in L5, decreased vibration sense up to the ankles bilaterally					

F – flexion, E – extension, DF – dorsi-flexion, PF – plantar flexion.

P: *There is clearly a sensory level so cord compression is very likely.*

I don't think this is a sensory level since sensation below L5 is normal. It is dermatomal loss with weakness of ankle dorsiflexion. Absent ankle jerks and vibration may be secondary to diabetes, but we can't be sure.

What other signs go against cord compression?

Activity 38.1

(Allow three minutes)

....

....

....

....

....

The neurology was discussed with the consultant who felt that there was a low probability of cord compression. He suggested dexamethasone and a spinal MRI in the morning which was normal. Dexamethasone was stopped. CT of the thorax, abdomen, and pelvis revealed extensive consolidation in the right upper lobe but no masses or metastases.

A bronchoscopy did not show any luminal tumour but washings from the right upper lobe were sent for cytology and microbiology. Meanwhile her temperature and inflammatory markers remained high. An atypical pneumonia screen (mycoplasma) and lyme serology was requested (which can cause meningo-radiculitis). On day 6 of her admission she developed a left sided wrist drop secondary to radial nerve palsy.

P: *I don't know what this could be.*

A neurologist's opinion was sought who diagnosed mononeuritis multiplex. Peripheral eosinophilia ($3 \times 10^9 \, l^{-1}$), positive anti-myeloperoxidase and positive nerve biopsy confirmed a diagnosis of Churg-Strauss syndrome. Microbiology and cytology (bronchial washings) were negative. She was treated with immunosuppressants with a good response.

Misinterpretation of clinical signs: Involvement of multiple peripheral nerves is called mononeuritis multiplex. Vasculitic neuropathy affects the longest nerves first thereby commonly presenting as foot drop. The initial examination findings were in keeping with right common peroneal nerve palsy. Eliciting preserved foot inversion would have confirmed this as opposed to L5, S1 radiculopathy. In hindsight it is clear that the normal tone, downgoing plantars, no sensory level, and normal PR all argued against cord compression. *Anchoring* is evidently seen in this example where the registrar is wedded to the idea that his initial suspicion (cord compression) is right. Again, the team seem to take on this diagnosis without question and a cascade of investigations are initiated, although one could argue that a bronchoscopy would still have been necessary to exclude infection prior to initiating immunosuppressants.

System failures are also seen in action where time pressures (shift pattern of work) and lack of continuity of care contributes to a 'new' patient assessment. Although this could be considered a 'second opinion' which is often beneficial, one does wonder if the diagnosis of asthma had been interrogated further, Churg Strauss might have come to light earlier. However, this is a point of conjecture.

Three main strategies are suggested to address system failures: prevention, making error visible, and mitigating the effects of error (Nolan 2000). From a clinical reasoning perspective, most of what we are doing in this book (drawing attention to cognitive errors and suggesting solutions) fits with the first strategy. Consulting with a specialist or having a consultant-led post-take ward round helps correct misdiagnosis by making the error visible. Planned follow-up and feedback with cognitive information (e.g. why an alternative diagnosis is correct) is another way of doing this although it relies on being aware of one's own limitations (Berner et al. 2008). Autopsies, the gold-standard of diagnosis have shown that doctors often lack insight into their performance, leading to overconfidence, and errors in clinical judgement (Podbregar et al. 2001). This knowledge should give us the humility to understand that we are not infallible and thus practice the rigours of planned follow-up and feedback to calibrate our future practice. Indeed, planned follow-up if done on time can even mitigate the effects of the error by changing the management plan before further harm occurs.

Example 38.2

A 28 year old woman was admitted with a 10 day history of worsening leg weakness. PMH: nil. Medications: OCP.

J: SQs – *young woman + acute leg weakness. Provisional diagnoses – vascular or inflammatory aetiology.*

She could feel the toilet paper on her bottom when she had been to the toilet. She denied any bowel/bladder symptoms. There was no history of recent diarrhoea or viral illnesses. Occupation: book shop assistant. Never smoked and denied recreational drug abuse.

J: *There are no features to suggest cord compression.*

O/E: Pulse 82 bpm, BP 110/70, RR 14 per minute, Temperature 37.3 °C, BMs 9, Saturations 97% on air. Systemic examination: normal. PR: normal anal tone and perianal sensation.

CNS – cranial nerves normal, no cerebellar, or meningeal signs.

			Upper limbs				Lower limbs	
			Right	Left			Right	Left
Tone			Normal	Normal			Normal	Normal
Power	Shoulder	F	5/5	5/5	Hip	F	5/5	5/5
		E	5/5	5/5		E	5/5	5/5
	Elbow	F	5/5	5/5	Knee	F	5/5	5/5
		E	5/5	5/5		E	5/5	5/5
	Wrist	F	5/5	5/5	Ankle	DF	1/5	1/5
		E	5/5	5/5		PF	3/5	3/5
Reflexes	Biceps		++	++	Knee		+	+
	Triceps		++	++	Ankle		–	–
	Supinator		++	++	Plantar		↓	↓
Sensation			Normal in all four limbs					

F – flexion, E – extension, DF – dorsi-flexion, PF – plantar flexion.

What is the pattern that you see?

Activity 38.2

(Allow three minutes)

....

....

....

....

....

....

J: *Bilaterally symmetrical distal muscle weakness.*

       I would qualify that further as predominantly motor polyneuropathy (no sensory abnormalities) + areflexia in the affected limbs.

J: *Provisional diagnoses – diabetic neuropathy, GBS, cord compression.*

       The lack of a sensory level makes cord compression less likely.

The admitting doctor diagnosed GBS and admitted the patient for observation/neurology opinion. The neurologist was more circumspect and ordered a series of investigations including an LP, nerve conduction studies (NCS) and an autoimmune screen. The patient was worried that she might be paralysed for life and wanted to be started on treatment immediately.

How would you respond to her concerns?

Activity 38.3

Activity 38.3

(Allow few seconds!)

Medical Uncertainty, an all pervasive phenomenon in clinical practice can generate tremendous anxiety in patients leading to seemingly unreasonable patient expectations. From a physician's perspective there are three types of uncertainty, the first stems from a personal lack of knowledge (no one can know everything), the second from limitations in current level of understanding of a disease process and third from a personal inability to discriminate between the two aforementioned (Fox 1980).

Understanding the patient's perspective (a valid concern of disability) is the first step in addressing their concerns. A personal lack of knowledge would hinder effective communication with the patient. This is not confined to medical students alone but seasoned clinicians too. Acknowledging personal knowledge gaps to patients does not automatically tarnish one's image but this should be followed by volunteering to find an answer or consult relevant specialists. Indeed, unexpectedly, patient satisfaction is higher with physicians who acknowledge uncertainty, which is often supplemented with more information given to patients (Gordon et al. 2000). On the other hand, physicians who are intolerant of uncertainty are more likely to order extra tests (Zaat and van Eijk 1992).

Often there may be a true lack of available evidence or a period of observation would help the disease evolve into something more recognisable. This should be communicated to the patient by starting with an explanation of the likely differentials, the tests needed to exclude the more worrisome diagnoses and emphasising the significant role of the patient in co-creating a management plan. A reasonable follow up should be scheduled to reassess the clinical picture with a fall back mechanism to address any unexpected clinical development (Hewson et al. 1996).

The neurologist posited the likely differentials to the patient with GBS being most likely. The LP, autoimmune screens were being ordered to confirm this but he also explained the need to exclude other polyneuropathies with NCS. He emphasised that the treatment for each of these diagnoses was different and given the stability of the patient's clinical condition it was crucial to get the diagnosis right, before initiating therapy.

LP: Serum: CSF glucose ratio 0.7, protein $1.5\,g\,l^{-1}$, WCC $5 \times 10^9\,l^{-1}$, red cell count $10 \times 10^{12}\,l^{-1}$, no oligoclonal bands. NCS showed features suggesting demyelinating polyneuropathy. Despite treatment with IV immunoglobulins she had a fluctuating clinical course. A spinal MRI was normal. She was eventually diagnosed with CIDP owing to disease progression two months later.

Clearly, explicating an open mind to the diagnostic possibilities right from the start, made it easy for the neurologist to change the diagnosis in keeping with disease evolution.

▼

Pattern recognition is a useful technique in neurology but misinterpretation of signs should be avoided.

Medical uncertainty should be embraced with all fervour and shared with the patient whilst giving adequate information at the same time.

Planned follow-up and feedback are useful to counter system failures.

▲

References

Berner, E.S. and Rraber, M.L. (2008). Overconfidence as a cause of diagnostic error in medicine. *The American Journal of Medicine* 121 (5): S2–S23.

Fox, R.C. (1980). The evolution of medical uncertainty. *The Milbank Memorial Fund Quarterly. Health and Society* 58 (1): 1–49.

Gordon, G.H., Joos, S.K., and Byrne, J. (2000). Physician expressions of uncertainty during patient encounters. *Patient Education and Counseling* 40 (1): 59–65.

Hewson, M.G., Kindy, P.J., Van Kirk, J. et al. (1996). Strategies for managing uncertainty and complexity. *Journal of General Internal Medicine* 11 (8): 481–485.

Nolan, T.W. (2000). System changes to improve patient safety. *British Medical Journal (Clinical research ed.)* 320 (7237): 771–773.

Podbregar, M., Voga, G., Krivec, B. et al. (2001). Should we confirm our clinical diagnostic certainty by autopsics? *Intensive Care Medicine* 27 (11): 1750–1755.

Zaat, J.O. and van Eijk, J.T. (1992). General practitioners' uncertainty, risk preference, and use of laboratory tests. *Medical Care* 30 (9): 846–854.

39 Unilateral Weakness

This chapter tells you how to approach unilateral weakness from a neurological perspective

Example 39.1

A 62 year old man presented with sudden onset right-sided weakness that started at 9 a.m. As the paramedics were assessing him he had generalised tonic-clonic seizures (GTCSs) which resolved with PR diazepam. PMH: HT, DM, IHD with a stent, CKD. Medications: aspirin, clopidogrel, atorvastatin, bisoprolol, losartan, vidagliptin, lantus insulin, co-codamol.

J: *SQs – middle aged man + acute right sided weakness and seizures + vascular risk factors. Provisional diagnoses – stroke, TIA, hypoglycemia, post epileptic Todd's palsy.*

Current smoker 40 py, alcohol 6 pints of lager/week. Baseline ET 300 yards. O/E: RR 16 per minute, Temperature 37.7 °C, HR 100 bpm, BP 180/90, Saturations 95% on air, BMs 12 mmol l⁻¹. CVS: No carotid bruits, irregular rhythm, RS, and PA: normal. CNS: Right handed. Cranial nerves: right UMN facial nerve palsy. Speech: expressive dysphasia. The National Institutes of Health Stroke Scale (NIHSS) score was 15 with right sided visual and sensory inattention, partial right hemianopia, no effort against gravity in the right arm and leg, and no sensory loss on the right. Plantars: up-going on the right with increased tone and hyper-reflexia.

J: *The examination confirms right sided hemiparesis – stroke. I take it that seizures can occur with stroke.*

Yes, of course but stroke is a very basic inference. How would you qualify this further?

Activity 39.1

(Allow three minutes)

Assuming the clinical picture represents a stroke (sudden onset with vascular risk factors), the following steps should be thought through:

• *Is this a cortical or subcortical (lacunar) stroke?* Using the associated signs, identify whether they subserve cortical function i.e. speech, visual field defects, inattention, or cortical sensory signs as discussed in Chapter 34. Here we have, expressive dysphasia,

The Hands-on Guide to Clinical Reasoning in Medicine, First Edition. Mujammil Irfan.
© 2019 John Wiley & Sons Ltd. Published 2019 by John Wiley & Sons Ltd.
Companion website: www.wiley.com/go/irfan/clinicalreasoning

visual and sensory inattention, and partial hemianopia, all representing cortical signs, in fact the dominant hemisphere (speech). The right UMN facial nerve palsy confirms our suspicions. This implies a large vessel occlusion/bleed.

- *Is this involving the anterior circulation (internal carotid artery territory) or posterior circulation (vertebro-basilar artery territory)?* Here, the signs seem to implicate parietal/temporal lobe involvement i.e. anterior circulation.
- *What is the pathological mechanism?* Occlusions can be intrinsic atherosclerosis and in situ thrombosis or from cardiac/carotid embolism. Haemorrhage is often secondary to hypertension, amyloid angiopathy, or rarely aneurysmal. In this case, AF suggests a cardio-embolic mechanism of stroke.

In summary we have, a left anterior circulation large vessel (MCA) cortical infarct or haemorrhage likely secondary to AF. Note that haemorrhage cannot be ruled out on clinical findings alone. Indeed, haemorrhagic conversion of an infarct is also known to occur.

> An urgent CT scan showed no evidence of haemorrhage or SOL.

> J: *So he does not have a stroke?*

How would you answer this question?

Activity 39.2

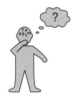

(Allow few seconds!)

Stroke is classically defined as a clinical diagnosis and indeed early thrombolysis may not show evidence of infarct on imaging. However, a higher index of suspicion (prior probability of disease) with a negative test (discrepant test – possible false negative) needs further investigations preferably with higher sensitivity. Sometimes treatment decisions may still have to be made in the absence of supportive evidence and stroke is a good example since this decision has a narrow therapeutic window for thrombolysis (4.5 hours to be precise). Obviously these decisions will have to be taken in concurrence with patients and/or their advocates.

There are several caveats for a CT scan in the context of stroke. A CT does not always show acute infarcts although there can be subtle features to suggest an infarct (Chalela et al. 2007). Posterior fossa lesions are better visualised on MRI than a CT making it the preferred investigation for posterior circulation strokes. Hence CT is more useful to rule out haemorrhage than confirm an infarct. The down-side of this approach is that stroke can be mimicked by other pathologies that are also inevitably thrombolysed. Fortunately life-threatening intracranial haemorrhages in stroke mimics are not common and are indeed three times less common than true strokes that have been thrombolysed (Zinkstok et al. 2013). However, this still exposes the patients to drugs with significant side-effects not to mention the costs, label of stroke, and the ethical aspects of it all. Hence the onus still lies with the clinician to ensure that the right pathology is thrombolysed.

> Following informed consent, he was thrombolysed and started on anticoagulation for AF two weeks later. He made good recovery and was discharged with short term carer support which was eventually terminated when he was self-caring.

Example 39.2

A 32 year old woman presents with a sudden onset left-sided weakness. PMH: Migraine, bipolar disorder. Medications: Ibuprofen, valproate, citalopram.

P: *SQs – Young woman + acute neurological deficit + history of migraines and depression + no vascular risk factors. Provisional diagnoses –* **hemiplegic migraine***, stroke,* **recreational drugs, cerebral venous thrombosis***, IIH, aneurysm, SAH.*

The term used in this context is 'young stroke.' Differentials include the ones that **are in bold** above and conditions such as vasculopathies (e.g. arterial dissections, vasculitis), haematologic disorders (e.g. essential thrombocythemia), and cardiac defects causing paradoxical embolism. IIH and SAH often do not present with focal neurology other than diplopia. Unruptured aneurysms and rarely mycotic aneurysms (e.g. causing intracerebral haemorrhage) can cause lateralising signs.
The weakness started two hours ago and was associated with a gradual onset headache.

This episode was dissimilar to her usual migraines. She had a recent flu-like illness. She denied recreational drugs or contraceptive pills. Current smoker of 20 py, alcohol 10 units/week.

O/E: Temperature 36.6 °C, Saturations 99% on air, RR 12 per minute, HR 92 bpm, BP 140/80, BMs 8 mmol l⁻¹. NIHSS = 8 with a partial hemianopia, some effort against gravity in affected left-sided limbs, mild-moderate sensory loss and sensory inattention, up-going plantar on left. Rest of the systemic and neural examination: normal. CT head: normal. Bloods: normal, except CRP 30 mg l⁻¹.

Would you thrombolyse this patient?

Activity 39.3

(Allow few seconds!)

P: *I would discuss with the stroke physician.*

You are absolutely right! Recognising one's limitations is an important attribute. However, it would be wise to look at the clinical reasoning processes behind this decision.

Is this a true stroke (vascular pathology)? An acute neurological deficit with few vascular risk factors (smoking) in a young patient makes it less likely that this is a true stroke (Saver and Barsan 2010). On the other hand, lateralising signs with an exact time of onset and history of migraines (associated with intracranial dissections) suggests a true stroke (Hand et al. 2006; Chaves et al. 2002). Of note, the clinical picture points to a right MCA territory infarct (inattention) which conforms to a vascular territory.

Assuming that this is a stroke mimic, the likely aetiology could be hemiplegic migraine or conversion disorder (factitious neurology) both of which are diagnoses of exclusion. We have also seen that the risk-benefit calculation of thrombolysis in stroke mimics favours thrombolysis although the potential risks remain (see Example 39.1). Counter-intuitively thrombolysis of cervical artery dissections does not worsen the clinical picture and thrombolysis has been attempted in patients who do not respond to anticoagulation in cerebral venous thrombosis (Zinkstok et al. 2011; Viegas et al. 2014).

One could argue that on balance, thrombolysis would be the preferred option however, this would have to be discussed with the patient to ascertain her views.

> She was thrombolysed and transferred to a stroke unit for observation. A CT angiogram performed the next day showed evidence of a right intracranial carotid artery dissection. She was managed with antithrombotic therapy in the long-term with good resolution of deficits.

This example illustrates 'discrimination between hypotheses' using clinical signs and symptoms in the backdrop of medical co-morbidities. Evidence based discussions on what the diagnosis is, could be construed as academic but the decision for thrombolysis is a real decision with real risks. Given the time-bound nature of thrombolysis it is imperative that we strive for a greater degree of confidence (if not absolute) in our diagnosis before embarking on treatment. This principle can be extended to other areas of medicine where the risk of short-term mortality/morbidity will have to be balanced against long-term mortality/morbidity.

▼

The pre-test probability of a diagnosis affects interpretation of test results.

Clinical signs and symptoms in the backdrop of medical co-morbidities help in discriminating between hypotheses.

▲

References

Chalela, J.A., Kidwell, C.S., Nentwich, L.M. et al. (2007). Magnetic resonance imaging and computed tomography in emergency assessment of patients with suspected acute stroke: a prospective comparison. *Lancet (London, England)* 369 (9558): 293–298.

Chaves, C., Estol, C., Esnaola, M.M. et al. (2002). Spontaneous intracranial internal carotid artery dissection: report of 10 patients. *Archives of Neurology* 59 (6): 977–981.

Hand, P.J., Kwan, J., Lindley, R.I. et al. (2006). Distinguishing between stroke and mimic at the bedside: the brain attack study. *Stroke* 37 (3): 769–775.

Saver, J.L. and Barsan, W.G. (2010). Swift or sure?: the acceptable rate of neurovascular mimics among IV tPA-treated patients. *Neurology* 74 (17): 1336–1337.

Viegas, L.D., Stolz, E., Canhão, P., and Ferro, J.M. (2014). 'Systemic thrombolysis for cerebral venous and dural sinus thrombosis: a systematic review. *Cerebrovascular Diseases* 37 (1): 43–50.

Zinkstok, S.M., Vergouwen, M.D., Engelter, S.T. et al. (2011). Safety and functional outcome of thrombolysis in dissection-related ischemic stroke: a meta-analysis of individual patient data. *Stroke* 42 (9): 2515–2520.

Zinkstok, S.M., Engelter, S.T., Gensicke, H. et al. (2013). Safety of thrombolysis in stroke mimics: results from a multicenter cohort study. *Stroke* 44 (4): 1080–1084.

PART VI
Geriatric Medicine

▼

This chapter tells you how to take a history from the perspective of Geriatric medicine

▲

F – Fatigue (Do you feel fatigued?)
R – Resistance (Can you climb one flight of stairs?)
A – Ambulation (can you walk one block?)
I – Illnesses > 5
L – Loss of weight > 5%

Geriatric medicine is unique in that, clinical presentation in the elderly transcends the boundaries of disease pertaining to a single organ system. The approach will thus have to be equally holistic in identifying and solving these problems. Additionally, collateral history will often be needed to ensure that the diagnosis is not missed.

In order to understand the principles of history taking in Geriatric medicine we would first have to get to grips with a few concepts. Ageing is a natural process that starts the moment we are born. With increasing age our physiological systems gradually decline from a functional stance. However, as clinical experience tells us, physiological age does not always correlate with chronological age. There are certain factors which interact with each other synergistically bringing about an accelerated decline leading to disability and death. Figure 40.1 illustrates these concepts and their interrelationships.

Intrinsic disease burden signifies the accumulated co-morbidities which commonly include IHD, DM, HT, etc.

Frailty is a state where an individual is burning maximal physiologic reserves *just* to maintain homeostasis. This accelerated decline in physiological reserve in combination with poor nutrition and functional disability increases their vulnerability to minor challenges; a state called 'frailty' (Clegg et al. 2013). Frailty ≠ age e.g. the prevalence of frailty in >85 year olds was estimated to be only 25% (Song et al. 2010). Screening tools such as Fatigue, Resistance, Ambulation, Illnesses, Loss of Weight 'FRAIL' where a score of ≥3 = frailty and 1–2 = pre-frailty, can be used to identify frail patients for formal assessment and intervention (Morley et al. 2012).

Disability is defined as the presence of restriction of at least one activity of daily living e.g. washing, dressing, having a meal, etc. (Fried et al. 2001).

These factors interact with each other in such a way that a minor precipitating event e.g. a UTI +/− an extrinsic factor (e.g. recently started on an ACEi) can result in a disproportionate response leading to any of the geriatric syndromes (e.g. delirium and falls), significant morbidity and even death. In other words, the geriatric giants represent the physical manifestation of all the events leading up to that point. Furthermore, these then interact with their precursors to bring about a vicious cycle.

The cumulative deficits model of frailty at the top of Figure 40.1 visually represents a gradation of cumulative deficits (signs, symptoms, laboratory values, and disease states) resulting in mild to severe frailty (Rockwood and Mitnitski 2007). It follows that intervention should be goal directed as illustrated. However, there is a threshold beyond which intervention is less likely to produce any benefits and palliation should be considered. Indeed, the frailty index predicts poor outcomes, dependency, and mortality. This is important since the recognition of frail patients would help clinicians in weighing up the risks and benefits or futility of invasive procedures or treatments, thereby enabling patients to make informed choices.

The Hands-on Guide to Clinical Reasoning in Medicine, First Edition. Mujammil Irfan.
© 2019 John Wiley & Sons Ltd. Published 2019 by John Wiley & Sons Ltd.
Companion website: www.wiley.com/go/irfan/clinicalreasoning

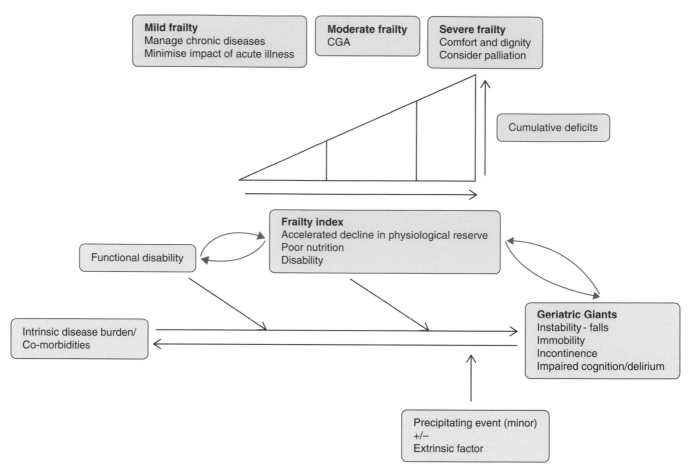

Figure 40.1 Schema showing intricate interactions between frailty and intrinsic disease burden precipitating 'geriatric giant' presentations

More often than not, intervention is directed at the extreme right of the equation neglecting the preceding ingredients that finally precipitated the presentation. This leaves patients vulnerable to recurrent hospital admissions, worsening morbidity, dependence, and death.

Comprehensive geriatric assessment (CGA) is the most evidence based intervention but is labour and resource intensive. It is a multi-disciplinary assessment and intervention that involves assessing the medical (including cognitive status and drug review), psychosocial, and functional limitations of frail older adults. The crux of CGA is that goal-directed holistic care that transcends organ systems can be negotiated with patients and their carers with a view to maintaining functional independence and minimising poor outcomes.

Falls – Risk factors:
1. Any condition or illness in medicine is more likely to happen again if it has happened before. Similarly, a history of falls increases the risk of falls.
2. Adverse drug reactions are a common cause of hospitalisation and this is true of falls too. In fact, polypharmacy is an independent risk factor for hip fractures and this is significant since it is easily modifiable (Lai et al. 2010).

The primary mechanism of falls is loss of postural control, an important cause of which is transient loss of consciousness (TLOC). Although I do not like referring you to pictures in other parts of the book, in the interests of avoiding repetition I shall have to refer you to Table 10.1 and Figure 10.1. If TLOC is elicited, questions should be asked in the order: pre-, during and post-episode characterising the TLOC. Importantly, cardiac syncope should not be missed in an emergency presentation since it carries a high mortality but is often easily treatable.

Assessment of falls should be undertaken in the backdrop of Figure 40.1. The injuries sustained should be dealt with and intervention directed to the entire equation. Use your imagination to fill in the ingredients of a fall by giving examples for each of the components starting with, the intrinsic disease burden. Figure 40.2 shows some examples superimposed on figure 40.1 and figure 40.3 shows the interventions in italics. Remember any similar combination can cause falls but this has to be elicited from the history.

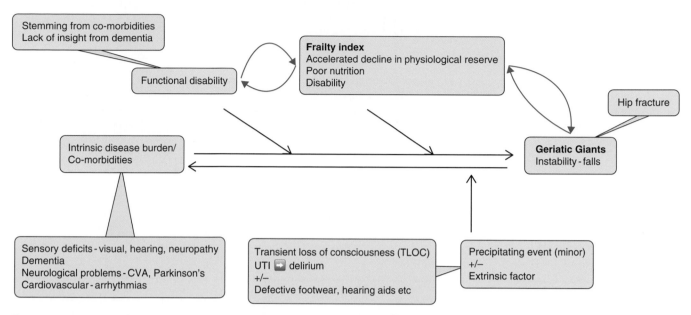

Figure 40.2 Assessment of geriatric presentations superimposed on the schema shown in figure 40.1

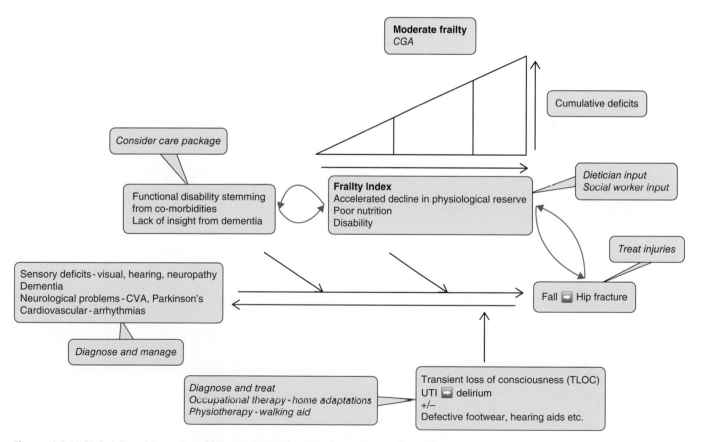

Figure 40.3 Multi-disciplinary intervention of falls superimposed on the schema shown in figure 40.1

40.1 INCONTINENCE

Urinary incontinence carries significant morbidity, impacts quality of life, and is associated with dependency. In older people, it is often the extraneous factors which follow Figure 40.1 that affect continence and their identification is essential before formally evaluating incontinence (Figure 40.4). The next step is to identify red flags indicating specialist referral e.g. associated pelvic pain, weight loss, PV discharge, haematuria (signalling malignancy), and most importantly acute incontinence signalling cord compression/neurological deficits. The last step is to classify the type of incontinence using history since treatment depends on the cause (Figure 40.5).

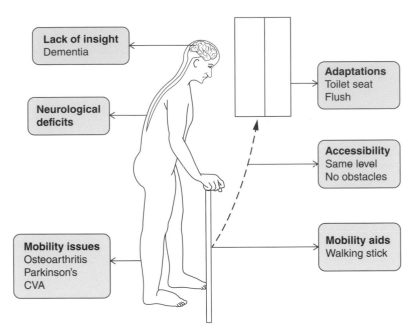

Figure 40.4 External factors causing incontinence

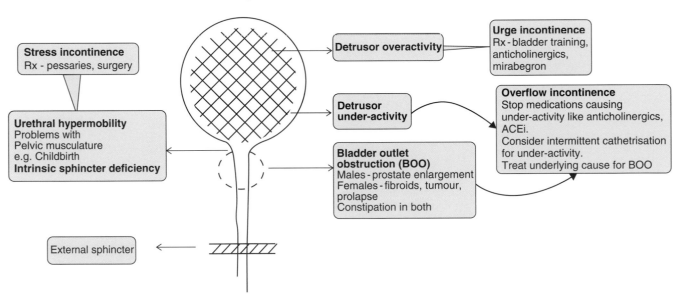

Figure 40.5 Aetiology of urinary incontinence

40.2 COGNITIVE IMPAIRMENT/DELIRIUM

30% of hospitalisations related to the elderly are complicated by delirium (Marcantonio 2017). It is under-diagnosed, difficult to tease out from other medical conditions and is often mistaken for dementia. Hence a collateral history is of vital importance. Figure 40.6

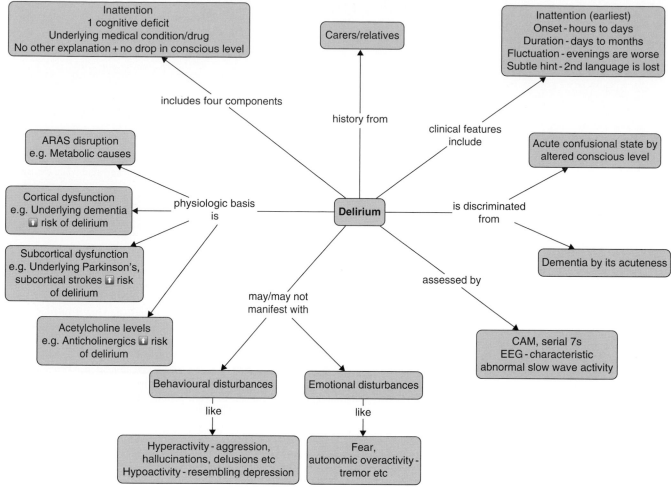

Figure 40.6 Assessment of delirium

shows a concept map for delirium where the history is interwoven into the various components. A characteristic finding in delirium is 'inattention'. Confusion assessment method (CAM) is a screening tool with the best positive likelihood ratio (LR) of 9.6. It focuses on four components, *a*cute onset and fluctuation, *i*nattention, *d*isorganised thinking and *a*ltered consciousness (AIDA) (Wong et al. 2010).

References

Clegg, A., Young, J., Iliffe, S. et al. (2013). Frailty in elderly people. *Lancet (London, England)* 381 (9868): 752–762.

Fried, L.P., Tangen, C.M., Walston, J. et al. (2001). Frailty in older adults: evidence for a phenotype. *The Journals of Gerontology. Series A, Biological Sciences and Medical Sciences* 56 (3): M146–M156.

Lai, S.-W., Liao, K.F., Liao, C.C. et al. (2010). 'Polypharmacy correlates with increased risk for hip fracture in the elderly: a population-based study. *Medicine* 89 (5): 295–299.

Marcantonio, E.R. (2017). Delirium in hospitalized older adults.' C.G. Solomon ed. *The New England Journal of Medicine* 377 (15): 1456–1466e.

Morley, J.E., Malmstrom, T.K., and Miller, D.K. (2012). A simple frailty questionnaire (FRAIL) predicts outcomes in middle aged African Americans. *The Journal of Nutrition, Health & Aging* 16 (7): 601–608.

Rockwood, K. and Mitnitski, A. (2007). Frailty in relation to the accumulation of deficits. *The Journals of Gerontology. Series A, Biological Sciences and Medical Sciences* 62 (7): 722–727.

Song, X., Mitnitski., A., and Rockwood, K. (2010). Prevalence and 10-year outcomes of frailty in older adults in relation to deficit accumulation. *Journal of the American Geriatrics Society* 58 (4): 681–687.

Wong, C.L., Holroyd-Leduc, J., Simel, D.L., and Straus, S.E. (2010). Does this patient have delirium?'. *Journal of the American Medical Association* 304 (7): 779.

41 Clinical Examination: Why Do I Keep Falling?

▼

This chapter tells you how to elicit relevant clinical signs from a Geriatric medicine perspective

▲

Clinical examination in the elderly often gets relegated to the background when clinical presentations are labelled as 'social' or UTI. As elsewhere in medicine, having preformed notions of what the diagnosis is, leads one to diagnose a 'UTI' and nothing else when the truth may be far from it.

Pitfalls of clinical examination in the elderly:

- Clinical presentations are atypical i.e. it is more likely to be a common diagnosis presenting atypically than a rare diagnosis e.g. pneumonia presenting as delirium instead of pyrexia, cough, and sputum.
- Incidental pathology is high which misleads the physician into making erroneous diagnoses. Always bear in mind the context of the inquiry and focus on the primary 'acute' problem.
- The elderly can be less mobile and slow in responding to instructions making clinical examination difficult. Enlisting the help of carers or nurses can help in appropriate positioning to enable an adequate examination. Mimicking the manoeuvre whilst standing parallel to them helps them mirror your actions. In difficult circumstances, one may have to return to complete the examination.
- Establishing the severity of illness can be tricky in atypical presentations. A sudden change from the baseline functional status should alert the clinician and a period of observation may help the signs to evolve facilitating localization of the problem. However, this must be balanced with the risk of precipitating delirium in unfamiliar hospital surroundings.
- Examination should be tailored to the context of the enquiry since problems are often multi-factorial as illustrated in the following sections.

There are a few findings which can be normal in the elderly as described below:

*Cardiovascular system (*CVS*)*: S4 is normal in people aged > 75 years since the left atrium enlarges to deliver a greater amount of blood into the stiffened LV from aortic stiffening. Difference in blood pressure (BP) between the two arms is more commonly due to ipsilateral subclavian artery atherosclerosis than aortic dissection and must be interpreted with the context.

*Respiratory system (*RS*)*: 30% of older adults have crackles in the lung bases.

Musculoskeletal: Sarcopenia is an independent risk factor for mortality. It is an age-related loss of muscle mass and strength > 2 standard deviations. Legs > arms, fast twitch fibres > slow.

Haematopoietic: D-dimer levels are raised twofold without underlying VTE and in hospitalised older patients (Isaia et al. 2011). Risk of VTE is higher in elderly.

The next section focuses on an examination strategy in common clinical presentations.

The Hands-on Guide to Clinical Reasoning in Medicine, First Edition. Mujammil Irfan.
© 2019 John Wiley & Sons Ltd. Published 2019 by John Wiley & Sons Ltd.
Companion website: www.wiley.com/go/irfan/clinicalreasoning

41.1 FALLS

With Figure 40.2 in mind, clinical examination should identify:

The *intrinsic disease burden* and how it could have impacted on the 'fall.' For example, treatment of hypertension with several anti-hypertensives can lead to a postural drop in BP. Parkinson's disease can cause decreased mobility (gait assessment) as well as orthostatic hypotension. Diabetes mellitus can cause peripheral neuropathy (glove and stocking sensory loss). All of these can precipitate a fall.

Precipitating factors such as UTI (suprapubic or renal angle tenderness) causing delirium can result in disorientation triggering a fall. Extrinsic factors such as visual or hearing impairment can contribute to the fall. Ensure that spectacles, hearing aids, and walking aids are in working condition.

Functional disability e.g. osteoarthritis where pain can be a significant factor affecting mobility leading to instability and falls. Difficulty in assessing pain in patients with dementia can be overcome by using validated scales like Pain assessment in cognitively impaired and unimpaired older adults (PAINAD) (Chibnall and Tait 2001). Patients are observed over a few minutes during activity e.g. turning in bed or transferring and scored. It is important to note that the trend is more useful than a single value.

Lack of insight secondary to dementia can result in an incorrect assessment of risk on the part of the patient thereby increasing the likelihood of falls. The Mini-Cog screening tool for dementia takes less time to administer and is unaffected by language and educational background (Borson et al. 2000). It can be used to identify at risk individuals ultimately affecting their rehabilitation potential and discharge destination.

Frailty can be assessed using simple screening tools like 'FRAIL' where ≥3 = frailty and 1–2 = pre-frailty, identifying individuals who would benefit from early intervention (Morley et al. 2012). Nutritional status can also impact muscle strength contributing to the fall e.g. signs of proximal myopathy from chronic steroid use, vitamin D deficiency.

To summarise, clinical examination should be undertaken starting with the individual patient's co-morbidities, drugs, and psychosocial circumstances in that order. Use your imagination to consciously visualise how all these factors singly and in conjunction with others precipitate a fall and look for those signs.

Mini-Cog = Clock drawing test (CDT) + uncued recall of three unrelated words.

All three words recalled – non-demented.
None recalled – demented.
one to two words recalled – intermediate.
Intermediate + abnormal CDT = demented.
Intermediate + normal CDT = Non-demented.

41.2 INCONTINENCE

Most causes of urinary incontinence in the elderly can be diagnosed by history alone. Red flag symptoms as mentioned in Chapter 40 should trigger the search for serious disorders.

New onset urinary incontinence especially urgency should raise the suspicion of cord compression. Sensory level, asymmetric UMN signs in lower limbs, loss of perianal sensation and rectal tone are in keeping with this diagnosis.

PR examination is useful in men to assess the prostate, in women to look for pelvic masses and constipation in both. A formal gynaecological examination is necessary in women with red flag symptoms.

Lastly, it cannot be emphasised enough that incontinence in the elderly is often due to extraneous factors e.g. painful osteoarthritis delaying quick access to the toilet. Managing these will treat most of the 'incontinence.'

41.3 DELIRIUM AND DEMENTIA

Prior knowledge of the types of dementia syndromes helps in directing the physical examination. Alzheimer's is the most prevalent (60–80%) followed by other syndromes such as vascular, Parkinson's, fronto-temporal, and Lewy-Body disease.

Patients with Alzheimer's do not have any focal signs; hence in the majority, physical examination will be normal. A thorough neurological examination is essential to identify other unusual forms of dementia as well as mimics such as normal pressure hydrocephalus (NPH) and structural brain lesions like SDH.

For instance, focal neurological deficits and vascular risk factors suggest vascular (multi-infarct) dementia. Similarly, variable confusion occurring with extra-pyramidal features and 'sweet' (non-threatening) hallucinations should suggest Lewy-Body disease. NPH can present with falls, urinary incontinence and/or dementia, three common geriatric giants.

Delirium can often complicate dementia in which case a collateral history of baseline cognitive impairment helps in identifying the 'delirium' component which is likely to be reversible. In difficult circumstances where there is no collateral history, the default should be 'delirium' which ensures no reversible element is missed.

Delirium is multi-factorial hence the initial approach should be to diagnose any treatable medical conditions like infections, structural brain lesions (e.g. SDH, stroke), and review medications which can often precipitate delirium.

References

Borson, S., Scanlan, J., Brush, M. et al. (2000). The mini-cog: a cognitive 'vital signs' measure for dementia screening in multi-lingual elderly. *International Journal of Geriatric Psychiatry* 15 (11): 1021–1027.

Chibnall, J.T. and Tait, R.C. (2001). Pain assessment in cognitively impaired and unimpaired older adults: a comparison of four scales. *Pain* 92 (1–2): 173–186.

Isaia, G., Greppi, F., Ausiello, L. et al. (2011). D-dimer plasma concentrations in an older hospitalized population. *Journal of the American Geriatrics Society* 59 (12): 2385–2386.

Morley, J.E., Malmstrom, T.K., and Miller, D.K. (2012). A simple frailty questionnaire (FRAIL) predicts outcomes in middle aged African Americans. *The Journal of Nutrition, Health & Aging* 16 (7): 601–608.

▼
This chapter tells you how to approach continence from a geriatric perspective
▲

Example 42.1

A 72 year old lady presented with a fall. PMH: Glaucoma, IHD, HT, CKD, and back pain. Medications: latanoprost eye drops, atenolol, aspirin, candesartan, co-dydramol, and atorvastatin.

P: *SQs – Elderly lady + fall + vascular risk factors + glaucoma + chronic back pain. Provisional diagnoses – fall is multi-factorial as depicted in Figure 40.1. I would need more information along the lines of this model.*

The paramedics noted that she had tripped over a rug with no TLOC and they described it as a 'mechanical fall.' Minor injuries including bruising on the right elbow were described. She was recently diagnosed by her GP with a UTI and was on trimethoprim for the last two days. She was living alone with carer support twice a day.

P: *Intrinsic disease burden – background history, extrinsic factors – drugs (orthostatic hypotension), poor vision from glaucoma or inappropriate mobility aids, precipitating event/-s – UTI, new drug – although trimethoprim is unlikely to cause falls.*

Unfortunately, we do not have corroborating evidence for confirming some of these hypotheses (e.g. poor vision, inappropriate mobility aids) but that is how you would proceed.

O/E: Pulse 82 bpm, BP 140/90, RR 18 per minute, Saturations 97% on air, Temperature 37.3 °C and blood sugars (BMs) 10 mmol l^{-1}. PA: no renal angle tenderness, soft, and non-tender. CNS: grossly intact, not formally examined; musculo-skeletal: bruises on right elbow; rest of systemic examination: normal. The SHO diagnosed mechanical fall with uncomplicated UTI and continued trimethoprim. He requested social care input in the management plan.

Bloods: Hb 100 g l^{-1}, MCV 72 fl, WCC 13 × 10^9 l^{-1}, platelets 250 × 10^9 l^{-1}, CRP 40 mg l^{-1}; LFTs: normal, except albumin 30 g l^{-1}, Na$^+$ 129 mmol l^{-1}, K$^+$ 3.7 mmol l^{-1}, urea 10 mmol l^{-1}, creatinine 140 μmol l^{-1} (baseline creatinine 130 μmol l^{-1}). Urine dipstick: protein 2+, leucocytes + and blood +. Urine MC&S sent. CXR: awaited.

P: *Severity of illness – ill. This is likely to be a UTI since she has a positive urine dipstick. The hyponatraemia is probably secondary to trimethoprim or SIADH due to the UTI.*

The Hands-on Guide to Clinical Reasoning in Medicine, First Edition. Mujammil Irfan.
© 2019 John Wiley & Sons Ltd. Published 2019 by John Wiley & Sons Ltd.
Companion website: www.wiley.com/go/irfan/clinicalreasoning

We are missing a lot of information in the history including infective symptoms related to the urinary tract. Remember that tests (urine dipstick) do not make the diagnosis (UTI), they only increase or decrease the probability of our initial diagnostic hypotheses. Although the causes of hyponatraemia are valid, we need to interpret it in light of the volume status which is again missing.

The Post-take ward round Consultant agreed with the management plan and asked the registrar to review the CXR when it was available and added haematinics. The CXR later showed a left upper lobe mass and a CT scan was ordered given the suspicion of malignancy.

The nursing staff reported that she had not opened her bowels since admission and was incontinent of urine. She was prescribed laxatives for the constipation and the incontinence was ascribed to the UTI.

P: *I think the suspected lung malignancy is causing the hyponatraemia. With the microcytic anaemia, history of back pain and renal impairment would you suspect multiple myeloma?*

It certainly is a possibility. How would you synthesise the information so far?

Activity 42.1

(Allow three minutes)

....

....

....

....

....

P: *Revised SQs – Elderly lady + fall with unclear aetiology + suspected lung malignancy + constipation + urinary incontinence + vascular risk factors + glaucoma + chronic back pain. Provisional diagnoses – oh! Could there be cord compression given the suspected malignancy?*

Well done! However, note how you ascribed 'chronicity' to the back pain quite possibly because it was listed in PMH. It is very important that we do not guess but confirm clinical information with the patient before we close the loop.

Day 3

She complained of severe low back pain and the on-call doctor prescribed opiate analgesia. The nurses reported that she was increasingly confused and was struggling to lift her right foot during transfers. O/E: Right foot drop, loss of ankle jerk, and bilaterally up-going plantars; sensory level to L5 on the right. PR: saddle anaesthesia with sparing of pinprick sensation and loss of anal tone. She was diagnosed with cord compression and an urgent MRI requested. Dexamethasone was started, and she was referred to oncology for possible emergency radiotherapy.

In retrospect, it was found that she had had worsening low back pain for the last six weeks which was worse at night, in keeping with cord compression. The next of kin confirmed the urinary incontinence was new. Bone profile revealed hypercalcaemia which accounted for the confusion and was treated accordingly. Unfortunately, she did not recover to her pre-morbid mobility despite the radiotherapy and was transferred to a care home facility for further care. She had a final diagnosis of metastatic lung cancer with cauda equina syndrome (CES) and received palliative care owing to her co-morbidities and frailty.

Why do you think the admitting team missed the diagnosis for so long?

Activity 42.2

(Allow a minute)

Hindsight, as we all know is a wonderful thing and we can see that the fall was very likely due to neurological weakness. Unfortunately, this was missed owing to a lack of complete neurological examination. The admitting SHO merely transferred the impression of the paramedics that this was a mechanical fall and excused himself from performing further clinical assessment. He succumbed to 'diagnosis momentum.' New findings like constipation and urinary incontinence continued to be seen through the prism of 'UTI' exhibiting 'anchoring' where the initial impressions were given undue weight despite evidence to the contrary (Croskerry 2002). Knee-jerk responses to various clinical problems e.g. constipation → laxatives without assessing the cause are to be avoided at all costs. In short, this case exemplifies a common course of delayed diagnosis of CES which has been described amply in literature (Fairbank et al. 2011). The next of kin can be a valuable resource since they can help confirm or refute chronicity of findings especially when the elderly are unable to give a good history.

Lastly, there is a lack of clearly defined signs and symptoms for CES. Traditional teaching describes conus medullaris lesion as mixed UMN and LMN and CES as LMN but the signs vary depending on the site of compression (Byrne et al. 2000). Indeed, experts have debated on the so-called red flags calling them 'white flags' instead, since they often represent irreversible deficits (Todd 2017). Of the varied presentations only bilateral signs (2.23) and post-void urinary volume > 500 ml (1.46) have the highest LR for CES (Domen et al. 2009). The only predictor of post treatment functional independence is pre-morbid ambulatory status which highlights the role of early diagnosis (Kim et al. 1990).

Example 42.2

An 82 year old man was seen in the clinic for symptoms of urinary urgency over two months. PMH: HT, DM, IHD. Medications: aspirin, simvastatin, frusemide, ramipril, losartan, bisoprolol, calcichew D3, and co-codamol prn.

J: *SQs – Elderly man + sub-acute urinary urgency + vascular risk factors. Provisional diagnoses – UTI, although seems less likely given the long duration, prostate problems, diabetic autonomic neuropathy causing urinary symptoms.*

Good! You have used contextual factors like age and diabetes mellitus to come up with possibilities. Remember to use the model in Figure 40.1 and explore all the factors therein. Accordingly, extrinsic factors which include access issues, defective mobility aids, etc. and precipitating events could be drugs or intercurrent illnesses.

He denied any other urinary symptoms such as hesitancy or dysuria but reported increased frequency. There were no other infective symptoms or red flags like haematuria, back pain, or malignancy. No symptoms suggestive of diabetic autonomic dysfunction were elicited.

O/E: Pulse 72 bpm, BP 110/70, Saturations 96% on air, RR 12 per minute and Temperature 36.5 °C. Systemic examination: normal; PR: normal tone and no saddle anaesthesia, asymmetric enlargement of prostate but smooth surface and no fixation or nodularity. A prostate specific antigen (PSA) was requested along with 'routine' bloods. It was raised at 7 ng ml^{-1} and the rest of the bloods were normal. He was referred to the urologists with a possible diagnosis of prostate cancer.

With a positive predictive value of 25% for this PSA level and an absolute risk reduction (ARR) in mortality of 0.02% with screening, how would you interpret his chances of having prostate cancer?

Activity 42.3

(Allow two minutes)

....

....

....

....

....

This means that he has a 25% chance of having prostate cancer. In other words, one in four people with this PSA level will have prostate cancer which seems well worth the effort. However, we cannot equate this to him having prostate cancer! Moreover, levels between 4 and 10 ng ml^{-1} are in the grey zone and the very low ARR of 0.02% means that finding prostate cancer may not have significant mortality benefits. The number needed to treat-NNT (1/ARR) of 50 implies that we have to treat 50 patients to prevent one death from prostate cancer – in short, a lot of anxiety for little gain.

Repeat PSA with the urologist remained high at 8 ng ml^{-1} and a prostate biopsy was recommended which was negative for malignancy. He remained anxious about the risk of prostate cancer and consulted his GP for sleeplessness for which he was prescribed zopiclone. During this visit it came to light that the recently prescribed frusemide by the GP had precipitated the urgency which had settled when he decided to come off it.

The unfortunate series of events continued when he had a fall secondary to the drowsiness and fractured his right hip. The surgery was complicated by post-operative pneumonia and multi-organ failure to which he sadly succumbed.

At what points in the patient journey do you think things went wrong?

Activity 42.4

(Allow a minute)

This is an all too familiar chain of events often seen in hospitalised older adults. Let us start with the rationale to do the PSA in the first place. A thorough history would have elicited the cause for the urgency which in itself was iatrogenic, without recourse to further tests. Correct interpretation of test results and communicating them to patients in an understandable way is also vital in reducing their anxiety.

This brings the concept of overdiagnosis to the fore. By definition, overdiagnosis is the correct diagnosis that results in more harm than benefits (Carter 2017). It is a socio-cultural construct that occurs as a matter of degree than dichotomously. Although PSA screening has increased the incidence of prostate cancer, PSA is unable to discriminate between aggressive prostate cancers from indolent, slow-growing tumours that are not life-threatening. Herein, screening leads to uncertainty as we do not know if the pre-cancerous condition can turn into cancer. It thereby predisposes to anxiety even when it is negative, and this has to be borne in mind when requesting these tests (McNaughton-Collins et al. 2004).

Indeed, the U.S. Preventive Services Task Force recommends not screening men of any age for prostate cancer but to individualise screening as a shared decision-making process (Moyer 2012). Several approaches have been recommended to reduce overdiagnosis in clinical practice, specifically viewing screening tests through the lens of absolute risk and only doing the test when this can be reduced by screening (Chiolero et al. 2015). The purpose of activity 42.3 was to show this in action.

▼

New onset urinary dysfunction in the right context should raise suspicion of cord compression.

Diagnostic hypotheses should be revised in light of new clinical findings and anchoring should be avoided.

Overdiagnosis especially in the elderly can lead to negative outcomes like polypharmacy and iatrogenic disorders causing mortality and morbidity.

▲

References

Byrne, T., Benzel, E., and Waxman, S. (2000). *Diseases of the Spine and Spinal Cord*. Oxford: Oxford University Press.

Carter, S.M. (2017). Overdiagnosis: an important issue that demands rigour and precision comment on "medicalisation and overdiagnosis: what society does to medicine"'. *International Journal of Health Policy and Management* 6 (10): 611–613.

Chiolero, A., Paccaud, F., Aujesky, D. et al. (2015). How to prevent overdiagnosis. *Swiss Medical Weekly* 145: w14060.

Croskerry, P. (2002). Achieving quality in clinical decision making: cognitive strategies and detection of bias. *Academic Emergency Medicine: Official Journal of the Society for Academic Emergency Medicine* 9 (11): 1184–1204.

Domen, P.M., Hofman, P.A., van Santbrink, H., and Weber, W.E. (2009). Predictive value of clinical characteristics in patients with suspected cauda equina syndrome. *European Journal of Neurology* 16 (3): 416–419.

Fairbank, J., Hashimoto, R., Dailey, A. et al. (2011). Does patient history and physical examination predict MRI proven cauda equina syndrome?'. *Evidence-Based Spine-Care Journal* 2 (4): 27–33.

Kim, R.Y., Spencer, S.A., Meredith, R.F. et al. (1990). Extradural spinal cord compression: analysis of factors determining functional prognosis – prospective study. *Radiology* 176 (1): 279–282.

McNaughton-Collins, M., Fowler, F.J. Jr., Caubet, J.F. et al. (2004). Psychological effects of a suspicious prostate cancer screening test followed by a benign biopsy result. *The American Journal of Medicine* 117 (10): 719–725.

Moyer, V.A. (2012). Screening for prostate cancer: U.S. preventive services task force recommendation statement. *Annals of Internal Medicine* 157 (2): 120.

Todd, N.V. (2017). Guidelines for cauda equina syndrome. Red flags and white flags. Systematic review and implications for triage. *British Journal of Neurosurgery* 31 (3): 336–339.

43 Falls

▼
This chapter tells you how to approach falls in the elderly
▲

The best way of not falling is to be immobile – quite an erroneous statement one might say, but that is what most older people do to prevent falls. Falls by their very nature are multifactorial; it follows that the treatment should be along similar lines.

Example 43.1

> A 78 year old lady was referred by A&E as a 'social admission' having been found by paramedics fallen under the stairs. PMH: HT, OA. Medications: candesartan, co-codamol.

> P: *SQs – elderly lady + fall + hypertension + OA. Provisional diagnoses – focusing on the cause of fall – postural hypotension, instability from OA or pain. I would ask questions based on the model in Figure 40.1.*

> She said that she was checking the settings on her boiler and as she turned, she lost her balance and fell. She denied LOC, vertigo, ear ache, or any preceding symptoms. There was no post-episode confusion. She hurt her right knee which was already bruised from a previous injury when she caught it under the stair-lift few weeks ago. An X-ray of the right knee showed no obvious fracture. There were no recent illnesses. This was her fourth fall in the last six months and the previous falls were similar in nature.

> P: *Severity of illness – ill. It sounds like a mechanical fall with no red flag symptoms.*

> Mechanical fall is a misnomer that results in bypassing critical thinking (Sri-on et al. 2016). If we do not find out the reason for the fall, we cannot prevent it in the future. She has fallen four times over the last six months hence, we need to dig a little deeper.

What questions would you ask?

Activity 43.1

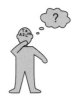

(Allow a minute)

We need to look for specific pre-syncopal symptoms, any change in social circumstances, functional impairment (activities of daily living – ADLs), mobility and instability issues due to OA.

She lived alone in a house with no next of kin close by. She was struggling to cope with ADLs on her own. No walking aids, carers, or adaptations at home. Bloods: Hb 110 g l⁻¹, WCC 14 × 10⁹ l⁻¹, platelets 350 × 10⁹ l⁻¹; clotting profile: normal; bilirubin 20 μmol l⁻¹, ALT 35 IU l⁻¹, ALP 200 IU l⁻¹, albumin 23 g l⁻¹, CRP 40 mg l⁻¹, Na⁺ 134 mmol l⁻¹, K⁺ 3.7 mmol l⁻¹, urea 10 mmol l⁻¹, creatinine 130 μmol l⁻¹ (baseline creatinine 120 μmol l⁻¹).

Given the mildly raised ALP, the registrar specifically enquired about episodic abdominal pain and infective symptoms related to cholecystitis which she denied. The low albumin prompted questions on loss of weight and appetite. She admitted to both and fatigue but could not quantify the weight loss. She had gone down by at least three dress sizes over last six months. There were no red flags of malignancy.

P: *It seems to be a significant weight loss.*

Indeed, I would search hard for signs of malignancy.

O/E: Pulse 86 bpm, BP 138/80, RR 14 per minute, Temperature 36.6 °C, Saturations 94% on air, BMs 8 mmol l⁻¹. PA: large, painless, nodular liver felt with the lower margin extending 10 cm below right costal margin; no free fluid. PR and breast examination: normal. Right knee: deformed secondary to OA; old bruise and diffuse tenderness with no effusion. Rest of the systemic examination: normal. FRAIL score: 4 (fatigue, unable to climb a flight of stairs or walk around a block and weight loss > 5%). ECG: normal.

P: *Is there an age cut off for assessing frailty?*

No, frailty ≠ age. We should endeavour to assess frailty score in all patient encounters thereby ensuring appropriate management strategies are formulated.

What factors would inform your decision to investigate further?

Activity 43.2

(Allow a minute)

Recognition of frailty helps in assessing risk/benefit ratios of investigations and treatments as poor outcomes, risks, and mortality are higher in a frail person. FRAIL score is a screening tool and cannot be used to diagnose 'frailty.' Instead, it should trigger a more comprehensive assessment such as CGA which can help tailor interventions. Finally, the patient's philosophy of life will also have a significant bearing on their informed decisions. These will have to be taken into consideration in addition to the routine factors that we have to balance when we formulate a management plan.

With her consent a contrasted CT scan thorax, abdomen, and pelvis was requested which showed likely colonic carcinoma with hepatic metastases and incidental large bilateral pulmonary emboli. She was started on therapeutic anticoagulation with LWMH and analgesia for the right knee. A CGA confirmed frailty and it was felt that further invasive investigations would not be in her best interests which concurred with

her decision. She received multi-disciplinary input with optimization of her environment including a walk-in shower, mobility aids, package of care and district nurse
input for administration of LMWH. Community palliative care was organised and
future care prospects explored with the patient with a view to nursing home care if
needed.

What helped the registrar to discover the underlying pathology despite the label of 'social
admission?'

Activity 43.3

(Allow a minute)

The first thing that strikes is the attention to detail. Subtle clues like the mildly elevated
ALP and low albumin were pursued relentlessly and diagnostic momentum was broken
(Croskerry 2002). A comprehensive assessment including frailty was undertaken and the
entire equation in Figure 40.1 was explored. Terms like 'mechanical fall,' 'social admission,'
etc. should set alarms off and trigger a comprehensive history and examination to uncover
underlying pathology since these terms lull the physician into a false sense of security and
absolve them of the sin of being lackadaisical with their clinical assessment.

Example 43.2

A 76 year old man was referred by his general practitioner for recurrent falls over six
months. PMH: Glaucoma, HT, and depression. Medications: timolol eye drops,
doxazosin, and olanzapine.

J: *SQs – Elderly man + recurrent falls + hypertension + glaucoma + depression. Provisional
       diagnoses – wide differential.*

Using the model in Figure 40.1, postulate the factors specific to our patient under the
headings shown:

Activity 43.4

Intrinsic disease burden..

....

Extrinsic factors...

Precipitating event...

(Allow three minutes)

J: *Intrinsic disease burden = background history, extrinsic factors = possible poor vision
       secondary to glaucoma, precipitating event could be anything depending on the history,
       but possibilities include drug-induced orthostatic hypotension (systemic absorption of
       timolol and doxazosin). The key would be to elicit any TLOC.*

He denied any TLOC or sensory issues (normal vision). The falls seemed to occur when
he suddenly turned or whilst walking. He blamed his walking stick for these falls. He
had bruised his arms and legs on a couple of occasions but no history of fractures or
head injuries. No symptoms suggestive of orthostatic hypotension i.e. no postural
symptoms. No recent infective symptoms. He was unable to climb a flight of stairs or
walk around a block. He was having difficulty in doing his ADLs.

O/E: Pulse 82 bpm, BP 110/60, Saturations 96% on air, RR 14 per minute, Temperature 37.2 °C and BMs 8 mmol l⁻¹. Systemic examination: normal. The admitting SHO asked for lying and standing BP and urine dipstick. Lying BP 110/60 and standing BP: 100/70 with no reproducible symptoms. Urine dipstick: protein +, ketones +, leucocytes +. She diagnosed a UTI based on these results and started trimethoprim. Bloods: normal with CRP 20 mg l⁻¹. ECG: normal.

J: *Severity of illness – ill. There is no evidence for orthostatic hypotension. The FRAIL score is 2 which is pre-frailty. I'm not sure if there is any hard evidence for a UTI.*

Good!

The consultant on the post-take ward round reviewed the history and discovered that he was having difficulty with ADLs, taking far too long to complete them. Upon direct questioning he admitted to difficulty in turning in bed whilst sleeping. On examination he had evidence of symmetrical rigidity and bradykinesia but no tremor. He diagnosed Parkinson's disease, started levodopa, and referred him to a Geriatrician.

Why do you think these signs were missed by the SHO?

Activity 43.5

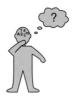

(Allow a minute)

Availability heuristic can explain the ease with which we hone in on a UTI for most geriatric presentations. We must strive to provide evidence for any diagnosis that we make which was lacking for a UTI. Although, knowledge deficits can contribute towards failure in triggering the right hypothesis the reasons can be varied and deep. Often neurological examination is short-changed during busy admissions and even when done is neither efficient nor complete. Bradykinesia in particular does not form part of 'routine neurological' examination and hence can be easily missed. Eliciting the reason for difficulty with ADLs triggered the right hypothesis which shows how the devil is in the detail.

The geriatrician diagnosed drug-induced Parkinson's secondary to olanzapine which was started a year ago (Thanvi and Treadwell 2009). Both levodopa and olanzapine were stopped in consultation with the patient's psychiatrist. The patient improved over the next eight months with resolution of symptoms.

Features that discriminate Idiopathic Parkinson's disease from other Parkinsonian syndromes

- Unilateral onset and persistent asymmetry
- Good response to dopaminergic therapy
- Postural instability and dementia is a late manifestation
- Progression of signs and symptoms over the years

J: *Why is this not Parkinson's disease?*

Clinical features that discriminate idiopathic Parkinson's from Parkinsonian syndromes are shown opposite. Indeed, evidence based reasoning cannot be applied for diagnoses which lack a technological gold standard e.g. a laboratory or radiological test. Unfortunately, Parkinson's disease is a clinical diagnosis and short of autopsy there is no definitive test *in vivo*. The LRs that can be computed from autopsy studies will be limited by their small numbers and verification and selection biases (Simel et al. 2009). In fact, the Movement Disorder Society has declared that the gold standard for diagnosing Parkinson's is an expert clinician.

▼

FRAIL score helps in screening for frailty which is very useful to guide decisions on patient management.

Terms such as mechanical fall and collapse query cause should ring alarm bells prompting a diligent search for pathology.

Evidence based reasoning cannot be applied for diagnoses that rest on empirical observation.

▲

References

Croskerry, P. (2002). Achieving quality in clinical decision making: cognitive strategies and detection of bias. *Academic Emergency Medicine: Official Journal of the Society for Academic Emergency Medicine* 9 (11): 1184–1204.

Simel, D., Rennie, D., and Keitz, S. (2009). *The Rational Clinical Examination*. New York: McGraw-Hill.

Sri-on, J., Tirrell, G.P., Lipsitz, L.A., and Liu, S.W. (2016). Is there such a thing as a mechanical fall?'. *The American Journal of Emergency Medicine* 34 (3): 582–585.

Thanvi, B. and Treadwell, S. (2009). Drug induced Parkinsonism: a common cause of Parkinsonism in older people. *Postgraduate Medical Journal* 85 (1004): 322–326.

44 Acute Confusion

▼
This chapter tells you how to approach delirium from a geriatric medicine perspective
▲

Example 44.1

A 70 year old woman was admitted with 'acopia' and recurrent falls. PMH: TIA (aphasia), three recent hospital admissions with UTI, cognitive impairment query Alzheimer's, IHD and COPD. Medications: bisoprolol, clopidogrel, symbicort and atrovent inhalers, nitrofurantoin, trospium, ramipril, and nitroglycerine (GTN) spray.

J: *SQs – Elderly woman + acopia and recurrent falls + vascular risk factors + possible Alzheimer's. Provisional diagnoses – along the lines of intrinsic disease burden (PMH), precipitating event (e.g. infection) and extrinsic factors (e.g. new drugs).*

Good! I would not use 'acopia' as an SQ though, since the term often harbours serious underlying pathology (Kee and Rippingale 2009). It is similar to terms such as 'social admission' and should in fact trigger a deeper search for reversible disease processes.

The nursing staff reported that this was a failed discharge from a recent hospital admission. The discharge letter mentioned a similar episode of confusion and fall with an eventual diagnosis of UTI. She lived alone, and her niece who helped with meals and shopping. She had carers coming in twice a day to help with personal activities of daily living (PADL) including bathing and cleaning. She could transfer with a Zimmer frame and mobilise to the toilet but was incontinent of urine and wore pads.

Today she was found by the carers having fallen on her way to the toilet. She had no recollection of the events. She was felt to be confused and had an episode when she stared with a blank expression lasting a few seconds prompting the admission. She denied any urinary or infective symptoms. There was no injury sustained. No recent head injuries.

J: *There could be transient loss of consciousness and I would keep the differentials of vasovagal, orthostatic, and cardiogenic syncope (IHD) or epilepsy (blank stare).*

O/E: Pulse 74 bpm, BP 130/80, Saturations 96% on air, RR 15 per minute, Temperature 36.6 °C and BMs 7 mmol l⁻¹. She seemed to answer questions in a tangent and was not oriented to time, place, or person. CNS: no lateralizing signs, no signs of meningeal irritation. Rest of systemic examination: normal.

Bloods: WCC $16 \times 10^9 l^{-1}$, platelets $350 \times 10^9 l^{-1}$, Hb $140 g l^{-1}$, U&Es, LFTs and bone profile: normal, CRP $50 mg l^{-1}$. Urine dipstick: protein 2+, blood +, leucocytes +, nitrites +. CXR and ECG: normal. The SHO diagnosed a UTI and gave her

The Hands-on Guide to Clinical Reasoning in Medicine, First Edition. Mujammil Irfan.
© 2019 John Wiley & Sons Ltd. Published 2019 by John Wiley & Sons Ltd.
Companion website: www.wiley.com/go/irfan/clinicalreasoning

trimethoprim whilst withholding her nitrofurantoin, and sent urine for MC&S. He requested social services input with physiotherapy and occupational therapy.

Do you agree with the diagnosis?

Activity 44.1

(Allow a minute)

J: *I'm not sure that there is good evidence for UTI. She seems to have delirium.*

I agree since she is exhibiting inattention, the hallmark of delirium.

She became agitated overnight and began thrashing around. She seemed to be enacting dreams and disrupted the ward. The nursing staff called in the on-call SHO to prescribe some night time sedation since they wanted to care for patients who were sicker. The SHO relented and prescribed haloperidol.

The SHO was asked to re-assess the patient three hours later as she had become more confused and had a Medical Early Warning Score (MEWS) of 4 (RR 20 per minute, heart rate 110 bpm, BP 150/90, apyrexial and responding to pain). The SHO assumed she might be septic and gave her empiric antibiotics and IV fluids.

The next morning, she was found to be quite lucid but was unable to recall anything. The consultant ward round continued the current management.

J: *This seems to be typical of delirium, but we do not know the cause yet.*

The following night, there was a repetition of psychomotor behavioural disturbances with visual hallucinations. She was given a further dose of haloperidol after which she slept. The next morning, the registrar noted the fluctuating BP on her charts and asked for postural BP which showed a fall in systolic blood pressure > 20 mm of Hg with symptoms of presyncope. She performed a detailed neurological examination and discovered symmetric bradykinesia and rigidity. Mini mental state examination (MMSE) was 20 with relative preservation of memory. The trospium (anticholinergic) was stopped since it was contributing to the delirium.

In retrospect, the fluctuating confusion (recurrent so-called 'UTI admissions'), cognitive impairment, dysautonomia (fluctuating BP, orthostatic hypotension, urinary incontinence), visual hallucinations, acting out dreams (REM sleep behaviour disorder), Parkinsonian features and antipsychotic (haloperidol) sensitivity all fitted with Lewy body dementia. A CT head excluded subdural haematoma. She was eventually discharged to a nursing home facility. Behavioural therapy and rivastigmine improved the hallucinations and confusion but the cognitive impairment persisted.

Why do you think the diagnosis was missed for so long?

Activity 44.2

(Allow a minute)

Attribution error – 'acopia' elicited negative connotations of a less deserving patient to be hospitalised (Croskerry 2002). Delirium was missed to start with and instead of finding out the cause, knee-jerk responses with drugs were used to treat 'disruptive behaviour' on the ward. We have a tendency towards 'action' where we desire to be seen doing something even when it may cause more harm than good (Foy and Filippone 2013). The statement 'Don't just do something, stand there!' would do us well when we feel the urge to act (Sinha 2017). Sometimes less is more as long as we are circumspect with our decisions. Obviously, this will have to be tied with a robust follow-up plan with more closer observation which can be seen to be more labour intensive than taking the easier route of 'just giving the drugs.'

Example 44.2

A 75 year old woman was admitted with agitation and acute confusion. PMH: Depression, chronic fatigue syndrome, mild cognitive impairment, history of alcohol excess, HT, OA. Medications: venlafaxine, co-dydramol, tramadol, losartan.

P: *SQs – Elderly woman + acute confusion + psychiatric issues + mild cognitive impairment (MCA) + alcohol excess + HT. Provisional diagnoses – encephalitis, alcohol withdrawal, intercurrent infection like UTI, CAP.*

The carer had found her in her assisted living flat this morning confused and agitated. This was new for her. No seizures or lateralizing signs (e.g. hemiparesis) were witnessed. Yesterday she complained of increasing aches in her body with her chronic fatigue syndrome for which she saw the out of hours GP who prescribed tramadol. There were no obvious infective symptoms or headache that she had complained of. The carers helped her with PADLs and visited her twice a day. She was fairly house bound owing to social anxiety. They confirmed that she had abstained from alcohol for nearly three years. She had a brother who lived in a nearby city.

O/E: Pulse 110 bpm, BP 160/90, Saturations 96% on air, RR 20 per minute, Temperature 38.6 °C and BMs 10 mmol l⁻¹. She was restless and disoriented. CNS: Glasgow coma scale (GCS) 12 (E3, M5, V4). No signs of meningeal irritation. No lateralizing signs. She had a tremor in her arms with bilaterally upgoing plantars. Rest of systemic examination: normal.

P: *The pyrexia, tachycardia, and altered mental status points to sepsis. The bilaterally upgoing plantars could represent encephalitis. The acute history makes the tremor unlikely to be Parkinsonian e.g. Lewy body dementia.*

The recent example of 44.1 seems to have made it easier for you to recall Lewy body disease (availability heuristic). Note the discrepancy of hypertension which does not fit with sepsis though.

What other hypotheses can you think of that can explain all the findings?

Activity 44.3

(Allow three minutes)

....

....

....

....

....

P: *I can't think of anything.*

Whenever, we are stuck for answers remember that up to 6.5% of hospital admissions are due to adverse drug reactions (ADRs) (Davies et al. 2010). 20–30% of hospital admissions in the elderly are due to ADRs (Chan et al. 2001).

P: *Could it be the tramadol?*

It can certainly cause confusion but doesn't explain the pyrexia. This is the point when it would be useful to consult the British National Formulary (BNF) or online tools for drug interactions and side effects. A quick search will reveal that venlafaxine interacts with tramadol to cause serotonin syndrome (Boyer and Shannon 2005).

The SHO prescribed tazobactam and piperacillin (broad-spectrum) antibiotics and IV fluids for presumed sepsis. The registrar notes hyperreflexia, hypertonia and clonus in the limbs and requests a CT head to exclude structural lesions like SDH, cerebral abscess, or stroke. Tramadol is stopped. CT head, urine dipstick, and CXR: normal. ECG: sinus tachycardia, slightly prolonged QTc 460 ms. Bloods: WCC $16 \times 10^9 \, \text{l}^{-1}$, CRP $60 \, \text{mg} \, \text{l}^{-1}$, CK $400 \, \text{IU} \, \text{l}^{-1}$; remainder: normal.

On the post-take ward round, the consultant asks for an LP to exclude encephalitis. IV acyclovir is started. The ward pharmacist highlights the drug interaction causing serotonin syndrome. She suggests stopping venlafaxine and giving benzodiazepines for agitation. The LP under anaesthetic supervision and sedation is reported normal and acyclovir is stopped. The agitation and tremor settle but she remains confused.

Delirium is often slow to resolve and can take several weeks to months (McCusker et al. 2003). In fact, unresolved delirium predicts discharge to skilled nursing facilities. However, it is worth excluding reversible conditions like intercurrent infections, drugs or underlying dementia. The presence of previous MCI can support a diagnosis of dementia but remember that this is a very heterogenous group with differing outcomes. Furthermore, underlying cognitive impairment can predispose individuals to delirium.

Over the next two weeks she gets bed-bound needing assistance to transfer and dependence for all PADLs. She displays aggression during routine care and a psychiatry assessment reveals persistent delirium with MMSE 20. The nursing staff question the lack of a do not attempt resuscitation (DNAR) form as she is felt to be deteriorating.

The team arranges a meeting with the brother and a discussion is had about DNAR and her long-term care needs. The brother is taken aback by the sudden mention of DNAR and disagrees with this decision despite explanation.

Activity 44.4

(Allow a minute)

Do you agree with the decision on DNAR?

P: *I agree since she has no quality of life.*

I don't think we can make accurate judgements on someone's quality of life unless we have a good grasp of their history over a long period of time. This cannot be the basis for making DNAR decisions.

This decision is a good example of balancing short-term benefits of intervention (successful cardio-pulmonary resuscitation – CPR) with long-term outcomes (functional independence). Studies have shown that isolated discussions on DNAR can evoke strongly negative reactions from patients and their families. Discussing overall goals of care, ascertaining patients' views/values on life and tailoring and facilitating therapy to achieve the shared goals sets the scene. Discussing DNAR as part of these shared goals in line with their life values as part of an emergency care plan has a better chance of being accepted (Pitcher et al. 2017; Fritz et al. 2017). Substantiating these discussions with objective evidence of their own chances of survival with good neurological recovery will truly inform them and help them see the rationale behind the decisions (Ebell et al. 2013). For example, her GOFAR score (good outcome following attempted resuscitation) is 12 giving her a 9.4% probability of survival to discharge with good neurologic status following CPR. Putting this in the context of a CPR success rate of 20% for in-hospital arrests will give a clear perspective of what we can achieve.

A second opinion was requested who agreed with the DNAR decision. This was subsequently challenged by the brother in a court when the decision was returned in favour of the medical team. She received supportive care and was discharged to a nursing home.

▼
Sometimes it is worth considering not intervening but always arrange robust follow-up in these instances!

Do not address DNAR decisions in isolation but set these decisions in the context of their overall goals of care.
▲

References

Boyer, E.W. and Shannon, M. (2005). The serotonin syndrome. *The New England Journal of Medicine* 352 (11): 1112–1120.

Chan, M., Nicklason, F., and Vial, J.H. (2001). Adverse drug events as a cause of hospital admission in the elderly. *Internal Medicine Journal* 31 (4): 199–205.

Croskerry, P. (2002). Achieving quality in clinical decision making: cognitive strategies and detection of bias.'. *Academic Emergency Medicine: Official Journal of the Society for Academic Emergency Medicine* 9 (11): 1184–1204.

Davies, E.C., Green, C.F., Mottram, D.R. et al. (2010). Emergency re-admissions to hospital due to adverse drug reactions within 1 year of the index admission. *British Journal of Clinical Pharmacology* 70 (5): 749–755.

Ebell, M.H., Jang, W., Shen, Y. et al. (2013). Development and validation of the Good Outcome Following Attempted Resuscitation (GO-FAR) score to predict neurologically intact survival after in-hospital cardiopulmonary resuscitation. *Journal of the American Medical Association: Internal Medicine* 173 (20): 1872–1878.

Foy, A.J. and Filippone, E.J. (2013). The case for intervention bias in the practice of medicine. *The Yale Journal of Biology and Medicine* 86 (2): 271–280.

Fritz, Z., Slowther, A.M., and Perkins, G.D. (2017). Resuscitation policy should focus on the patient, not the decision. *BMJ (Clinical research ed.)* 356: j813.

Kee, Y.-Y.K. and Rippingale, C. (2009). The prevalence and characteristic of patients with 'acopia.'. *Age and Ageing* 38 (1): 103–105.

McCusker, J., Cole, M., Dendukuri, N. et al. (2003). The course of delirium in older medical inpatients: a prospective study. *Journal of General Internal Medicine* 18 (9): 696–704.

Pitcher, D., Fritz, Z., Wang, M., and Spiller, J.A. (2017). Emergency care and resuscitation plans. *British Medical Journal (Clinical research ed.)* 356: j876.

Sinha, P. (2017). Don't just do something, stand there! *Journal of the American Medical Association: Internal Medicine* 177 (10): 1420.

45 Dementia

▼

This chapter tells you how to approach dementia from a Geriatric medicine perspective

▲

Example 45.1

An 86 year old woman is admitted via the GP with a three month history of weight loss. PMH: COPD, HT, stroke (minimal residual right sided weakness), MCI, IHD hypercholesterolemia, PVD, CKD stage 2, appendicectomy, cholecystectomy, and OA. Medications: ropinirole, bendrofluazide, clopidogrel, aspirin, simvastatin, carvedilol, enalapril, amlodipine, seretide and ventolin inhalers, and dihydrocodeine.

J: *SQs – Elderly woman + sub-acute weight loss + vascular risk factors + COPD + OA. Provisional diagnoses – malignancy, cachexia associated with severe COPD, mesenteric ischemia (vascular risk factors), poor diet, polymyalgia rheumatica.*

The history was primarily obtained from the niece. She reported that her aunt was becoming increasingly frail, but no falls or red flag symptoms were noted. The ET of 100 yards was fairly constant over the last year with stable COPD. There were no symptoms suggestive of mesenteric ischemia. Her niece felt that she was increasingly forgetful and gave examples of leaving food in microwave and not eating. At this point the patient exclaimed 'oh … my memory is awful!'

She lived alone and mobilised using a stick. Her niece helped with shopping. She was independent with her ADLs. No history of alcohol excess. Ex-smoker 40 py.

J: *Severity of illness – ill. The significant memory dysfunction with the history of MCI points to dementia.*

O/E: Pulse 84 bpm, BP 130/76, Saturations 97% on air, RR 16 per minute, Temperature 37.7 °C and BMs 10 mmol l^{-1}. The mini-cog was abnormal indicating dementia. Systemic examination including breast and per-rectal examination with consent was normal.

Bloods: FBC, U&Es, LFTs and bone profile: normal. ESR 45 mm h^{-1}; CXR and urine dipstick: normal. The registrar suggested formal cognitive assessment, a CT thorax, abdomen, and pelvis to exclude malignancy and a dietician review.

J: *The mini-cog also points to dementia. I think she has dementia +/– malignancy.*

Remember that the diagnosis of dementia rests on an equal weighting of all cognitive domains and not just memory dysfunction. Furthermore, it has to affect function with impairment of ADLs.

The Hands-on Guide to Clinical Reasoning in Medicine, First Edition. Mujammil Irfan.
© 2019 John Wiley & Sons Ltd. Published 2019 by John Wiley & Sons Ltd.
Companion website: www.wiley.com/go/irfan/clinicalreasoning

Activity 45.1

(Allow a minute)

What other differentials can you think of that can present with weight loss?

J: *GI malabsorption states* (but no diarrhoea), *peptic ulcer disease* (on aspirin and clopidogrel). *Endocrine disorders like Addison's or diabetes mellitus.*

Well done, I would add chronic infections like TB drugs and psychiatric disorders like depression since the latter is often under-recognised in the elderly.

On the post-take ward round, her niece had left and the history was reviewed with the patient. Having noticed poor eye contact, the consultant enquired about how she fills her time at home. She reported having lost interest in the games that she used to watch when her husband was alive. She admitted to sleeplessness when she would lie awake wondering why? She screened positive on the patient health questionnaire – 9 (PHQ-9) questionnaire making depression likely (Kroenke et al. 2001).

Her medications were rationalised to reduce polypharmacy. A formal assessment confirmed depression and she was started on an anti-depressant by a Geriatrician. Her symptoms had improved, and she had gained weight upon follow up in three months.

What made us focus on dementia at the start?

Activity 45.2

(Allow a minute)

The predominant memory dysfunction and the history of MCI seem to have misled us. Although the mini-cog was in keeping with dementia, people with depression can also perform poorly owing to poor effort. On the contrary people with dementia try really hard but fail. Subtle clues like poor eye contact and interaction can be missed when we are focused on filling in a clerking proforma which although is a useful tool in itself, can detract from the very purpose it serves. Here we see how a single unspoken cue can yield a new hypothesis. Activity 45.1 shows how we can pause and evaluate before we stick a diagnostic label.

This example also throws medicalisation into sharp relief (Hofmann 2016). The diagnosis of MCI is controversial with one camp claiming medicalisation of the normal ageing process whilst the opposition claiming that this helps in recognising individuals at risk for developing dementia. We will have to temper this last claim with the fact that there is no evidence at present supporting drug therapy to prevent progression to dementia. Furthermore it stigmatises individuals leading to further isolation and dependence especially when a fair percentage improves over a period of time (Ritchie et al. 2001). Indeed, if the final diagnosis happens to be depression, its recognition will be delayed. All this will have to be balanced against the late recognition of dementia in clinical practice which can also be detrimental.

Example 45.2

An 82 year old man with known Alzheimer's dementia was brought to A&E having collapsed during a meal with an unresponsive episode. PMH: IHD, HT, history of treated colon cancer, TIA, and right carotid endarterectomy 10 years ago. Medications: clopidogrel, nitroglycerine (GTN) spray, Isosorbide mononitrate, lisinopril, amlodipine, donepezil, and prn paracetamol.

P: *SQs – Elderly man + collapse query Cause + vascular risk factors + Alzheimer's and history of colon cancer. Provisional diagnoses – carotid artery stenosis, TIA, intercurrent infection, brain metastases.*

Collapse query Cause is neither a diagnosis nor a symptom. The presence of TLOC implies syncope which is a better term to give us the right context in which we can frame our hypotheses.

Can you revise the hypotheses based on this being syncope?

Activity 45.3

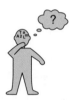

(Allow a minute)

P: *The main differentials are vaso-vagal or cardiogenic syncope and epilepsy.*

Perfect! As for the TIA, the only subtype that can result in TLOC is vertebro-basilar artery territory TIA (posterior circulation) which is quite rare.

He was unable to give any history but the carer who witnessed the episode reported no warning, followed by TLOC and spontaneous recovery within a minute or so. There were no other symptoms during or after the episode. He had had an anterior wall MI six years ago and was stable with his ET of 20–30 yards. Physically he was largely limited to the residential home, socially he enjoyed a good conversation. He needed assistance with ADLs but could feed himself. He was continent and used a stick to mobilise.

O/E: pulse 50 bpm, BP 120/70, saturations 97% on air, RR 14 per minute, temperature 37 °C, and BMs 8 mmol l⁻¹. Bruises on right arm from the fall. No carotid bruits or murmurs. Rest of the systemic examination – normal.

Bloods: FBC, U&Es, LFTs, bone profile normal. CRP 40 mg l⁻¹. Urine dipstick normal. CXR – cardiomegaly, no pulmonary oedema. ECG: sinus bradycardia.

What would you suggest at this point?

P: *Given the bradycardia, I would put him on a cardiac monitor and add TFTs to the bloods.*

The story fits with cardiogenic syncope. The previous anterior wall MI (possible scar tissue involving AV node) and donepezil (cholinergic activity) make heart blocks a real possibility.

The admitting registrar requested telemetry and postural BP, the latter being normal. She stopped donepezil and amlodipine. It came to light that he also had a DNAR order with him.

Five days into admission he continued to be symptomatically bradycardic with a heart rate of 20–30 bpm and had unresponsive episodes with significant pauses >three seconds that responded to atropine. The consultant cardiologist pondered over the decision for a permanent pacemaker (PPM). The nursing staff did not feel that this was appropriate citing the DNAR order and advocated comfort care with a view to palliation.

Do you think he is a candidate for a PPM? Give reasons.

Activity 45.4

(Allow a minute)

P: *Since he has a DNAR order I feel that palliation would be in his best interests.*

Unfortunately, this is a common misconception amongst healthcare professionals. We conflate DNAR decisions with decisions to treat when the two are separate. For example, patients with heart failure with a DNAR are less likely to receive optimal care than those without (Chen et al. 2008). DNAR decisions should sit within the wider constraints of 'overall goals of care' where the emphasis can lie anywhere between active treatment and comfort care or palliation.

Concepts such as frailty can help us objectively predict adverse outcomes helping us make decisions instead of basing them on age and quality of life (Kim et al. 2016). Importantly, patient preferences should be explored if they have capacity or their families consulted when they lack capacity. The threshold to intervene would be lower in the case of reversible pathologies but the risks of intervention will have to be balanced against the benefits.

The alternative option of not doing anything would expose the patient to immediate risk of death. This example illustrates how we balance immediate risk of death against long-term risk of complications from the PPM in a pre-frail older person.

The team assessed his capacity and concluded that he did indeed understand the implications of his slow heart beat and the poor prognosis without treatment. The FRAIL score was 2 and the cardiologist decided to proceed with a PPM insertion after having explained the rationale to the patient and his family. Risks of intervention were highlighted, and a PPM was inserted with consent. He remained well on follow up in three months with no recurrence of syncope.

▼

Non-verbal cues can yield new hypotheses, look for them!

Do not conflate DNAR decisions with decisions to treat.

▲

References

Chen, J.L.T., Sosnov, J., Lessard., D., and Goldberg, R.J. (2008). Impact of do-not-resuscitation orders on quality of care performance measures in patients hospitalized with acute heart failure. *American Heart Journal* 156 (1): 78–84.

Hofmann, B. (2016). 'Medicalization and overdiagnosis: different but alike. *Medicine, Health Care and Philosophy* 19 (2): 253–264.

Kim, D.H., Kim, C.A., Placide, S. et al. (2016). Preoperative frailty assessment and outcomes at 6 months or later in older adults undergoing cardiac surgical procedures: a systematic review. *Annals of Internal Medicine* 165 (9): 650–660.

Kroenke, K., Spitzer, R.L., and Williams, J.B.W. (2001). The PHQ-9: validity of a brief depression severity measure. *Journal of General Internal Medicine* 16 (9): 606–613.

Ritchie, K., Artero, S., and Touchon, J. (2001). 'Classification criteria for mild cognitive impairment: a population-based validation study. *Neurology* 56 (1): 37–42.

46 History Taking: Where is the Pain?

As illustrated in previous chapters, history taking becomes easier when symptom aetiologies are borne in mind. This can be done on an anatomical or patho-physiologic basis which does not tax the brain!

46.1 ABDOMINAL PAIN

There are three types of pain in the context of the gastro-intestinal tract (GIT).

Visceral pain: The hollow viscera and mesenteries respond to mechanical stretch (colic), inflammatory, and chemical stimuli. Visceral pain from solid organs arises when the capsule gets stretched e.g. liver. Figure 46.1a shows that the visceral pain is poorly localised in the midline since it is bilaterally represented in the spinal cord via sympathetic nerves. Since these pain pathways utilise the autonomic nervous system, reflex nausea, vomiting, salivation, and sweating accompany the pain.

Somatic pain: The parietal peritoneum is innervated by somatic nerves that enter the spinal cord unilaterally on either side. Therefore, somatic pain is sharply localised to the area where the inflamed structure comes into contact with it. Since the overlying abdominal wall is innervated by the same nerves, there is cutaneous hyperalgesia and reflex contraction of the wall muscles called guarding.

For example, acute appendicitis starts with a poorly localised peri-umbilical pain (visceral pain) that then migrates to the right iliac fossa (RIF) classically to the McBurney's point (somatic pain) accompanied by nausea, vomiting, and later guarding.

Referred pain: Both visceral and somatic structures can produce referred pain if they share the same spinal cord segments as the cutaneous dermatomes. For instance, acute cholecystitis initially causes vague visceral pain over T5-9 dermatomes in lower chest and upper abdominal wall antero-posteriorly. As inflammation proceeds, either the peripheral (intercostal nerves T7-11) or central (phrenic nerve C3-5) diaphragmatic peritoneum gets involved resulting in somatic pain. This pain is perceived either in the right upper-quadrant (RUQ) through to the back involving the inferior angle of the scapula (T7-11 dermatomes) or the ipsilateral shoulder tip (supraclavicular nerves C3-4) respectively (Figure 46.1b,c).

Using this knowledge and anatomy of course, one can predict the pattern of pain that occurs in conditions such as renal colic, bowel obstruction, myocardial infarction, pleurisy, etc.

46.2 DIARRHOEA

Figure 46.2a shows a concept map of acute diarrhoea. It is defined as ≥3 loose stools/day but practically is an increase in frequency or change in stool consistency. In general, invasive micro-organisms cause constitutional symptoms such as fever. Chronic diarrhoea is defined as a decrease in faecal consistency for >4 weeks. The aetiology of diarrhoea varies with the settings (resource rich or poor).

The Hands-on Guide to Clinical Reasoning in Medicine, First Edition. Mujammil Irfan.
© 2019 John Wiley & Sons Ltd. Published 2019 by John Wiley & Sons Ltd.
Companion website: www.wiley.com/go/irfan/clinicalreasoning

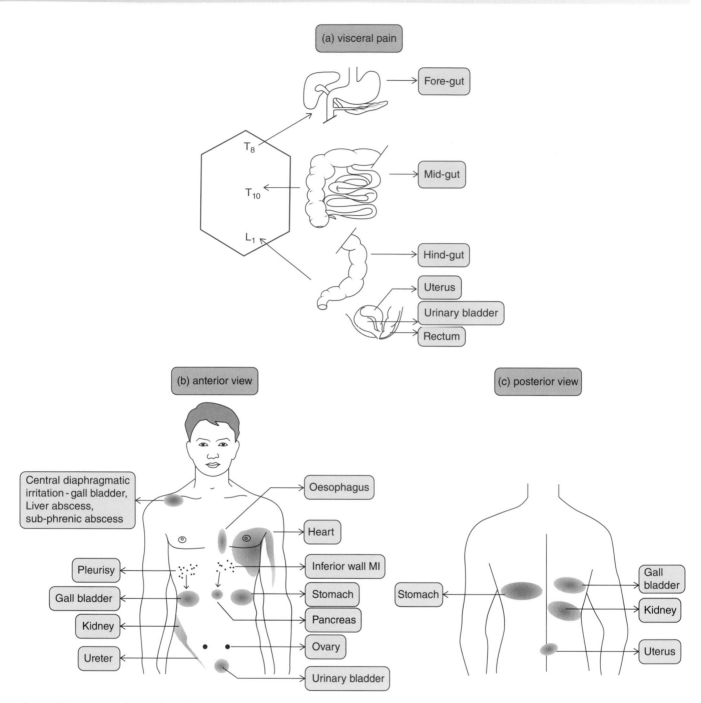

Figure 46.1 Aetiology of abdominal pain

46.3 CONSTIPATION

As with other symptoms, acute and chronic constipation should make you think of different aetiologies. Acute constipation especially obstipation (constipation + not passing flatus) is often due to surgical causes like bowel obstruction. Chronic constipation on the other hand has varied aetiology which can be pathophysiologically classified into local colonic causes (tumour, ischaemia, stenosis), neurologic, endocrine, metabolic, or drug induced – especially opiates. It is important to first clarify what the patient means by

(a)

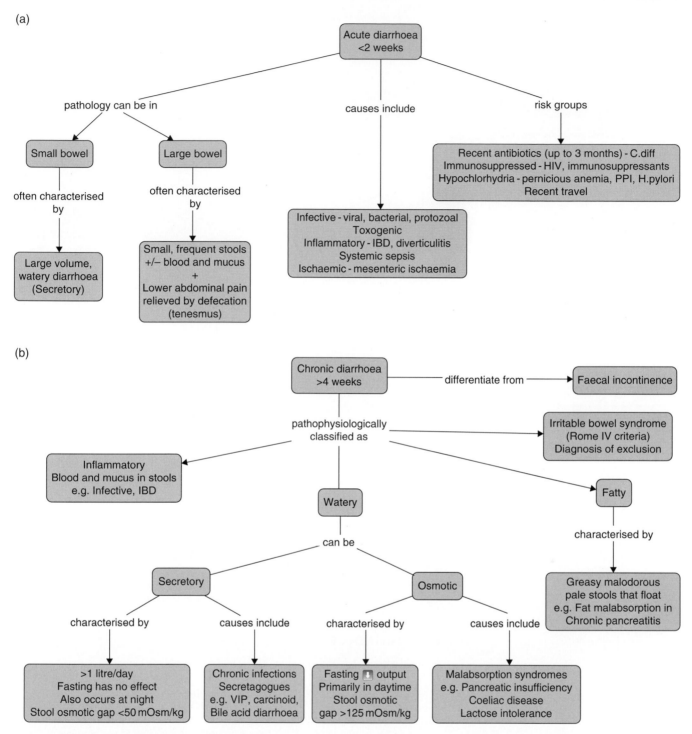

(b)

Figure 46.2 Aetiology of acute and chronic diarrhoea

constipation. Constipation is commonly defined as <3 bowel movements/week but this has been challenged. Symptoms commonly associated with it include reduced frequency, hard stools, and unsatisfactory defaecation. Alarm symptoms like blood or mucus per rectum, change in bowel habits, weight loss, and family history of bowel cancer especially in the elderly should trigger further investigations.

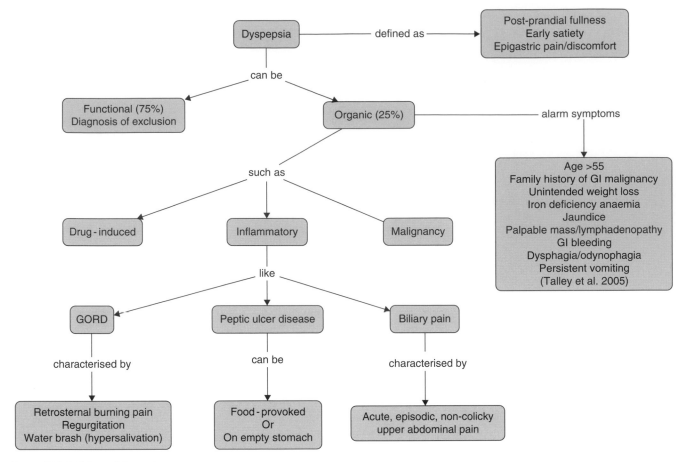

Figure 46.3 Aetiology of dyspepsia

46.4 DYSPEPSIA/INDIGESTION

The organic causes of dyspepsia can be classified anatomically into those arising from oesophagus, stomach, duodenum, or biliary tract. Patho-physiologically they can be considered under the headings: inflammatory, neoplastic, and drug-induced. Remember to look for associated alarm symptoms as described in the concept map (Figure 46.3).

46.5 JAUNDICE

Serum hyperbilirubinaemia ($>34\,\mu\text{mol}\,l^{-1}$) is clinically visible as jaundice/icterus in the sclera, under the tongue and skin. Figure 46.4 shows the physiology of bilirubin with the different types of jaundice superimposed. Disease processes that affect the hepatic architecture can easily spill over from the hepatocytes to the biliary canaliculi resulting in a mixed picture (unconjugated/conjugated) depending on the degree of involvement of the two components. Figure 46.5 shows the concept map of the aetiology of jaundice.

Although this is a history taking chapter, I have included the history, examination findings, and investigations in the different types of jaundice in Table 46.1 to aid understanding. Think through the information provided in Figures 46.4 and 46.5 and fill in the missing information in Table 46.1.

Of note, in the laboratory, conjugated bilirubin reacts directly with the reagent in an aqueous solution and is therefore called direct bilirubin. In the presence of methanol both conjugated and unconjugated bilirubin react with the reagent yielding the total bilirubin concentration. The unconjugated bilirubin is then calculated as total bilirubin – conjugated bilirubin and is normally around 4% of the total bilirubin.

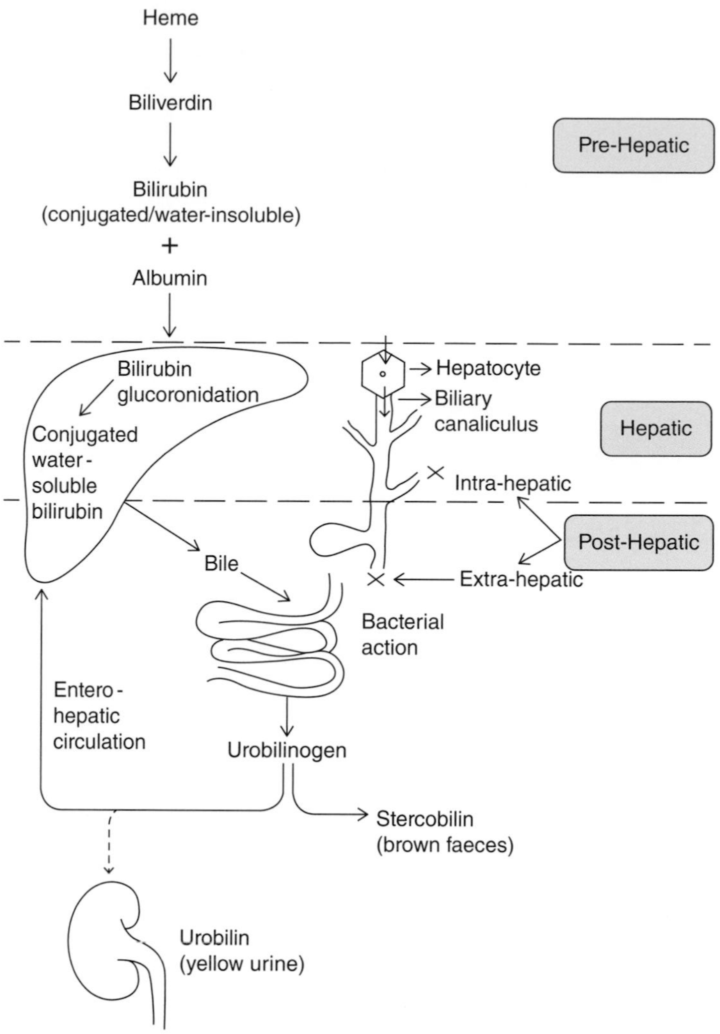

Heme

↓

Biliverdin

↓

Bilirubin
(conjugated/water-insoluble)
+
Albumin

↓

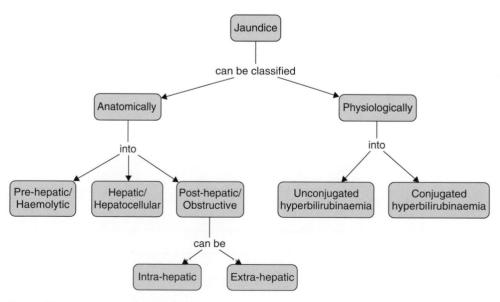

Bilirubin
glucoronidation

Conjugated
water-
soluble
bilirubin

→ Hepatocyte
→ Biliary
canaliculus

× Intra-hepatic

× ← Extra-hepatic

Pre-Hepatic

Hepatic

Post-Hepatic

Bile

Bacterial
action

Entero-
hepatic
circulation

Urobilinogen

→ Stercobilin
(brown faeces)

Urobilin
(yellow urine)

Figure 46.4 Pathophysiology of jaundice

Jaundice

can be classified

Anatomically   Physiologically

into   into

Pre-hepatic/   Hepatic/   Post-hepatic/   Unconjugated   Conjugated
Haemolytic   Hepatocellular   Obstructive   hyperbilirubinaemia   hyperbilirubinaemia

can be

Intra-hepatic   Extra-hepatic

Figure 46.5 Concept map of aetiology of jaundice

Table 46.1 Discriminatory features of types of jaundice. Fill in the missing information to make the table your own.

		Pre-hepatic/haemolytic	Hepatic/hepatocellular	Post-hepatic/obstructive
History		Personal/family history of jaundice Drugs Infections		Weight loss, biliary colic, Charcot's triad Drugs Infections Pale stools, dark urine
Examination		Hepato-splenomegaly Lymphadenopathy	Signs of acute liver failure/ chronic liver disease	
Investigations	Hyperbilirubinaemia	Unconjugated/indirect	Mixed	Conjugated/direct
	ALT, AST	Normal	+++	+
	ALP, GGT	Normal	+	+++
	Urine bilirubin	–		↑
	Urine urobilinogen	↑		↓/–

ALT – alanine transferase; AST – aspartate aminotransferase; ALP – alkaline phosphatase; GGT – gamma glutamyl transpeptidase.

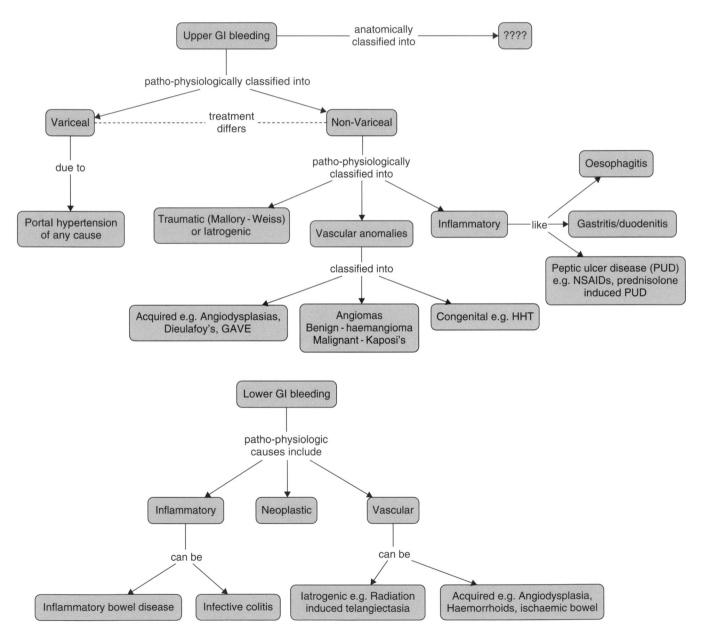

Figure 46.6 Aetiology of gastro-intestinal bleeding

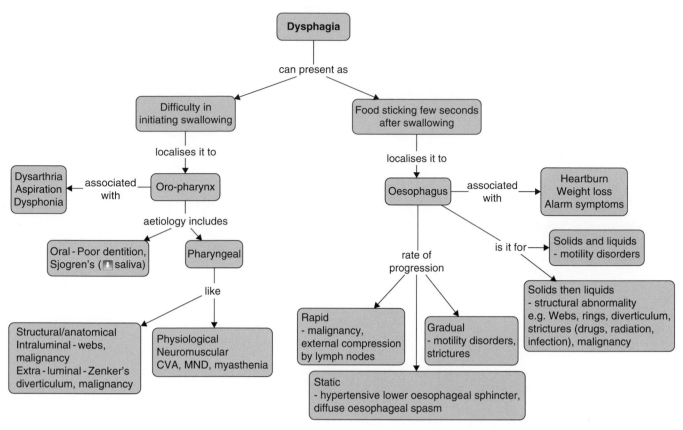

Figure 46.7 Aetiology of dysphagia

46.6 GASTROINTESTINAL BLEEDING (GIB)

A slow trickling bleed can present as iron deficiency anaemia whilst a large volume bleed is more dramatic with haematemesis, melena, or haematochezia. Figure 46.6 classifies GIB into upper and lower where the former indicates a source of bleeding proximal to the ligament of Treitz (attached to the duodeno-jejunal flexure) and the latter distal to it.

Upper gastrointestinal bleeding (UGIB) typically results in haematemesis and melena, the latter owing to bacterial degradation of haemoglobin into hematin and other haemachromes in the gut. Small volume bleed can cause a coffee ground vomitus due to oxidation of iron by gastric acid whereas a large volume bleed can even result in haematochezia (fresh per rectal bleeding). Lower gastrointestinal bleeding (LGIB) often presents as haematochezia but a slow bleed with reduced gut motility can still result in melena. As you can see the presentation does not always help in localising the source.

46.7 DYSPHAGIA

Dysphagia can be mapped onto the physiology of swallowing and anatomically classified into oropharyngeal and oesophageal dysphagia. Oropharyngeal dysphagia correlates to the first two phases of deglutition – oral preparatory phase and pharyngeal phase whilst the latter correlates to the oesophageal phase. Figure 46.7 shows the questions that need to be asked in this setting.

Reference

Talley, N.J., Vakil, N.B., and Moayyedi, P. (2005). American gastroenterological association technical review on the evaluation of dyspepsia. *Gastroenterology* 129 (5): 1756–1780.

▼
This chapter focuses on relevant clinical features and their interpretation from a Gastroenterology perspective
▲

As illustrated before, clinical examination is best visualised in a systematic manner. An end of the bed assessment should lead to the hands, working your way up the arms, face, down the neck, chest, abdomen, and legs.

47.1 ACUTE LIVER FAILURE

It is defined as deranged LFTs (representing acute liver injury) + hepatic encephalopathy + prolonged PT/INR ≥ 1.5 over a duration of <26 weeks. As you can see the definition includes laboratory features with clinical findings. Examination is directed at unravelling the cause (Figure 47.1) and excluding stigmata of chronic liver disease (Figure 47.2). Occasionally there could be acute decompensation of chronic liver disease.

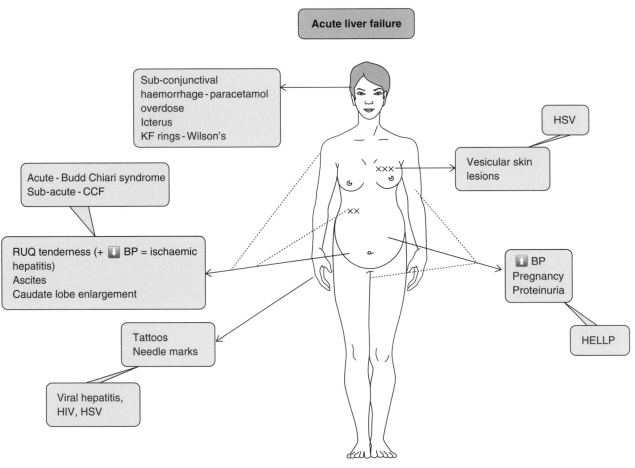

Figure 47.1 Clinical examination in acute liver failure

The Hands-on Guide to Clinical Reasoning in Medicine, First Edition. Mujammil Irfan.
© 2019 John Wiley & Sons Ltd. Published 2019 by John Wiley & Sons Ltd.
Companion website: www.wiley.com/go/irfan/clinicalreasoning

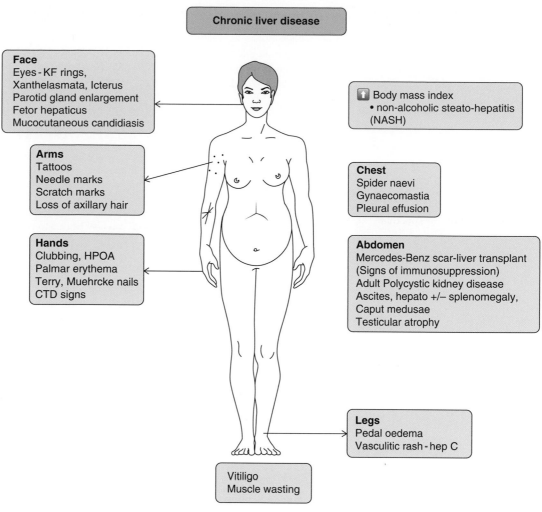

Figure 47.2 Clinical examination in chronic liver disease

47.2 CHRONIC LIVER DISEASE

Stigmata of chronic liver disease help in identifying long-standing liver derangement (Figure 47.2). Unfortunately, not all signs are present in all cases making it difficult to be confident about the chronicity. Understanding the patho-physiologic basis will help in etching the clinical signs into memory. Of note, the liver can be normal, shrunken, or enlarged in cirrhosis. Examination should also be purposefully directed at eliciting the aetiology.

47.3 ORGANOMEGALY

Upon finding hepatomegaly it is wise to ensure that the liver span (normal < 18 cm) is actually increased and you are not palpating a liver that has just been pushed down secondary to emphysema, for instance. In resource rich countries, the major causes of hepatomegaly are three Cs (cirrhosis, carcinoma, CCF) and three Is (infectious, immune, infiltrative) (Hoole et al. 2015). Cirrhosis commonly results in a shrunken liver but cardiac cirrhosis, Budd-Chiari syndrome, and NASH can cause hepatomegaly.

Drawing upon this observation, you can see that the examination should be directed at uncovering any of these possibilities. Describing the liver edge, surface and presence, or absence of tenderness can help narrow the aetiology. Tender hepatomegaly signals CCF, infective hepatitis (viral hepatitis), or drug toxicity (paracetamol overdose).

If splenomegaly is detected, one should look for concurrent lymphadenopathy since the spleen is essentially made up of lymphoid tissue. This would point to haematological (myelo-/lymphoproliferative disorders) and infectious (Epstein Barr Virus – EBV, viral hepatitis, infective endocarditis, malaria, leishmaniasis) conditions. Infiltrative conditions (Gaucher's, amyloidosis) often tend to involve both the liver and the spleen. Thinking anatomically, portal hypertension from any cause can result in splenomegaly. Remember that cirrhosis often results in functional hypersplenism rather than true splenomegaly causing thrombocytopenia and other haematological disturbances.

47.4 INFLAMMATORY BOWEL DISEASE

IBD has an auto-immune pathogenesis and a known association with spondyloarthropathies. The latter implies that we have to look for associated joint, eye, and skin signs (Figure 47.3). Gallstones and renal stones occur due to malabsorption related metabolic disturbances. Entero-cutaneous fistula formation can be perianal or abdominal. The clue for underlying IBD in an OSCE setting is the presence of colectomy scar ± stoma bag, although the latter can also be due to colonic carcinoma or diverticular perforation.

47.5 ACUTE ABDOMEN

A complete treatise on the surgical causes of acute abdomen is beyond the scope of this book. However, it is important to appreciate that patients do not respect the boundaries of a 'medical ward.' A patient admitted with a medical problem can still end up having surgical issues and it is up to the physician to identify them.

Special populations like the elderly, immunosuppressed, and women of child-bearing age can present with common surgical diagnoses as well as population specific conditions like

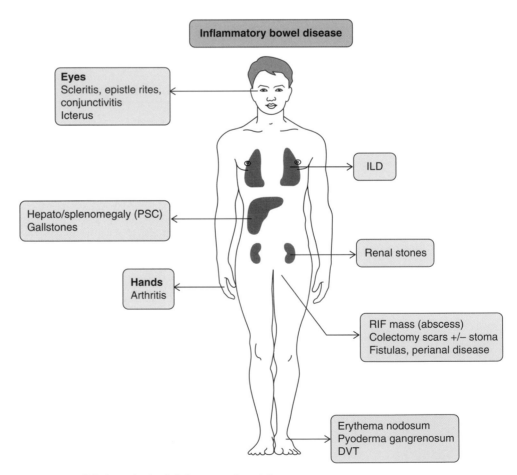

Figure 47.3 Clinical examination in inflammatory bowel disease

opportunistic infections. The elderly, can often lack physical signs and with their co-morbidities, present an even greater challenge.

Medical conditions like diabetic ketoacidosis (DKA), alcoholic ketoacidosis, hypercalcemia, herpes zoster, and pseudo-obstruction secondary to metabolic disturbances can mimic an acute abdomen. Thoracic pathologies can also present with upper abdominal pain from referred pain as seen in Chapter 46.

47.6 SKIN SIGNS IN GI PROBLEMS

It is often quite helpful to look for cutaneous features in specific GI presentations which give clues to the aetiology as illustrated below:

GI bleeding – Hereditary haemorrhagic telangiectasia (telangiectasias in nail beds, palms, and feet), Pseudoxanthoma elasticum (yellow plaques, papules in flexural areas – plucked chicken skin appearance in axilla).

Peptic ulcer disease – Systemic mastocytosis (Darier's sign).

Malignancy – Peutz-Jeghers syndrome (pigmented macules on lips, hands, and feet), acanthosis nigricans (often axillary brown to black skin papillomas), Gardner's syndrome (multiple cysts, fibromas, and lipomas).

Diarrhoea with per rectal bleeding – IBD – skin signs include erythema nodosum, pyoderma gangrenosum, clubbing). Severe Crohn's can sometimes cause zinc deficiency presenting with red, scaly, crusty lesions around eyes, mouth, genitalia, and white patches on tongue.

Chronic diarrhoea (think malabsorption) – Carcinoid (flushing, telangiectasias, wheeze, right sided murmurs), systemic mastocytosis, systemic sclerosis (CREST syndrome), celiac disease (dermatitis herpetiformis with pruritic vesicles on extensor surfaces of knees and elbows).

Reference

Hoole, S., Fry, A., and Davies, R. (2015). *Cases for Paces*, 3e. Chichester: Wiley Blackwell.

▼
This chapter tells you how to interpret tests from the perspective of Gastroenterology
▲

This chapter discusses some important blood tests and radiological investigations from a clinical stance.

48.1 LIVER FUNCTION TESTS (LFTS)

The pattern of LFT dysfunction is more important than individual tests. Figure 48.1 shows the major clinical patterns: hepatitic picture, cholestatic picture, mixed (with one being predominant), and isolated hyperbilirubinemia. These are superimposed on a schematic diagram of a hepatocyte.

ALT is found in the hepatocellular cytosol whilst AST is found in the cytosol and mitochondria. Hepatocyte injury (hepatitic picture) results in the release of these enzymes into the circulation.

The degree of transaminase elevation can give clues to the aetiology e.g. viral hepatitis, toxin induced hepatitis, and ischemic hepatitis cause levels in their 1000s whilst chronic hepatitis B and C can have normal levels. LDH can help discriminate between ischemic hepatitis (↑) and viral hepatitis. A ratio of AST/ALT > 2:1 points to alcoholic liver disease, hepatitis C induced cirrhosis, non-alcoholic steatohepatitis (NASH), or Wilson's disease.

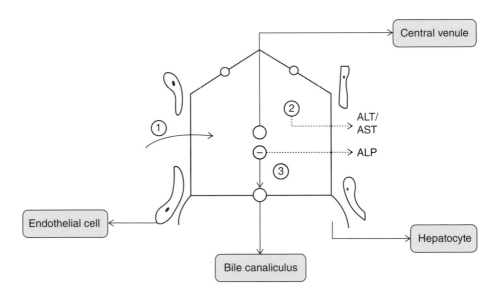

1. Isolated hyperbilirubinaemia 2. Hepatitic picture 3. Cholestatic picture 4. Mixed picture = 2 + 3

Figure 48.1 Pathophysiology of patterns of liver function test dysfunction

ALP is found in the cell membranes of hepatobiliary tissue including hepatocytes. Cholestasis (impaired bile flow) from any cause results in the accumulation of bile acids in the hepatocytes triggering increased synthesis of ALP which is then regurgitated into the circulation by the hepatocytes.

GGT and 5′ nucleotidase are other cholestatic enzymes that can be used to confirm the hepatic origin of the raised ALP. However, GGT is similarly non-specific (false positives with alcohol and drugs). Although 5′ nucleotidase is primarily released into the circulation by hepatobiliary tissue it can be discordant with ALP rise. Therefore, a normal 5′ nucleotidase in the face of raised ALP still does not exclude a hepatic source.

Isolated hyperbilirubinemia can be conjugated or unconjugated. The former occurs in rare genetic disorders like Rotor syndrome but can be seen in combination with other LFT abnormalities in cholestatic jaundice.

Isolated unconjugated hyperbilirubinemia is seen in haemolytic anaemias including ineffective erythropoiesis where red cells are not maturing 'effectively' owing to the absence of raw materials like iron, folate, or vitamin B12. Other causes of ineffective erythropoiesis include myelodysplastic syndrome, thalassemia, and sideroblastic anaemia. The immature red cells die in the bone marrow resulting in unconjugated hyperbilirubinemia and iron overload as bowel absorption of iron continues (except iron deficiency anaemia). A haemolytic screen consisting of LDH, serum haptoglobin, peripheral blood smear and reticulocyte count will help in identifying haemolysis. Drugs like rifampicin can also prevent hepatic uptake of unconjugated bilirubin causing its levels to rise. Rare inherited conditions like Gilbert syndrome can cause asymptomatic mild unconjugated hyperbilirubinemia when stressed e.g. unrelated disease process, fasting.

Measurement of serum bilirubin and bile acids gives us an insight into the liver's ability to take up and detoxify metabolites and drugs. LFTs can thus also be grouped from a functional stance into: tests that reflect hepatocyte injury, tests of the liver's ability to transport organic anions and metabolise drugs, tests that reflect biosynthetic function and tests that detect chronic hepatic inflammation (e.g. viral hepatitis, autoimmune liver disease).

Limitations of LFTs:

• They can be raised in non-hepatic conditions i.e. they are non-specific.
• They can be normal in end-stage liver disease.

Although LFTs give us a handle on hepatic dysfunction other biochemical and haematological parameters help in completing the picture (Figure 48.2).

For instance, given the synthetic function of liver, acute liver failure (ALF) can manifest in a prolonged PT (short half-life of clotting factors of a few hours) whilst serum albumin remains normal (half-life 20 days). This reflects the prognostic significance of PT in ALF. In end-stage liver disease the urea can be subnormal, again owing to the same reason. Similarly, the degree of hyponatremia closely correlates to the severity of chronic liver disease giving it prognostic value.

48.2 HAEMATOLOGICAL ABNORMALITIES IN HEPATIC DYSFUNCTION

Contrary to popular thinking widely prevalent in clinical practice, liver disease patients are not auto-anticoagulated.

Current clotting profile indices (PT, APTT) do not predict bleeding risk since they all measure procoagulant factors alone. While we are on this topic, cirrhotic coagulopathy has a different pathophysiologic basis than warfarin anticoagulation hence INR cannot be used as a target but it is useful in prognosticating scores such as MELD (model for end-stage liver disease).

Figure 48.3 shows that all stages of clot formation and dissolution are abnormal with the end-result (prothrombotic or fibrinolytic) differing between individual patients

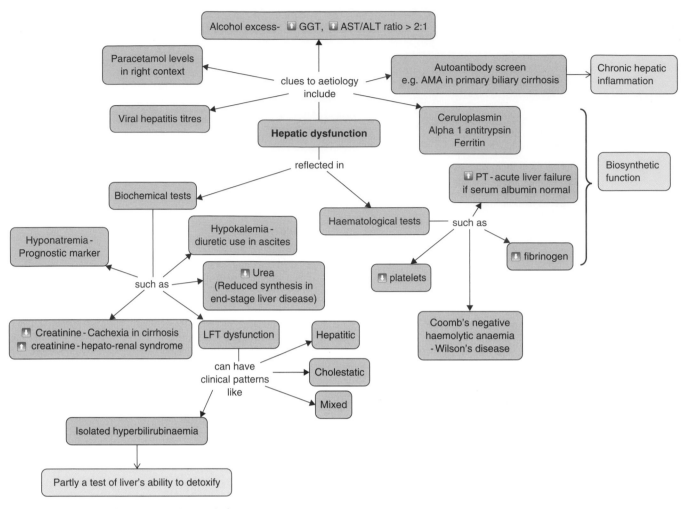

Figure 48.2 Overview of blood tests in hepatic dysfunction

depending on which process is dominant. Weeder et al. (2014) call this 'rebalanced haemostasis'. Hence, we cannot automatically preclude liver disease patients from thromboprophylaxis.

With this in mind a global test of haemostasis such as thromboelastography (TEG) is more useful to assess all stages of coagulation and fibrinolysis. Although such tests still need standardisation, a small study found that less blood products were used in the TEG group compared to the group managed using standard clotting profile results (De Pietri et al. 2016).

48.3 ASCITIC FLUID ANALYSIS

The serum: ascites albumin gradient (SAAG) ≥11 g l⁻¹ points to portal hypertension (of any aetiology) as the cause of ascites i.e. a transudate. It performs better than the ascitic fluid protein classification for transudates and exudates. Of note, both cardiac ascites and cirrhotic ascites have a SAAG >11 g l⁻¹ but in cardiac ascites the total fluid protein is ≥25 g l⁻¹.

Ascitic fluid corrected neutrophil count ≥250 cells mm⁻³ indicates a high likelihood of spontaneous bacterial peritonitis (SBP) and should prompt initiation of antibiotic cover.

48.4 ABDOMINAL RADIOGRAPHS (AXR)

Abdominal radiographs (AXRs) are frequently requested in the evaluation of acute abdominal pain but this has been shown to have a very low yield (Eisenberg et al. 1983). This is in keeping with what we have learnt so far, that unsuspected diagnoses do not get

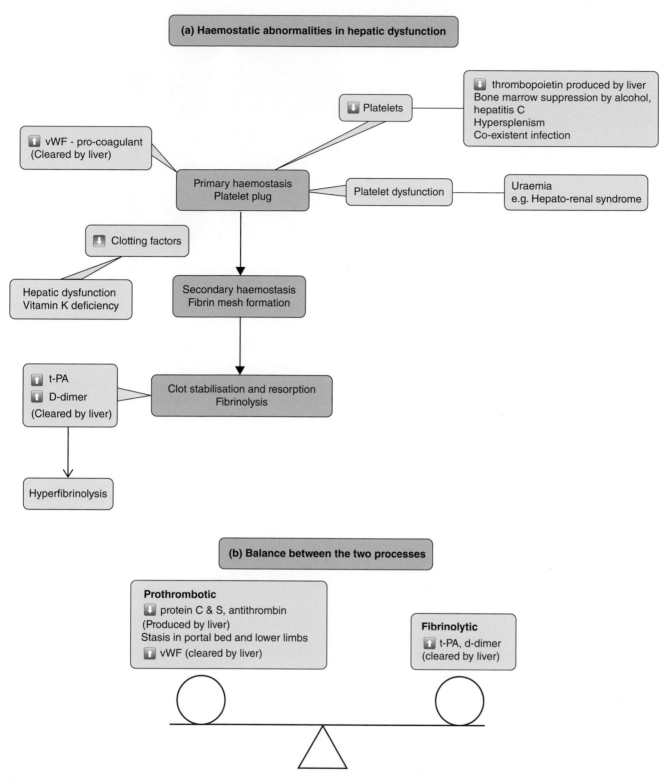

Figure 48.3 Figure showing a) the range of haemostatic abnormalities in hepatic dysfunction and b) factors affecting the 'rebalanced haemostasis' in hepatic dysfunction

revealed by tests. The highest yield is when the following diagnoses are suspected from clinical assessment i.e. significant pre-test probability.

- Bowel obstruction (BO), perforation
- Renal-ureteric calculi
- Ischaemia

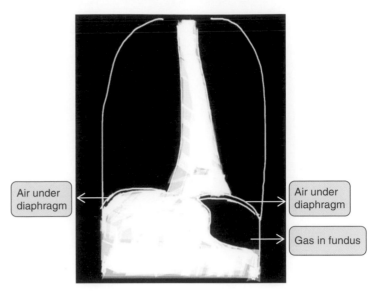

Figure 48.4 Pneumoperitoneum

- Trauma
- In addition, a 'surgical abdomen' with moderate to severe tenderness can be initially assessed with an AXR.

Various mnemonics like BBC or *Go* through the AXR *Slowly But Calmly* (*Gas* pattern, *Soft* tissues, *Bones* and *Calcification*, and artefacts) can help in ensuring that no pathology is missed. As always don't stop at finding the first glaringly obvious abnormality ('search satisficing'), search for more.

Pneumoperitoneum (Figure 48.4)

Suspected pneumoperitoneum should trigger an erect CXR, abdominal examination – PA or lateral view, or if the patient is too ill to sit up/move a left lateral decubitus AXR should be used to detect Rigler's sign (air on both sides of bowel wall), air fluid levels or free air above the liver edge. Ideally one must sit upright for at least 5–10 minutes for small leaks to be identified on erect films. A significant pneumoperitoneum can manifest with the 'double wall/Rigler's' sign on a supine film too. Gastro-duodenal perforations declare themselves with a pneumoperitoneum in ⅔ of cases whilst distal small/large bowel perforations do so in only ⅓.

Pneumoretroperitoneum (Figure 48.5) occurs when there is retroperitoneal viscus perforation (duodenum or rectum). Dark gas highlights retroperitoneal structures like the kidneys, spleen, and psoas muscles. There may not be concurrent air under the hemidiaphragms given the retroperitoneal perforation. Note that normally the kidneys and psoas muscles are highlighted by fat surrounding them which is paler than gas.

Bowel Obstruction - BO (Figure 48.6)

The following points need to be remembered while looking for bowel obstruction:

- Only an erect film can show air-fluid level.
- The 3, 6, 9 rule gives you a rule of thumb for normal size (in centimetres) of small bowel, transverse colon, and caecum respectively.
- The jejunum has valvulae conniventes (complete mucosal folds across the lumen), ileum is featureless, and colon has haustrae (incomplete folds).
- The small bowel is central, filled with fluid and gas whilst the large bowel is peripheral, filled with faeces and gas.
- The more distal the obstruction, the more the number of loops seen.
- Adhesions are a common cause of bowel obstruction in the west whilst hernias commonly cause BO in the resource poor settings.
- Don't forget to look for pneumoperitoneum co-existing with obstruction (a rare complication).

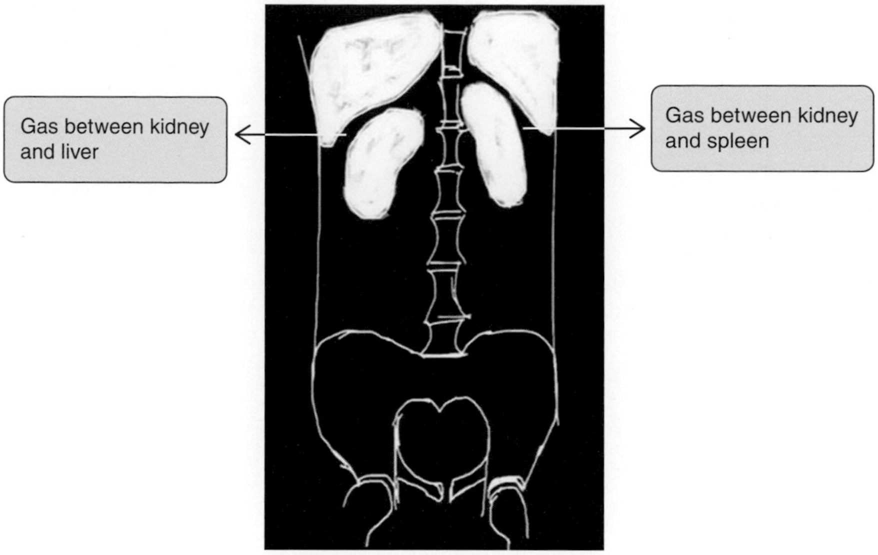

Gas between kidney and liver

Gas between kidney and spleen

Figure 48.5 Pneumoretroperitoneum

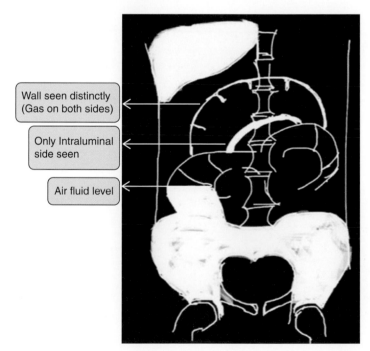

Wall seen distinctly (Gas on both sides)

Only Intraluminal side seen

Air fluid level

Figure 48.6 Bowel obstruction

48.5 ULTRASOUND ABDOMEN

Normal measurements

- Gall bladder wall in fasting state – 2 mm.
- Common hepatic duct (inner wall to inner wall) – <7 mm in <60 years old, and <10 mm in >60 years old.
- Common bile duct – 4 mm in < 40 years old + 1 mm per decade thereafter.

In suspected acute cholecystitis, one is looking for downstream obstruction in the biliary tree and gall bladder wall thickening. USG has a sensitivity of >95% in detecting gallstones. It is also useful in diagnosing cirrhosis (transient elastography) and detecting complications such as ascites, portal hypertension, and hepatocellular carcinoma. Another use of USG is in screening for abdominal aortic aneurysms.

References

Eisenberg, R.L., Heineken, P., Hedgcock, M.W. et al. (1983). Evaluation of plain abdominal radiographs in the diagnosis of abdominal pain. *Annals of Surgery* 197 (4): 464–469.

De Pietri, L., Bianchini, M., Montalti, R. et al. (2016). Thrombelastography-guided blood product use before invasive procedures in cirrhosis with severe coagulopathy: a randomized, controlled trial. *Hepatology (Baltimore, MD)* 63 (2): 566–573.

Weeder, P.D., Porte, R.J. & Lisman, T., 2014. Hemostasis in liver disease: implications of new concepts for perioperative management. *Transfusion medicine reviews,* 28(3), pp.107–13.

49 Weight Loss and Diarrhoea

▼
This chapter tells you how to approach weight loss and diarrhoea from a gastroenterological perspective
▲

Example 49.1

A 70 year old lady was referred for a medical opinion for a six week history of intermittent diarrhoea and weight loss. She was an in-patient in the psychiatry ward for depression and cognitive impairment with behavioural issues. Preliminary investigations had revealed Hb 100 g l⁻¹, MCV 79, LFTs, U&Es and TFTs were normal.

> J: SQs – *Elderly woman + chronic diarrhoea and weight loss + mild normocytic anaemia + background of psychiatric issues. Provisional diagnoses – malignancy or iatrogenic (drugs).*

PMH: IHD, hypothyroidism, hypercholesterolemia, previous ischemic stroke with residual right sided weakness and peripheral vascular disease (PVD). Medications: citalopram, aspirin, atorvastatin, thyroxine, lisinopril, and olanzapine.

What questions would you ask in the history?

> J: *Using the concept map (46.2b), the questions would primarily be aimed at discriminating inflammatory, watery or fatty stools (malabsorption).*

That is a good place to start, however, remember that patients do not follow textbooks. Some can have mild symptoms despite significant pathology. Distinguishing organic from inorganic causes of diarrhoea is important, and the concurrent weight loss lends credence to the organic nature of the problem in this case. Framing the questions in the context (working space) of vascular disease (IHD, stroke, PVD), autoimmune disease (thyroid disease) and medications in use would be particularly important.

What gastroenterological diagnoses could cause chronic diarrhoea with this background history?

Activity 49.1

(Allow two minutes)

....
....
....
....
....

- Vascular disease – mesenteric ischemia
- Autoimmune disease – coeliac disease
- Medications – iatrogenic diarrhoea
- Age – malignancy

The Hands-on Guide to Clinical Reasoning in Medicine, First Edition. Mujammil Irfan.
© 2019 John Wiley & Sons Ltd. Published 2019 by John Wiley & Sons Ltd.
Companion website: www.wiley.com/go/irfan/clinicalreasoning

Given the neuropsychiatric issues it was difficult to elicit a comprehensive history but the diarrhoea had been noticed since admission. She was reported to have limited mobility with significant dependence on activities of daily livings (ADLs). Nonetheless, the nurses reported that the stools were not greasy or malodourous but were semi-formed, intermittent with no blood or mucus. There were no suggestions of abdominal pain precipitated by meals (peptic ulcer disease, mesenteric ischemia), and no new medications had been started except olanzapine. No antibiotics received in last three months (Clostridium difficile).

O/E: Cachectic. Pulse 82 bpm, BP 140/90, Saturations 97% on air, RR 14 per minute, Temperature 36.8 °C, BMs 10. PA: soft, non-tender, no bruits or organomegaly. Rest of the systemic examination: normal, except residual right-sided weakness.

J: *Severity of illness – ill. I suspect the primary concern is GI malignancy. Since she is frail with co-morbidities, would you consider a faecal occult blood test?*

A screening test cannot be used as a diagnostic test. If the FOB is positive, it should prompt a colonoscopy which is not possible in our patient. Furthermore, FOB has not been validated in the setting of chronic diarrhoea.

The registrar requested iron studies along with vitamin B12 and folate, stool MC&S and coeliac serology, which reported iron saturation 15%, normal B12 and folate, positive tTG with normal IgA levels and negative stool MC&S. She was diagnosed with coeliac disease and a gluten free diet settled the diarrhoea and stabilised the weight loss and neuropsychiatric manifestations (Hu et al. 2006).

Can you explain the rationale behind the frugality of the tests requested?

Activity 49.2

(Allow a minute)

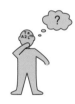

Knowledge perspective: the combination of anaemia, chronic diarrhoea, weight loss, co-existent autoimmune disease (hypothyroidism), and neuropsychiatric issues triggers the possibility of coeliac disease. This example illustrates that one should focus on the wider spectrum of disease presentation rather than the typical textbook descriptions. Discrepant data like normocytic anaemia is explained by causal reasoning based on sound pathophysiologic principles where the natural progression of iron deficiency anaemia follows the pattern of initially preserved haematological indices. Moreover, a combination of iron, vitamin B12 and folate deficiency can preserve the haematological indices which is quite possible in malabsorption states like coeliac disease.

Test decision perspective: Test decisions start with deciding on appropriate differential diagnoses in order to establish pre-test probability which dictates the order in which we test. We would then need to think of her overall status (patient factors) before we embark on invasive and expensive investigations. She is frail with significant co-morbidities and this along with her choices (or views of next of kin/best interests) will have a bearing on her management.

Amongst the differentials that we are considering, coeliac disease is the only pathology that is reversible. On the other hand, malignancy in our patient, would be very unlikely to be amenable to curative treatment. However, this should not detract from confirming the diagnosis since it would give us the prognosis helping the patient plan their next steps from a psychosocial perspective.

This thinking will then have to be balanced against the risks and accuracy of the test. Subjecting the patient to risky endoscopies with limited treatment opportunities may sway a patient to decide on conservative management focusing on quality of life.

Based on the above one could argue that the registrar went for what is more likely to be reversible.

Example 49.2

> A 42 year old lady from the Indian sub-continent presented to the hospital with a two month history of intermittent right lower quadrant abdominal pain associated with fatigue, weight loss of 7 kg and diarrhoea. PMH – non-smoker, hypertension, hypercholesterolemia. Medications – candesartan, atorvastatin.

> P: *SQs – middle aged Asian lady + chronic diarrhoea + weight loss + intermittent right iliac fossa (RIF) abdominal pain + vascular risk factors. Provisional diagnoses – inflammatory/ watery or malabsorption diarrhoea, infection, malignancy, chronic mesenteric ischemia.*

> She was born in the UK and had no significant travel history (infective enteritis) apart from visiting India annually, the most recent visit being a year ago. She reported semi-solid stools with no history of blood or mucus (inflammatory diarrhoea) or steatorrhea. No history of sexually transmitted disease, skin, joint, or eye disease (IBD). She gave a history of feeling hot and cold intermittently but denied night sweats. No personal or family history of TB and she had never smoked.
>
> O/E: Pulse 94 bpm, BP 110/80, Temperature 38 °C, Saturations 98% on air, RR 18 per minute and BMs 9. BCG scar on left arm; no lymphadenopathy. PA: RIF mass, mildly tender with no peritonism, ascites or organomegaly; PR: no evidence of perianal disease. Rest of the systemic examination: normal.

> P: *Severity of illness – ill. The pyrexia points to an inflammatory process. Clostridium difficile is a possibility although the RIF mass and weight loss goes against it.*

> Bloods: Hb 90 g l^{-1}, MCV 72 fl, WCC 11 × 10^9 l^{-1}, platelets 400 × 10^9 l^{-1}, CRP 80 mg l^{-1}, ESR 120 mm per hour., U&Es and LFTs: normal. The admitting team felt that the possibility of ileocecal TB was high and requested a CXR which was normal and an IGRA test which was positive.

Would you test further or treat her at this point?

Activity 49.3

(Allow a minute)

IGRA is intended to diagnose latent TB rather than active TB. The differential remains wide at this stage: ileocecal TB, Crohn's, infective colitis, malignancy (lymphoma) or inflammatory colitis with the treatment vastly differing. Hence further investigations are warranted given that she is relatively stable although ill.

Stool MC&S: negative. CT abdomen: asymmetric thickening of ileocecal region with proximal bowel dilatation, small volume pericecal lymphadenopathy and no ascites. Colonoscopy: diffusely inflamed mucosa with multiple deep ulcers in the ileocecal region with no rectal involvement. Histology confirmed granuloma formation in mucosal and submucosal regions with no acid-fast bacilli on ZN staining, mycobacterium tuberculosis (MTB) PCR was negative. Gram stain: negative (actinomycosis). No neoplastic cells were seen. Cultures were awaited. HIV, CMV serology: negative. The team felt this was TB and started antituberculous chemotherapy.

Given that the findings are non-discriminatory, how will you decide on treatment?

Activity 49.4

(Allow a minute)

Multiple authors have tried to come up with discriminatory features between these two conditions, but they do not occur consistently in all patients and especially not in combination to edge you to the diagnosis. Bayesian analysis can be used to quantify the probability of a particular diagnosis but again these models have not been validated in all populations (Limsrivilai et al. 2017).

The differentials of Crohn's and TB enteritis remain on the table. The delay of six weeks for the culture results is unacceptable since she is ill and not treating her would expose her to complications with their attendant morbidity and mortality. This often happens in medicine where the diagnosis can be a tie between two competing hypotheses. How do we decide on therapy at this juncture? If the treatment options for the two conditions are relatively safe we sometimes treat both at least initially e.g. frusemide and antibiotics for possible heart failure and CAP. However, this is not feasible in this instance as the treatment options are fairly toxic.

One way of embarking on therapy is to look at the risks of the two treatment approaches. Immunosuppressants for presumed Crohn's in the setting of TB would be disastrous but anti-TB therapy might subject the patient to disease progression with complications if it turns out to be Crohn's. If the culture results are negative in the latter scenario, it would be difficult to reason the cause of disease progression i.e. worsening Crohn's or drug-resistant TB? Furthermore, anti-TB therapy has its own side effects and risks of hepatitis.

We then weigh this against the pros and cons of further invasive investigations like laparoscopic resections which can give us insights into transmural involvement. Should we be subjecting our patient to these surgical risks?

Part of the answer lies in how clinicians deal with diagnostic uncertainty. Intolerance to diagnostic uncertainty makes clinicians over-investigate and over-diagnose. Clinicians tend to respond to it through an interplay of cognitive, emotional and ethical reactions (Alam et al. 2017). From a cognitive perspective, heuristics and intuitive reasoning based on stereotypes of gender, age or occupation are often used to minimise diagnostic uncertainty. It is possible that our patient's Indian background weighed in heavily in favour of TB. Attempts to achieve certainty in this way can precipitate premature closure leading to diagnostic errors.

On the ethical front, conveying this diagnostic uncertainty to patients is equally important since this influences shared-decision making. Several key strategies have been identified to manage uncertainty (Hewson et al. 1996; Griffiths et al. 2005). Those applicable to this scenario would be focusing on certainty for now based on current investigations results, providing evidence base for risks and benefits of management options and acknowledging uncertainty both in outcome and available evidence. Provisional decisions should be followed by appropriate safety netting (follow-up) with contingency planning if the initial tactic fails in collaboration with the patient. Patient expectations and tolerance to uncertainty will also have to be taken into account and a fine balance struck in deciding on the level of detail to communicate with the patient.

Culture results were negative for MTB. Anti-TB therapy was completed as per guidelines. One year later she re-presented with recurrent persistent symptoms and fistula formation. A right hemicolectomy confirmed a pathological diagnosis of Crohn's disease and she was started on immunosuppressants with a good result on follow-up.

▼

Always remain circumspect of patient factors when requesting tests.

Managing tolerance to diagnostic uncertainty will help in patient management.

▲

References

Alam, R., Cheraghi-Sohi, S., Panagioti, M. et al. (2017). Managing diagnostic uncertainty in primary care: a systematic critical review. *BMC Family Practice* 18 (1): 79.

Griffiths, F., Green, E., and Tsouroufli, M. (2005). The nature of medical evidence and its inherent uncertainty for the clinical consultation: qualitative study. *British Medical Journal (Clinical research ed.)* 330 (7490): 511.

Hewson, M.G., Kindy, P.J., Van Kirk, J. et al. (1996). Strategies for managing uncertainty and complexity. *Journal of General Internal Medicine* 11 (8): 481–485.

Hu, W.T., Murray, J.A., Greenaway, M.C. et al. (2006). Cognitive impairment and celiac disease. *Archives of Neurology* 63 (10): 1440–1446.

Limsrivilai, J., Shreiner, A.B., Pongpaibul, A. et al. (2017). Meta-analytic Bayesian model for differentiating intestinal tuberculosis from Crohn's disease. *The American Journal of Gastroenterology* 112 (3): 415–427.

50 Jaundice

▼

This chapter tells you how to approach jaundice, abdominal pain and distension from a gastroenterological perspective

▲

Example 50.1

A 56 year old man presented with bilateral shoulder pain over a week. PMH: Hypertension, diabetes mellitus type 2. Medications: candesartan, aspirin, rosuvastatin, glibenclamide, and sitagliptin.

> J: *SQs – middle aged man + acute bilateral shoulder pain + vascular risk factors. Provisional diagnoses – local causes like musculoskeletal problems but the bilateral nature makes them less likely, statin induced myopathy, c-spine compression is another possibility. I can't think of anything else.*

He reported an intense pain in his shoulders with difficulty in moving them. The statin was started ten years ago and had never given side effects. He was a current smoker of 40 py with occasional alcohol consumption of 10 units per week. He denied any systemic symptoms but complained of nausea and fatigue intermittently.

> J: *Severity of illness – ill. It could still be statin induced myopathy.*

That is true.

O/E: Pulse 86 bpm, BP 130/78, Temperature 37.8 °C, Saturations 98% on air, RR 14 per minute, BMs 12 mmol l⁻¹. PA: soft and non-tender, no ascites or organomegaly. Shoulders: tender and painful to move. Rest of the systemic examination: normal.

The examining registrar felt that this could be polymyalgia rheumatica and requested additional ESR and CRP. The consultant physician on call noted hyperesthesia in both shoulders and subtle weakness (4/5) of right shoulder abduction beyond 90°. There were no other features suggestive of cord compression. In particular there was no winging of the scapula. The history was re-visited. There was no significant trauma, travel history, exotic pets, blood transfusions, tattoos, over the counter medications including herbal supplements or risky sexual behaviour. No joint, skin symptoms (autoimmune). No family history of liver disease (α_1 antitrypsin deficiency, Wilson's). No red flag symptoms of malignancy were noted (paraneoplastic syndromes). An MRI brachial plexus, CK and LFTs were requested.

Activity 50.1

(Allow a minute)

Why did the consultant add LFTs to the bloods?

<table>
<tr><td>

</td></tr>
</table>

The Hands-on Guide to Clinical Reasoning in Medicine, First Edition. Mujammil Irfan.
© 2019 John Wiley & Sons Ltd. Published 2019 by John Wiley & Sons Ltd.
Companion website: www.wiley.com/go/irfan/clinicalreasoning

By ascribing a medical term (i.e. assigning a more specific SQ) to the constellation of clinical findings we can direct our mind in asking the right questions. Neuropathic pain + asymmetric shoulder weakness (axillary nerve involvement) gives us an SQ of brachial neuritis or neuralgic amyotrophy. Furthermore, the weakness makes polymyalgia rheumatica (PMR) less likely. We can only surmise that this combined with the knowledge of extrahepatic manifestations of viral hepatitis made the consultant add LFTs to the bloods and review the risk factors for liver disease. Note that other causes of inflammatory neuritis were also explored (malignancy, autoimmune, and drugs).

Bloods: Hb 120 g l⁻¹, platelets 350 × 10⁹ l⁻¹, WCC 14 × 10⁹ l⁻¹, CRP 40 mg l⁻¹, ESR 60 mm per hour., albumin 32 g l⁻¹, ALT 1000 IU l⁻¹, ALP 250 IU l⁻¹, bilirubin 35 μmol l⁻¹, PT 16 seconds, CK 100 IU l⁻¹, U&Es: normal. Rest of the clotting profile, CXR and ECG: normal. In hindsight the sclerae were noted to be icteric. There were no features of encephalopathy. The statin was withheld.

Viral hepatitis serology (A, B, C, and E), HIV, syphilis, cytomegalovirus, EBV, parvovirus B 19, lyme serology, autoimmune screen and stool hepatitis E RNA was requested. Hepatitis E IgG, IgM and stool RNA were positive, and the rest were negative. MRI brachial plexus: normal. EMG revealed denervation of axillary nerve supporting the diagnosis of neuralgic amyotrophy secondary to hepatitis E.

Supportive care with physiotherapy alleviated the symptoms. On follow up he was found to have no residual symptoms in 6 months.

This example highlights the importance of a detailed clinical examination. Pain can often limit neurological examination but careful examination to discriminate this from objective muscle weakness is essential to avoid missing the diagnosis. The use of SQs in generating the right hypotheses is also well illustrated. Hepatitis E in the western world presents more commonly with extrahepatic features and a higher index of suspicion is required in pregnant and immunosuppressed populations (e.g. HIV, diabetes mellitus) (Cheung et al. n.d.; Dartevel et al. 2015).

Example 50.2

A 65 year old man with known alcoholic cirrhosis presents with worsening jaundice and abdominal swelling. PMH: hypertension, diabetes mellitus, OA. Medications: aspirin, atorvastatin, ramipril, gliclazide, co-codamol.

P: *SQs – Middle aged man + alcoholic cirrhosis + ascites (decompensated cirrhosis) on a background of vascular risk factors and OA. Provisional diagnoses – infection, upper GI bleeding, drugs, alcohol excess precipitating decompensated cirrhosis.*

He reported worsening abdominal swelling and breathlessness over three weeks and that his friends had pointed out yellowing of his skin. He had been diagnosed with alcoholic cirrhosis five years ago and had remained stable until recently. He confirmed complete abstinence from alcohol over the last year. He denied any haematemesis, melaena or infective symptoms. No significant travel, pets, over the counter medications, risky lifestyle.

P: *There are no obvious precipitating factors for the decompensation.*

The admitting SHO documented the examination as: pulse 110 bpm, BP 96/80, saturations 96% on air, RR 22 per minute, temperature 37.5 °C, BMs 9 mmol l⁻¹. Cachectic with tattoos over left arm, no intravenous injection marks. Icteric. PA: non-tender, distended abdomen with shifting dullness – moderate ascites, multiple spider naevi on chest, no distended veins. No signs of hepatic encephalopathy. Bilateral pitting oedema up to the knees. Rest of the systemic examination: normal.

P: severity of illness – ill.

Bloods: Hb 130 g l⁻¹, MCV 104 fl, WCC 15 × 10⁹ l⁻¹, platelets 100 × 10⁹ l⁻¹, CRP 40 mg l⁻¹, Na⁺ 130 mmol l⁻¹, K⁺ 3 mmol l⁻¹, urea 5 mmol l⁻¹, creatinine 80 μmol l⁻¹, albumin 30 g l⁻¹, ALT 60 IU l⁻¹, AST 55 IU l⁻¹, bilirubin 40 μmol l⁻¹, ALP 100 IU l⁻¹, PT 14 seconds, aPTT 38 seconds, fibrinogen 1.5 g l⁻¹.

The SHO diagnosed decompensated alcoholic cirrhosis secondary to worsening liver disease.

How would you interpret the bloods?

Activity 50.2

(Allow 3 minutes)

....

....

....

....

....

He has macrocytosis with thrombocytopenia. The LFTs show hyperbilirubinaemia with mildly elevated transaminases, a low albumin and hypofibrinogenaemia. The thrombocytopenia suggests hypersplenism potentially secondary to portal hypertension given the ascites. U&Es show hyponatraemia and hypokalaemia with a low urea in keeping with cirrhotic pathophysiology. The low grade CRP with the mild leukocytosis should prompt a search for infection (e.g. SBP) although this could just be a stress response.

A diagnostic ascitic tap revealed clear fluid and treatment for SBP was withheld for the time-being. Urine and blood cultures were sent. Urine dipstick: protein+, no blood or nitrites. CXR: evidence of mild pulmonary congestion with bibasal atelectasis, heart size could not be assessed as it was an anter-posterior film. ECG: atrial ectopics, HR 110 bpm. Spironolactone was started and daily weights and U&Es monitored. Ramipril was stopped as low BP in cirrhosis decreases survival rates (Llach et al. 1988).

Would you have withheld antibiotics?

P: The lack of pyrexia or signs of hepatic encephalopathy with a non-tender abdomen makes SBP less likely.

The low BP with a low-grade CRP and leukocytosis should be borne in mind and the patient closely followed if you elect not to give antibiotics.

Day 2: Ascitic fluid: protein 28 g l⁻¹, albumin 16 g l⁻¹, glucose 5 mmol l⁻¹, PMN < 250 cells/mm³. On the consultant ward round, the patient lamented that his breathlessness had prevented him from doing anything at home making him bed bound. On revisiting the history, orthopnea and paroxysmal nocturnal dyspnoea were noted. O/E: JVP was elevated. Although the serum: ascites albumin gradient (SAAG) was >11 g l⁻¹, the fluid protein was noted to be >25 g l⁻¹, in keeping with cardiac ascites.

Echo confirmed LV systolic dysfunction with an EF of 30% and alcoholic cardiomyopathy was diagnosed. In light of the GGT being 150 IU l⁻¹ the patient admitted to ongoing alcohol excess. He was strongly advised abstinence as this was the single most important intervention that could reverse the heart failure (Masani et al. 1990). Ascitic fluid culture was negative. On follow up in six months the EF had improved to 45% with resolution of breathlessness.

Why do you think the diagnosis was missed on admission?

Activity 50.3

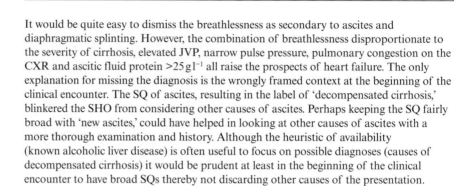

(Allow a minute)

It would be quite easy to dismiss the breathlessness as secondary to ascites and diaphragmatic splinting. However, the combination of breathlessness disproportionate to the severity of cirrhosis, elevated JVP, narrow pulse pressure, pulmonary congestion on the CXR and ascitic fluid protein $>25\,\mathrm{g\,l^{-1}}$ all raise the prospects of heart failure. The only explanation for missing the diagnosis is the wrongly framed context at the beginning of the clinical encounter. The SQ of ascites, resulting in the label of 'decompensated cirrhosis,' blinkered the SHO from considering other causes of ascites. Perhaps keeping the SQ fairly broad with 'new ascites,' could have helped in looking at other causes of ascites with a more thorough examination and history. Although the heuristic of availability (known alcoholic liver disease) is often useful to focus on possible diagnoses (causes of decompensated cirrhosis) it would be prudent at least in the beginning of the clinical encounter to have broad SQs thereby not discarding other causes of the presentation.

▼
Using specific medical terms as SQs will help in formulating the right hypothesis.

Framing a broad context helps in asking the right questions in the initial phases of the patient encounter.
▲

References

Cheung, M.C.M., Maguire., J., Carey, I. et al. (n.d.). Review of the neurological manifestations of hepatitis E infection. *Annals of Hepatology* 11 (5): 618–622.

Dartevel, A., Colombe, B., Bosseray, A. et al. (2015). Hepatitis E and neuralgic amyotrophy: five cases and review of literature. *Journal of Clinical Virology* 69: 156–164.

Llach, J., Ginès, P., Arroyo, V. et al. (1988). Prognostic value of arterial pressure, endogenous vasoactive systems, and renal function in cirrhotic patients admitted to the hospital for the treatment of ascites. *Gastroenterology* 94 (2): 482–487.

Masani, F., Kato, H., Sasagawa, Y. et al. (1990). An echocardiographic study of alcoholic cardiomyopathy after total abstinence. *Journal of Cardiology* 20 (3): 627–634.

▼

This chapter tells you how to approach haematemesis and melaena from a gastroenterological perspective

▲

Example 51.1

A 65 year old man was admitted with ascites and decompensated alcoholic liver disease. On day 3 of admission he had a 'coffee ground vomitus'. The nurse was concerned about a possible upper gastrointestinal bleed (UGIB) and used a urine dipstick to test the vomitus for blood which was positive. The on-call Senior House Officer (SHO) was asked to review the patient.

P: SQs – *middle aged man + decompensated alcoholic liver disease (ALD) + ascites + new coffee ground vomitus positive for blood. Provisional diagnoses – UGIB from varices, peptic ulcer disease.*

Urine dipstick uses peroxidases found in erythrocytes in the urine to oxidise reduced colourless phenolphthalein to purple phenolphthalein. Gastric peroxidases present in the vomitus can also do this thereby giving a false positive result. In other words, this is the wrong test to use for UGIB. However, given the background we will have to keep an open mind whilst assessing the patient.

The SHO dismissed the possibility of UGIB given that it was based on a positive urine dipstick result. The patient reported nausea and abdominal discomfort and had opened his bowels earlier in the day. He denied any melaena. No past history of UGIB or varices was noted.

O/E: NEWS 4, Pulse 120 bpm, BP 96/70, RR 16 per minute, Saturations 96% on air, Temperature 36.6 °C, BMs 7 mmol l⁻¹. Baseline observations over the last 48 hours: HR ranged from 90–100 bpm and the systolic blood pressure between 110–120 mm of Hg. Slightly confused but alert. Tattoos on left arm, spider naevi on the chest and muscle wasting in the limbs were noted. PA: Mildly distended with shifting dullness, caput medusae with flow away from umbilicus, non-tender and no organomegaly. Bowel sounds heard. Per rectal (PR): no melaena or masses. Rest of the systemic examination: normal. He initiated IV fluids to maintain the BP.

P: *Severity of illness – ill, provisional diagnosis – possible UGIB, decompensated ALD with signs of portal hypertension (ascites, caput medusae).*

Four hours later

Bloods: Hb 80 g l⁻¹, MCV 110 fl, platelets 120 × 10⁹ l⁻¹, WCC 14 × 10⁹ l⁻¹, Hct 0.3, PT 15 seconds, aPTT 40 seconds, fibrinogen 1 g l⁻¹, CRP 40 mg l⁻¹, albumin 26 g l⁻¹, ALP 200 IU l⁻¹, ALT 70 IU l⁻¹, bilirubin 50 μmol l⁻¹, Na⁺ 130 mmol l⁻¹, K⁺ 3.3 mmol l⁻¹, urea 7 mmol l⁻¹, creatinine 120 μmol l⁻¹. Previous bloods from day 1: Hb 100 g l⁻¹, MCV 110 fl, platelets 126 × 10⁹ l⁻¹, WCC 13 × 10⁹ l⁻¹, Hct 0.4, PT 18 seconds, aPTT 50 seconds, fibrinogen 1.5 g l⁻¹, albumin 28 g l⁻¹, ALP 225 IU l⁻¹, ALT 80 IU l⁻¹, bilirubin 60 μmol l⁻¹, Na⁺ 133 mmol l⁻¹, K⁺ 2.7 mmol l⁻¹, urea 6 mmol l⁻¹, creatinine 130 μmol l⁻¹ (baseline creatinine six months ago 90 μmol l⁻¹).

The Hands-on Guide to Clinical Reasoning in Medicine, First Edition. Mujammil Irfan.
© 2019 John Wiley & Sons Ltd. Published 2019 by John Wiley & Sons Ltd.
Companion website: www.wiley.com/go/irfan/clinicalreasoning

How would you interpret the bloods?

Activity 51.1

(Allow three minutes)

....
....
....
....
....

P: *Coagulopathy and macrocytic anaemia with a drop in Hb and HCT, thrombocytopenia, resolving mixed LFT derangement with electrolyte disturbances (↓Na+, ↓K+) and AKI.*

Next morning

The nurse queried whether he needed a blood transfusion but the SHO attributed the marginal drop in Hb to haemodilution following IV fluids he had received over the last 48 hours to correct the potassium and hypotension (note the low Hct).

The nurses informed the team on arrival that the patient was feeling dizzy and appeared more confused. On assessment the patient looked very ill and upon reviewing the observation chart it was clearly evident that there was a marked decline in the observations over the last 24 hours. Upper limbs: cool to touch from the elbow down. PA: diffusely tender. Repeat PR: fresh blood and clots. Aggressive fluid management and red cell transfusion was initiated whilst waiting for repeat blood tests.

How would you manage fluid balance in this scenario?

P: *Stat fluids?*

It is very likely that our patient has underlying oesophageal varices. Aggressive IV fluids can increase portal pressures potentiating further bleeding. Hence bolus fluids to maintain MAP whilst monitoring renal perfusion with urine output (UOP) would be a simple way forward.

He was given IV vitamin K (PT 15 seconds), IV antibiotics (ascites, confusion, abdominal tenderness = possible SBP, prophylaxis in variceal bleeding), terlipressin (portal hypertension, possible variceal haemorrhage) and PPI. He continued passing clots PR and was therefore given cryoprecipitate (less volume and low fibrinogen levels). Following haemodynamic stabilisation, an urgent endoscopy revealed bleeding oesophageal varices which were banded. A diagnostic ascitic tap performed when the patient was stable was negative.

Why do you think the overnight doctor missed the bleed?

Activity 51.2

(Allow a minute)

The on-call doctor exhibited 'premature closure' when he dismissed the possibility of UGIB because it was based on the faulty premise of a positive dipstick test. However, the background history of decompensated ALD should have alerted him to the possibility of variceal haemorrhage especially in the setting of deranged physiological observations although the NEWS was only 4.

In the setting of shock (hypovolaemia, sepsis, etc.), the trend of the observations is more important than a single reading. NEWS are only as useful as we make them to be. They cannot replace clinical judgement but instead should trigger a more thorough assessment. Secondly, restrictive transfusion policy of transfusing only when the Hb is <70 g l⁻¹ is not applicable in the setting of underlying co-morbidities like coronary artery disease, stroke or massive haemorrhage (Jairath et al. 2015). Physiological instability outweighs laboratory results since there can be a delay in the drop of Hb following a large bleed. It is important to recognise the limitations of scoring systems and clinical guidelines and use judgement where necessary to deviate from protocols.

Lastly, the preserved urea: creatinine ratio of <100 : 1 despite an UGIB can be explained by the chronic liver disease which affects urea metabolism with the cachexia contributing to the reduced creatinine levels (Mortensen et al. 1994).

Example 51.2

> A 75 year old lady was referred by the GP with iron deficiency anaemia and weight loss. PMH: depression, hypertension, osteoporosis. Medications: citalopram, atenolol.

J: *SQs – elderly lady + iron deficiency anaemia and weight loss + history of depression and hypertension. Provisional diagnoses – wide differential including GI malignancy, other malignancies, peptic ulcer disease.*

I see that you are limiting yourself to gastroenterology since we are on that placement. Always cast a wider net – other possibilities include endocrinopathies, malabsorption, chronic inflammatory conditions like rheumatoid arthritis (normocytic anaemia), chronic infections like human immunodeficiency virus (HIV), chronic system-wide diseases like COPD and drugs.

J: *Can depression cause this picture?*

It certainly is a possibility.

What questions would you ask her?

Activity 51.3

(Allow three minutes)

....

....

....

....

....

J: *I would start with the weight loss, its duration and associated symptoms especially related to the gastrointestinal tract.*

> She was recently bereaved following her husband's death six months ago and was started on citalopram two months ago for symptoms of depression. She had complained of persistent fatigue and loss of appetite when her GP discovered that she had microcytic anaemia and weight loss of 10 kg over the last six months. On specific questioning she reported dysphagia to solids and liquids over the last two months. She denied any blood, mucus or black stools per-rectally. There were no other red flag symptoms. She felt that the citalopram had improved her low mood.
>
> Bloods done by GP: Hb 90 g l⁻¹, MCV 70 fl, platelets 300 × 10⁹ l⁻¹, WCC 11 × 10⁹ l⁻¹, ESR 70 mm per hour, TFTs, U&Es and LFTs: normal.

Red flag symptoms for malignancy

- Haemoptysis
- Haematemesis, bowel habit changes, PR bleed
- Haematuria
- Generalised lymphadenopathy, B symptoms (night sweats, itching) for lymphoma
- Breast masses
- Non-physiological per vaginal bleed or discharge in women and
- Hesitancy/frequency of urination in men.

J: *Severity of illness – ill. She has an elevated ESR for her age and with her microcytic anaemia, would you consider multiple myeloma?*

Certainly!

J: *I would enquire about bone pains and symptoms of hypercalcaemia. Coeliac disease is another possibility.*

I think we should re-frame the SQs.

J: *Revised SQs – elderly lady + microcytic anaemia + weight loss + dysphagia + background of depression, hypertension and osteoporosis. Provisional diagnoses – oesophageal carcinoma is very likely.*

The registrar noticed osteoporosis on the GP referral letter and asked the patient whether she was on any medications that she took once a week or any injectables once a month or so. She admitted that she was on something starting with 'A' and nodded when prompted with alendronate. She had been on it for the past three months.

O/E: Pulse 78 bpm, BP 130/70, RR 18 per minute, Saturations 97% on air, Temperature 36.6 °C and BMs 8 mmol l⁻¹. No signs of hyperthyroidism or lymphadenopathy. Systemic examination: normal. PR: normal.

J: *Could it still be dietary given the recent bereavement? Perhaps we should ask about her diet, but malignancy would certainly remain on the cards.*

The registrar picked up on the temporal association of alendronate with the dysphagia and advised the patient of its side effects including oesophageal inflammation and ulceration which could account for her presentation. She was advised to stop alendronate for the time-being and started on a PPI. She was discharged with gastroenterology follow-up, an out-patient OGD and CT abdomen and pelvis.

She was found to have alendronate induced oesophageal ulceration and appropriate treatment was initiated. Alternative IV bisphosphonate therapy was arranged when her clinical condition improved.

Why do you think Jenny got side-tracked by the raised ESR?

Activity 51.4

(Allow a minute)

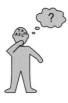

Pattern recognition distracted Jenny with the raised ESR, microcytic anaemia and weight loss prompting the diagnostic hypothesis of myeloma. Sub-consciously our brain can focus on selective data that confirms our suspicions (confirmation bias) (Croskerry 2002). We inadvertently miss other pertinent data like dysphagia and get side-tracked.

We also see how significant information can be lost in referral letters (obviously not on purpose). We must develop skills to decipher PMH from medications and vice-versa although this cannot be assumed to be accurate and will require subsequent confirmation.

▼

Understand the limitations of scoring systems and guidelines and learn when to over-ride them.

Pausing to re-frame the SQs can help avoid succumbing to confirmation bias derived from pattern recognition.

▲

References

Croskerry, P. (2002). Achieving quality in clinical decision making: cognitive strategies and detection of bias. *Academic Emergency Medicine: Official Journal of the Society for Academic Emergency Medicine* 9 (11): 1184–1204.

Jairath, V., Kahan, B.C., Gray, A. et al. (2015). Restrictive versus liberal blood transfusion for acute upper gastrointestinal bleeding (TRIGGER): a pragmatic, open-label, cluster randomised feasibility trial. *The Lancet* 386 (9989): 137–144.

Mortensen, P.B., Nøhr, M., Møller-Petersen, J.F., and Balslev, I. (1994). The diagnostic value of serum urea/creatinine ratio in distinguishing between upper and lower gastrointestinal bleeding. A prospective study. *Danish Medical Bulletin* 41 (2): 237–240.

52 Abdominal Pain

▼
This chapter tells you how to approach abdominal pain from a gastroenterological perspective
▲

Example 52.1

A 37 year old lady attended A&E with a three day history of left iliac fossa (LIF) pain on a background of Crohn's disease. She was referred by A&E as exacerbation of Crohn's.

P: SQs – Young lady + acute LIF pain + history of Crohn's colitis. Provisional diagnoses – Crohn's exacerbation, ectopic pregnancy, constipation, diverticulitis, infective colitis.

She was treated with IV fluids and co-codamol for the pain in A&E. Bloods: Hb 130 g l⁻¹, platelets 300 × 10⁹ l⁻¹, WCC 15 × 10⁹ l⁻¹, CRP pending, Clotting profile: normal, U&Es and LFTs: normal.

On review by the medical team she was noted to be on depot medroxyprogesterone acetate. The pain was initially intermittent but last evening it worsened and became constant. When questioned further about the characteristics of the pain she reported that the pain radiated to the back on the left. It occurred in waves and was associated with nausea and vomiting. She declined a pregnancy test. The pain had slightly improved with the co-codamol but her oral intake was poor owing to the nausea.

P: Severity of illness – ill. Revised SQs – Young lady + acute LIF colicky pain + nausea and vomiting + history of Crohn's on progestin only contraception. Provisional diagnoses – bowel obstruction secondary to Crohn's stricture.

What further questions would you ask to refine the hypotheses?

Activity 52.1

(Allow a minute)

P: Symptoms pertaining to Crohn's exacerbation and bowel obstruction.

I agree, but I would like to point out that the LIF colicky pain with radiation to the back associated with nausea and vomiting raises the possibility of renal colic which could be due to a calculus, infection or clot colic (tumour or gross haematuria). In view of this, further questions pertaining to urinary tract like dysuria, haematuria, frequency, previous renal stones, systemic symptoms including fever should also be explored.

The Hands-on Guide to Clinical Reasoning in Medicine, First Edition. Mujammil Irfan.
© 2019 John Wiley & Sons Ltd. Published 2019 by John Wiley & Sons Ltd.
Companion website: www.wiley.com/go/irfan/clinicalreasoning

She denied any dysuria, previous renal stones or infective symptoms. The Crohn's colitis had remained stable over the last five years with no exacerbations. There were no bowel symptoms in keeping with Crohn's exacerbation.

O/E: Pulse 88 bpm, BP 130/80, RR 18 per minute, Temperature 37.3 °C, Saturations 96% on air, BMs 9 mmol l⁻¹. PA: soft and non-tender, mild left renal angle tenderness but no organomegaly. PR: declined by patient. Rest of the systemic examination: normal.

The admitting registrar requested a urine dipstick for haematuria and an AXR which showed blood 3+ and no obvious urinary tract stones respectively; CRP 20 mg l⁻¹. Following consultation with Urologists, a CT urinary tract was requested, which showed left hydronephrosis and hydroureter with a left ureteric stone. She was referred to the urologists for further management.

What enabled the medical registrar to circumvent the A&E diagnosis of exacerbation of Crohn's?

Activity 52.2

(Allow a minute)

Discrepant data including normal temperature, lack of bowel symptoms consistent with exacerbation of colitis, no recent exacerbations and normal platelet count and fibrinogen (acute phase reactants) made the medical registrar question the A&E diagnosis. He used the unpacking principle to good effect where directed questions aimed at characterising the pain and its location enabled him to entertain other diagnoses.

System factors like busy A&E department, frequent interruptions and competing demands on the attending physicians adding to the cognitive load can contribute to short-cuts taken towards making a quick diagnosis. Unfortunately, Peter here fell into the trap of anchoring and confirmation bias despite evidence to the contrary, something which we should be wary of - having an open mind without preconceptions helps in arriving at the right diagnosis.

Example 52.2

A 72 year old man walked into A&E with a two day history of persistent abdominal pain and an episode of black stools. PMH: HT, DM, hypercholesterolemia. Medications: losartan, aspirin, glibenclamide, atorvastatin, and atenolol.

> J:　SQs – elderly man + acute abdominal pain + vascular risk factors. Provisional
> diagnoses – wide differential, peptic ulcer disease (PUD), GI malignancy to start with.

Two days ago he developed non-specific abdominal pain followed by an episode of melaena which did not recur since. He reported an episode of light headedness a day before when he briefly lost consciousness but denied any nausea/vomiting, weight loss or other red flag symptoms. No similar episodes in the past. No use of NSAIDs, bisphos-phonates or steroids. No GI infective symptoms.

O/E: Pulse 110 bpm, BP 150/94, Saturations 95% on air, RR 18 per minute, Temperature 37.6 °C, BMs 13. PA: soft, non-tender, no signs of peritonism, bowel sounds heard; PR: normal. The rest of the systemic examination: normal.

J: *Severity of illness – ill. Revised SQs – Acute non-specific abdominal pain + melaena + possible syncope + vascular risk factors. Provisional diagnoses – likely UGIB with syncope. Still thinking of PUD.*

Bloods: Hb 110 g l^{-1}, WCC 13 × 10^9 l^{-1}, platelets 250 × 10^9 l^{-1}; clotting profile: normal; Na$^+$ 137 mmol l^{-1}, K$^+$ 4 mmol l^{-1}, urea 9 mmol l^{-1}, creatinine 130 μmol l^{-1}, LFTs: normal, CRP 18 mg l^{-1}. Erect CXR no free air under the diaphragm. AXR: normal. ECG: sinus tachycardia, non-specific ST/T wave changes which were ascribed to long-standing hypertension.

He was admitted for observation with a working diagnosis of bleeding PUD. Losartan and aspirin were withheld. He was made nil by mouth, started on a PPI and analgesia and an in-patient OGD was requested.

J: *Was an AXR indicated in this instance?*

Not really, it is a low yield investigation given the presentation.

Day 2

He developed more severe abdominal pain with hypotension (110/80) and tachycardia (100 bpm) but the examination remained non-specific. No further melaena was reported. IV fluids were started, antihypertensives withheld and repeat bloods sent. The same evening, the on-call doctor was called to see him for a possible stroke. O/E: There was dense left hemiparesis with left homonymous hemianopia. An urgent CT head showed cerebral infarction in the right internal carotid artery territory. Thrombolysis was discussed but on balance felt to be too risky given the recent GI bleed. Clopidogrel was withheld for the same reasons.

ECG: similar to previous. Repeat bloods: Hb 100 g l^{-1}, WCC 15 × 10^9 l^{-1}, platelets 230 × 10^9 l^{-1}, Na$^+$ 138 mmol l^{-1}, K$^+$ 3.8 mmol l^{-1}, urea 8 mmol l^{-1}, creatinine 140 μmol l^{-1}, LFTs: normal, CRP 26 mg l^{-1}. IV fluids were continued.

J: *That was an unfortunate turn of events. Do you think that stopping aspirin precipitated a stroke?*

Not necessarily, it could just be coincidence.

Day 3

He continued to deteriorate with persistent hypotension and dropped his saturations to 84% on air. O/E: Pulse 120 bpm, BP 90/70, RR 24 per minute, apyrexial. Respiratory system (RS): reduced breath sounds on left with few crackles. CXR: bi-basal atelectasis with small left pleural effusion. He arrested shortly after and died following an unsuccessful resuscitation attempt. An autopsy revealed aortic dissection as the cause of death.

How would you synthesise the findings thus far?

Activity 52.3

(Allow three minutes)

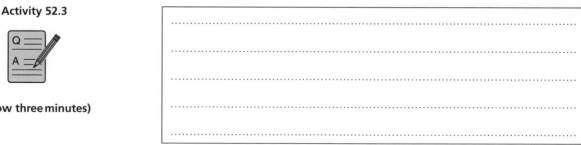

J: *SQs – acute abdominal pain and one off melaena + acute neurological deficit + AKI + persistent hypotension and tachycardia + desaturation. Working diagnosis – the findings are very disconnected; I'm not sure how I can put them together.*

You've done a good job so far. Although the findings are seemingly disconnected the key is to always go back to how we validate a diagnosis. A valid diagnosis needs to be coherent, adequate, and parsimonious (Kassirer and Gorry 1978). A working diagnosis of UGIB and stroke cannot explain all the findings especially in the absence of an ongoing active bleed.

Discrepant data where a presumed UGIB co-exists with hypertension and AKI in someone with vascular risk factors should trigger an alternative hypothesis. The subsequent stroke and desaturation with left pleural effusion with the persistent hypotension and abdominal pain could well be connected to the initial presentation. It is of course, easy to be glib about the diagnosis with hindsight bias but in the heat of the moment how do we string the data together?

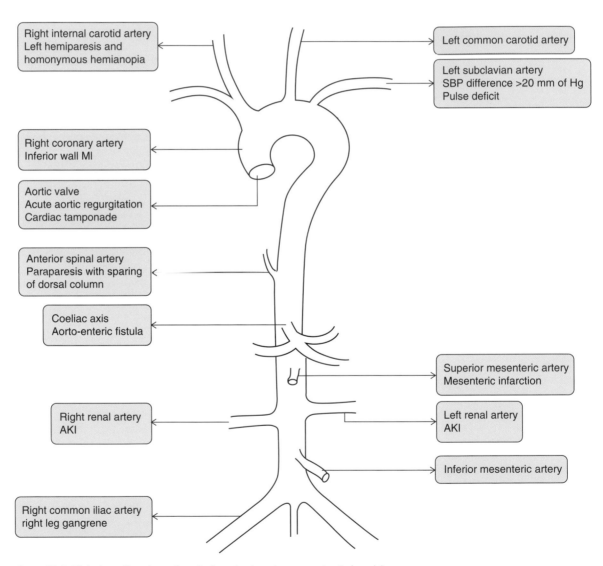

Figure 52.1 Clinical manifestations of aortic dissection based on an anatomical model

Research has shown that a combination of non-analytical and analytical reasoning can help clinicians overcome misdiagnosis (Eva et al. 2007). Re-framing the SQs brings non-analytical reasoning into the fore where heuristics are employed to decipher a working diagnosis. Since we have failed to satisfy the three elements of a 'valid diagnosis,' we can employ a pathophysiological model of causal reasoning (analytical) to do the same. Thinking broadly, one anatomical structure that traverses the neurological, abdominal (gut), renal and cardiovascular territories is the aorta. Aortic dissection can explain all the clinical manifestations seen in this example as shown in Figure 52.1. This principle should be used in all patient encounters and not just the difficult scenarios.

Clinical findings that are commonly found in patients with aortic dissection in whom the right diagnosis is missed include: perceived mildness of presentation, e.g. patient walking into A&E, clinical and laboratory findings mimicking another disease, e.g. ACS and lack of typical symptoms and findings, e.g. widened mediastinum on CXR (Kurabayashi et al. 2011).

▼
We can avoid anchoring by searching for discrepant data between the ascribed diagnosis and the clinical findings.

A combination of non-analytical and analytical reasoning can help overcome misdiagnosis.
▲

References

Eva, K.W. Hatala, R.M., Leblanc, V.R. and, Brooks, L.R. 2007. Teaching from the clinical reasoning literature: combined reasoning strategies help novice diagnosticians overcome misleading information. *Medical Education* 41(12), pp. 1152–8.

Kassirer, J.P. and Gorry, G.A. (1978). Clinical problem solving: a behavioral analysis. *Annals of Internal Medicine* 89 (2): 245–255.

Kurabayashi, M., Miwa, N., Ueshima, D. et al. (2011). Factors leading to failure to diagnose acute aortic dissection in the emergency room. *Journal of Cardiology* 58 (3): 287–293.

53 History Taking: My Joints Hurt

The Hands-on Guide to Clinical Reasoning in Medicine, First Edition. Mujammil Irfan.
© 2019 John Wiley & Sons Ltd. Published 2019 by John Wiley & Sons Ltd.
Companion website: www.wiley.com/go/irfan/clinicalreasoning

▼

This chapter focuses on history taking from a Rheumatological perspective integrated within the systems review

▲

Rheumatological diseases can be broadly considered under the following headings:

- Musculoskeletal diseases: muscle – e.g. polymyalgia rheumatica and polymyositis. Skeletal – e.g. monoarthritis, oligoarthritis and polyarthritis presentations.
- Systemic inflammatory diseases involving multiple organ systems – e.g. connective tissue disorders (CTDs).
- Regional and diffuse pain syndromes – soft tissue and myofascial pain syndromes, e.g. back pain, fibromyalgia.

General principles of rheumatological evaluation

1. Most rheumatological diagnoses rely on their phenotypic expressions. Hence pattern recognition narrows down the differential but the diagnosis rests on history, clinical examination and laboratory criteria together with disease evolution over time.
2. Often clinical presentations do not neatly fit into a specific rheumatological condition. In fact, half of autoimmune rheumatic disease presentations are termed 'undifferentiated' with some of them resolving spontaneously over time, some evolving into a recognisable entity that can be treated and the majority remaining undifferentiated with generally a good prognosis (Goldblatt and O'Neill 2013). Hence, a balance should be struck between giving potent therapy with side effects against giving time for the disease to evolve with a possible risk of joint destruction. A lot of this depends on the severity of illness and its impact on the functional status from the patient's perspective.
3. There is significant overlap between seemingly distinct clinical entities. For instance, psoriatic arthritis can present with features in keeping with rheumatoid arthritis or spondyloarthritis. Treatment is directed at the dominant phenotype in overlap syndromes.
4. Most rheumatological conditions are chronic in nature requiring long-term treatment with significant side effects which one needs to be aware of e.g. infection with immunosuppressants.
5. Older adults are often affected by musculoskeletal diseases that impact ADLs with resultant loss of independence in the later stages of life. Hence screening questions should always be part of the systems review.
6. More than one rheumatological disease can occur in the same patient, e.g. septic arthritis in a patient with pre-existing rheumatoid arthritis. It takes a high index of suspicion to diagnose this which implies that premature closure of hypotheses is to be avoided.

Figure 53.1 shows a concept map that gives a broad overview of how to take a history in rheumatology. Personalise the concept map to yourself by adding any other facts that you might learn in this chapter or on your placement.

The GALS (Gait, Arms, Legs, and Spine) screen is a useful strategy to identify a musculoskeletal problem (Doherty et al. 1992). The first three screening questions in GALS should be incorporated into the systems review of history taking as a routine:

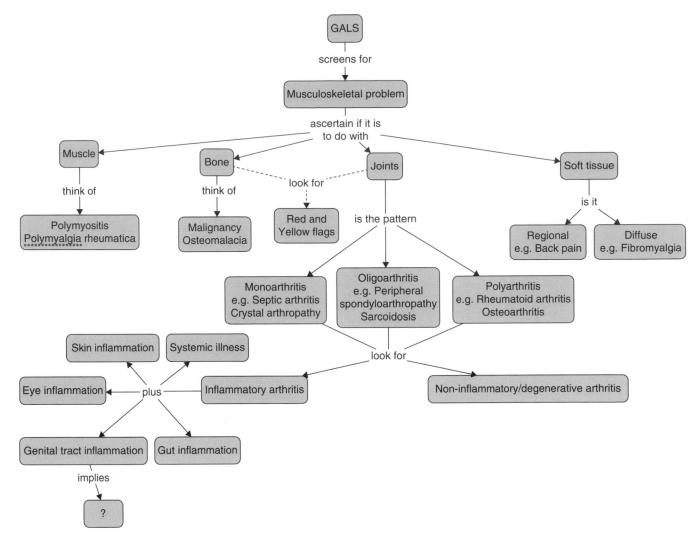

Figure 53.1 History taking in Rheumatology

'Do you suffer from any pain or stiffness in your muscles, joints or back?'

'Do you have any difficulty in dressing yourself?'

'Do you have any difficulty in walking up and down the stairs?' } Functional impact

Once a problem has been identified, the next step is to clarify if it is a problem with the muscles, bones, joints or soft tissues, e.g. rotator cuff injury of the shoulder joint can present with referred pain at the deltoid insertion mimicking bone or muscle pain.

Pain, stiffness, swelling, and loss of function are the most common symptoms that musculoskeletal problems present with. As with history taking in general, the past medical history (previous uveitis, preceding diarrhoea – reactive arthritis), drugs (loop diuretics – gout) and psychosocial history including recreational drugs (IV drugs – septic arthritis), travel (Lyme's), sexual history (urethritis – reactive arthritis), and the impact of the symptoms on their functional status need to be ascertained.

Joint pain will have to be characterised by the pattern of involvement i.e. mono (single), oligo (up to 5 joints) or polyarthritis (>5 joints). Again, the patient may present with a single joint complaint, but the history and examination might pick up that several joints are swollen making it polyarticular. Premature closure is to be avoided at all costs.

The next step is to differentiate inflammatory arthritis from non-inflammatory/ degenerative arthritis by recalling the five signs of inflammation: pain – worse with rest, e.g. worse in the morning with stiffness lasting >one hour implies inflammatory whereas worse on movement implies degenerative. Other inflammatory signs like swelling (synovial thickening or joint effusion), heat, redness, and loss of function and marked improvement with NSAIDs also imply inflammatory arthritis. Pain lasting all day and at rest implies chronic pain.

Once inflammatory arthritis is identified concurrent features should be looked for. For example, inflammatory arthritis plus:

- Systemic illness → rheumatoid arthritis, HIV, sepsis or CTDs.
- Oral, nasal, genital ulcers + Raynaud's, sicca symptoms and serositis → CTD.
- Concurrent or preceding gut inflammation → enteropathic arthritis, e.g. inflammatory bowel disease, celiac disease.
- Skin inflammation → sarcoidosis, reactive arthritis, psoriatic arthritis.
- Eye inflammation → rheumatoid arthritis, spondyloarthritis.

Associated red and yellow flags should always be elicited as part of any musculoskeletal problem especially bone and joint disease. Red flag symptoms include weight loss, fever, neurological deficits (with back pain), scalp tenderness, or visual disturbance (giant cell arteritis). These should prompt detailed examination and further investigation to exclude underlying malignancy or organ threatening disease. Yellow flags point to the psychosocial impact of the disease i.e. job dissatisfaction, loss of job, depression, loss of independence, etc. These factors interact with each other and also influence the prognosis of the disease. For example, they can perpetuate chronic pain which can take a life of its own.

Finally, a word of caution: 'classification criteria' for various systemic autoimmune rheumatic diseases (SARDs) abound but these are often misused by clinicians as 'diagnostic criteria' and this should be avoided.

References

Doherty, M., Dacre, J., Dieppe, P., and Snaith, M. (1992). The 'GALS' locomotor screen. *Annals of the Rheumatic Diseases* 51 (10): 1165–1169.
Goldblatt, F. and O'Neill, S.G. (2013). Clinical aspects of autoimmune rheumatic diseases. *Lancet (London, England)* 382 (9894): 797–808.

▼
This chapter focuses on relevant clinical features and their interpretation from a rheumatological perspective
▲

The handbook published by 'Arthritis Research UK' (2011) serves as a useful guide to the standardised clinical assessment of the musculoskeletal system. The examination is tailored along the lines of 'look, feel, move and functional assessment' of the Regional examination of the musculoskeletal system (REMS) (Coady et al. 2004). Once a problem has been identified using the GALS screening assessment the problem area is explored in detail using REMS. I suggest that you read this valuable resource to have an overview of musculoskeletal examination.

For the purpose of this chapter six important conditions are described highlighting pattern recognition and mimics. Although pattern recognition has been stressed it is with the caveat that disease phenotypes are not immutable since there can be a lot of overlap. Remember that clinical signs are often sensitive enough to pick up an abnormality but not specific enough to identify the cause. Examination in rheumatology also encroaches into other systems notably, neurology, dermatology, ophthalmology, vascular system and genito-urinary system. Hence in order to recognise the clinical manifestations one has to look at the person as a whole. Figures 54.1 to 54.4 show the clinical features of classic rheumatological disorders.

The trick to diagnosing autoimmune rheumatic disease is to recognise concurrent multisystem involvement. Given that each aspect is often looked after by an '–ologist' summarising the affected organ systems helps in recognising the phenotype.

Start with hand examination and work your way up the arm to the face and down to the legs. Use this template to flesh out any other autoimmune conditions that you know of in activity 54.1.

Activity 54.1

(Allow five minutes)

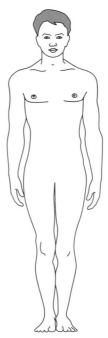

The Hands-on Guide to Clinical Reasoning in Medicine, First Edition. Mujammil Irfan.
© 2019 John Wiley & Sons Ltd. Published 2019 by John Wiley & Sons Ltd.
Companion website: www.wiley.com/go/irfan/clinicalreasoning

54.1 RHEUMATOID ARTHRITIS (RA) SEE FIGURE 54.1

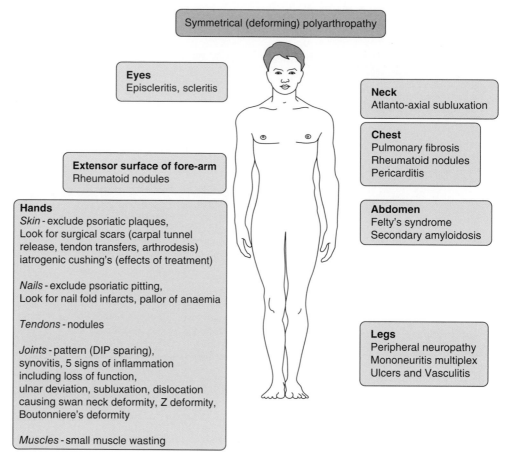

Symmetrical (deforming) polyarthropathy

Eyes
Episcleritis, scleritis

Neck
Atlanto-axial subluxation

Chest
Pulmonary fibrosis
Rheumatoid nodules
Pericarditis

Extensor surface of fore-arm
Rheumatoid nodules

Abdomen
Felty's syndrome
Secondary amyloidosis

Hands
Skin - exclude psoriatic plaques,
Look for surgical scars (carpal tunnel
release, tendon transfers, arthrodesis)
iatrogenic cushing's (effects of treatment)

Nails - exclude psoriatic pitting,
Look for nail fold infarcts, pallor of anaemia

Tendons - nodules

Joints - pattern (DIP sparing),
synovitis, 5 signs of inflammation
including loss of function,
ulnar deviation, subluxation, dislocation
causing swan neck deformity, Z deformity,
Boutonniere's deformity

Muscles - small muscle wasting

Legs
Peripheral neuropathy
Mononeuritis multiplex
Ulcers and Vasculitis

Figure 54.1 Clinical examination in Rheumatoid arthritis

54.2 PSORIATIC ARTHROPATHY (PSA) SEE FIGURE 54.2

Psoriatic arthropathy (PsA) was previously classified into five patterns
(Moll and Wright 1973):

- Asymmetrical oligo or monoarthritis
- RA like arthropathy but seronegative
- Ankylosing spondylitis like arthropathy with sacroiliitis
- OA like inflammatory arthropathy with predominant distal inter-phalangeal (DIP) joint
  involvement
- Arthritis mutilans with severely deforming polyarthropathy

However, it has been found that these patterns change with time and treatment.
Hence, there has been a drive to describe PsA in the following clinical domains
(Ritchlin et al. 2009):

- Peripheral arthritis
- Axial disease
- Dactylitis
- Enthesitis
- Skin and nail plate abnormalities.

Although the previous classification has been discredited it is useful to bear it in mind as
this would make us think of PsA when we encounter these patterns. Nevertheless, the clue
to the diagnosis is in finding the skin and nail plate abnormalities.

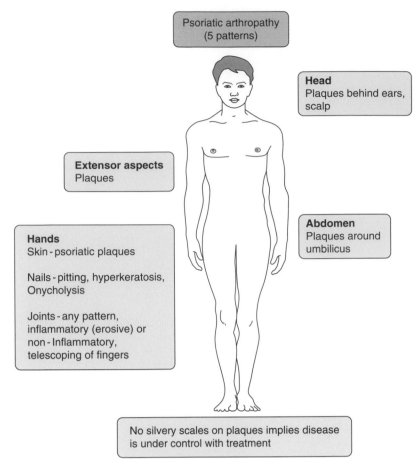

Psoriatic arthropathy
(5 patterns)

Head
Plaques behind ears,
scalp

Extensor aspects
Plaques

Abdomen
Plaques around
umbilicus

Hands
Skin - psoriatic plaques

Nails - pitting, hyperkeratosis,
Onycholysis

Joints - any pattern,
inflammatory (erosive) or
non - Inflammatory,
telescoping of fingers

No silvery scales on plaques implies disease
is under control with treatment

Figure 54.2 Clinical examination in psoriatric arthropathy

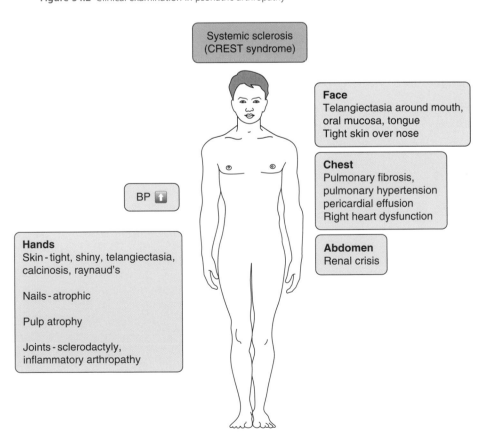

Systemic sclerosis
(CREST syndrome)

Face
Telangiectasia around mouth,
oral mucosa, tongue
Tight skin over nose

Chest
Pulmonary fibrosis,
pulmonary hypertension
pericardial effusion
Right heart dysfunction

BP ⬆

Abdomen
Renal crisis

Hands
Skin - tight, shiny, telangiectasia,
calcinosis, raynaud's

Nails - atrophic

Pulp atrophy

Joints - sclerodactyly,
inflammatory arthropathy

Figure 54.3 Clinical examination in Systemic Sclerosis

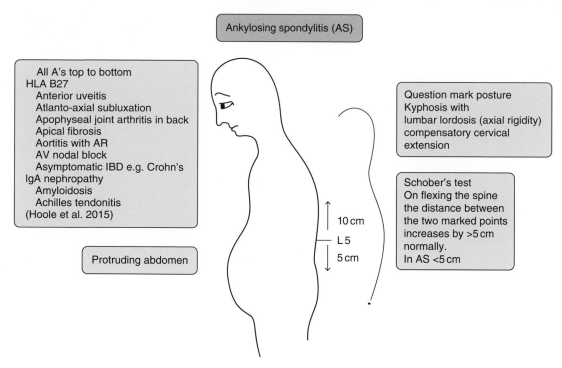

Ankylosing spondylitis (AS)

All A's top to bottom
HLA B27
    Anterior uveitis
    Atlanto-axial subluxation
    Apophyseal joint arthritis in back
    Apical fibrosis
    Aortitis with AR
    AV nodal block
    Asymptomatic IBD e.g. Crohn's
IgA nephropathy
    Amyloidosis
    Achilles tendonitis
(Hoole et al. 2015)

Protruding abdomen

Question mark posture
Kyphosis with
lumbar lordosis (axial rigidity)
compensatory cervical
extension

Schober's test
On flexing the spine
the distance between
the two marked points
increases by >5 cm
normally.
In AS <5 cm

10 cm
L5
5 cm

Figure 54.4 Clinical examination in Ankylosing Spondylitis

54.3 OSTEOARTHRITIS (OA)

Pattern – predominant distal interphalangeal joint – DIP (Heber den's nodes), proximal interphalangeal joint – PIP (Bouchard's nodes), first carpometacarpal (CMC), metacarpophalangeal (MCP) and PIP of the thumb are commonly involved. Erosive OA is different to nodal OA where MCP joint involvement is less frequent and functional impairment is unsurprisingly more likely. Secondary OA can occur in any inflammatory arthritides as well as metabolic diseases like haemochromatosis, diabetes mellitus and crystal arthropathies.

54.4 CRYSTAL ARTHROPATHIES

Gout: Pattern – monoarthritis, e.g. big toe (podagra) is seen in acute attacks. Untreated gout can present as acute polyarticular arthritis. Mimics include RA, psoriatic arthropathy especially in the chronic stages. Gouty tophi are subcutaneous urate deposits in a mesh of lipids, protein and debris. They give a clue to the aetiology and are often found in the pinna, bursae of upper and lower limbs.

Pseudogout: pattern – a heterogenous group of disorders that mimics other arthritides like RA, OA and gout and is most reliably distinguished by finding calcium pyrophosphate crystals in the synovial fluid of the affected joint.

References

Arthritis Research UK. 2011. *Clinical assessment of the musculoskeletal system. Arthritis Research UK, 2011* [online]. http://www.arthritisresearchuk.org/health-professionals-and-students/student-handbook.aspx. [Accessed: 29 January 2017]

Coady, D., Walker, D., and Kay, L. (2004). Regional Examination of the Musculoskeletal System (REMS): a core set of clinical skills for medical students. *Rheumatology (Oxford, England)* 43 (5): 633–639.

Hoole, S., Fry, A., and Davies, R. (2015). *Cases for PACES*, 3e. Chichester: Wiley Blackwell.

Moll, J.M. and Wright, V. (1973). Psoriatic arthritis. *Seminars in Arthritis and Rheumatism* 3 (1): 55–78.

Ritchlin, C.T., Kavanaugh, A., Gladman, D.D. et al. (2009). Treatment recommendations for psoriatic arthritis. *Annals of The Rheumatic Diseases* 68 (9): 1387–1394.

▼

This chapter focuses on the interpretation of radiographs and blood tests from a rheumatological perspective

▲

55.1 SEROLOGICAL TESTS

Multi-system disease implies concurrent signs and symptoms in multiple organ systems. Its identification is often followed by tests to exclude infections (e.g. infective endocarditis) and malignancy (e.g. local and distant metastases, paraneoplastic syndromes) since their treatment and prognosis varies. The diagnostic pathway then goes down the route of systemic autoimmune rheumatic diseases (SARDs). SARDs include conditions like rheumatoid arthritis (RA), ankylosing spondylitis (AS) and connective tissue diseases (CTDs) like systemic lupus erythematosis (SLE), mixed connective tissue disease (MCTD), Sjogren's syndrome, systemic sclerosis, anti-nuclear cytoplasmic antibody (ANCA) associated vasculitides etc. This diagnosis often involves treatment with potent immunosuppressive drugs which, if an infection has not been excluded can cause serious harm.

Once a clinical phenotype for a SARD has been deduced an autoimmune screen is requested. Quite frequently however, this screen is requested in the absence of the clinical context which makes its interpretation very difficult. The following points serve in guiding the right actions:

1. Autoantibodies are immunoglobulins produced against self antigens which can be cell components, proteins, carbohydrates, lipids or nucleic acids.
2. Autoantibodies can be found in 'normal' individuals and be falsely positive in a different clinical disease thereby misleading the clinician, e.g. antinuclear antibody (ANA) can be positive in hepatitis C.
3. The clinical context, prior probability of the disease, sensitivity and specificity of the test and the expected response to the outcome of the test should all be considered before requesting the test.
4. Immunological tests can be used in diagnosis (anti Sm antibody for SLE), assess disease activity (ESR in PMR), predict end-organ involvement (anti dsDNA predicts renal involvement in SLE), prognosis (positive RF in RA predicts erosive arthritis) and response to treatment (Table 55.1).
5. Remember that high sensitivity tests are useful for screening ('sensitive enough' to pick up the disease in the patient population e.g. ANA) and high specificity tests are then used to confirm the disease (disease specific autoantibodies, e.g. ds-DNA). The caveat is that if the clinical suspicion remains high, a negative screening test should still be followed up with a disease specific autoantibody test.
6. Autoantibodies may or may not be positive in clinical disease, i.e. their presence adds another layer of evidence to support the diagnosis, but their absence does not exclude the disease. A clinical diagnosis of SARD is still possible.
7. Disease specific autoantibodies can pre-date a SARD by several years but the factors that lead to phenotype expression (disease) are unclear.

55.2 ANTINUCLEAR ANTIBODIES (ANA)

Antinuclear antibodies encompass antibodies to extractable nuclear antigens and cytoplasmic antigens. The prevalence of ANA in healthy Caucasians is 5% at a dilution titre of 1 : 160 and increases with age (Lyons et al. 2005). Although the pattern of

The Hands-on Guide to Clinical Reasoning in Medicine, First Edition. Mujammil Irfan.
© 2019 John Wiley & Sons Ltd. Published 2019 by John Wiley & Sons Ltd.
Companion website: www.wiley.com/go/irfan/clinicalreasoning

Table 55.1 Disease specific antibodies and their significance in SARD specificity and disease activity

Disease specific autoantibodies	SARD specificity	End-organ specificity and disease activity
Anti Ds-DNA (double stranded DNA) Anti Sm (Smith), Ribosomal P protein	Relatively high specificity to SLE Pathognomonic of SLE	If positive in SLE predicts lupus nephritis and disease activity
Anti-centromere	Limited Systemic sclerosis	CREST (calcinosis, Raynaud's phenomenon, oesophageal dysmotility, sclerodactyly and telangiectasia) and pulmonary hypertension
Anti Scl-70, RNAP I/III, fibrillarin	Diffuse Systemic sclerosis	Anti Scl-70 – pulmonary fibrosis RNAP III – renal disease
Anti Jo 1 SRP (signal recognition peptide)	Antisynthetase syndrome Polymyositis	Pulmonary fibrosis
Anti Ro, La	Sicca symptoms Can be seen in many SARDs but most commonly seen in Sjogren's, SLE	Neonatal lupus (congenital complete heart block) Seropositivity in Sjogren's is associated with extra glandular complications and more frequent parotitis
U1RNP (ribonucleoprotein)	A diagnostic criterion for MCTD Also seen in systemic sclerosis	
ANCA	Small vessel vasculitdes (see under ANCA section 55.3)	Disease activity

immunofluorescence staining has traditionally been given importance, it is clear that more than one pattern can co-exist and the antigens are not very clearly compartmentalised into the various cell organelles. Figure 55.1 shows the ANA directed against specific cell antigens and their disease associations.

A positive ANA titre of >1:160 is considered to be significant. It is used as a screening test owing to its high sensitivity and a positive ANA should be followed up by a more disease specific autoantibody if the clinical suspicion remains high.
The prevalence of most autoantibodies in individual disease states is low to moderate and hence assessing pre-test probability prior to requesting the tests is vital in interpreting the results.

Sample clinical scenarios when an ANA (high sensitivity) should be requested:

- Clinical phenotype of a specific SARD
- Undifferentiated inflammatory arthritis
- Unexplained multisystem disease
- Unexplained neurological disease
- Haematological conditions like immune cytopenias
- Polyserositis

55.3 ANCA

There are two patterns seen on immunofluorescence, cytoplasmic anti-nuclear cytoplasmic antibody (C-ANCA) and perinuclear-ANCA (P-ANCA). C-ANCA represents the presence of anti-PR3 antibodies whilst P-ANCA represents the presence of anti-MPO. PR3 and MPO are normal antigens on lysosomal granules in neutrophils and monocytes. In disease states they migrate to the cell surface triggering an inflammatory cascade and tissue damage.

ANCA is found in vasculitides. Anti-PR3 is seen in granulomatosis with polyangiitis (GPA – formerly Wegener's) where it predicts disease activity but not always. Anti-MPO is seen in microscopic polyangiitis and eosinophilic granulomatosis with polyangiitis (EGPA) formerly Churg-Strauss syndrome.

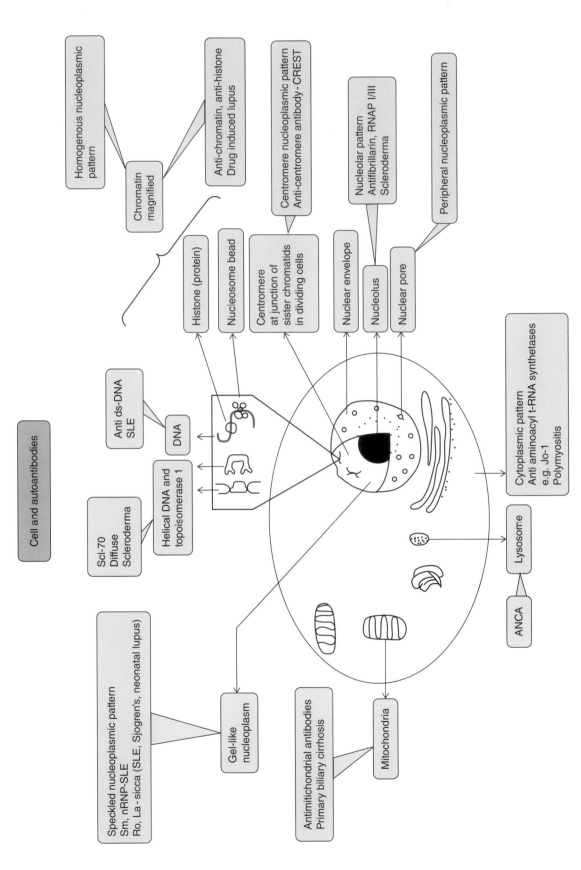

Figure 55.1 Auto-antibodies directed against various cell components correlated to disease states

55.4 ANTI-PHOSPHOLIPID SYNDROME

Antibodies are directed against phospholipids and phospholipid binding proteins namely, anticardiolipin antibodies and anti-beta 2 glycoprotein 1 (β2GP1) respectively. They are often requested in the following scenarios:

- Recurrent arterial/venous thromboses
- Recurrent fetal loss

Since antiphospholipid antibodies are non-specific (can occur in other conditions like infections, malignancy) they should always be repeated in 12 weeks if positive. Lupus anticoagulant another antibody found in anti-phospholipid syndrome causes a prolonged clotting time (e.g. APTT) in the laboratory but is a misnomer since it is prothrombotic *in vivo*.

55.5 RHEUMATOID ARTHRITIS (RA)

Rheumatoid factor (RF): Chronic inflammation and oxidative stress in an inflamed joint can result in a conformational change in the structure of IgG antibodies exposing 'cryptic carbohydrate epitopes' on its molecule. IgM antibodies produced against these exposed carbohydrate structures are called RF. The immune complexes formed between the RF and IgG molecules trigger a cascade of further inflammation and tissue damage. The prevalence of RF in Caucasians is 4% and increases with rising age (Newkirk 2002).

Antibodies to citrullinated protein antigens (ACPAs): During cell apoptosis in an inflamed joint, enzymes produced by activated neutrophils and monocytes substitute citrulline instead of arginine (citrullinate) in various peptides which serve as a neoantigen for antibodies called ACPAs. They are highly specific for RA with a specificity of 95% compared to a specificity of 85% for RF (Nishimura et al. 2007).

55.6 ACUTE PHASE REACTANTS

Autoantibodies are not the only biomarkers of SARD. Other laboratory measures include CRP and ESR. CRP is not affected by age and gender unlike ESR but both have half-lives of several days although CRP changes more rapidly than ESR. They are useful to assess disease activity in established SARD and will also help in diagnosing other inflammatory conditions like infection.

$$ESR = [age + 10\ (women)] / 2$$

Discrepant values of ESR and CRP are clinically useful. Minor or no elevation of CRP but high ESR points to hypergammaglobulinemia which occurs in SLE and Sjogren's. Serum electrophoresis can tell us if this is polyclonal (SLE, Sjogren's) or monoclonal (e.g. myeloma).

C3 and C4 are also acute phase proteins that can be raised in any inflammatory condition. They are particularly useful in renal disease. Low C3 points to alternative complement pathway activation, e.g. post-streptococcal glomerulonephritis whilst low C4 points to classical pathway activation e.g. SLE, C1 inhibitor deficiency, cryoglobulinemia, rheumatoid vasculitis and any chronic infection with immune complex formation.

55.7 RADIOLOGY IN RHEUMATOLOGY

The ABCDS (Alignment, Bones, Cartilage, Distribution (pattern) and Soft tissue changes) mnemonic can be used to interpret musculoskeletal radiographs. Focusing on the bones, one will have to look for evidence of demineralisation, erosions, joint space narrowing and new bone formation, e.g. osteophytes. Cartilage destruction can cause joint space narrowing which is often seen in inflammatory arthritis.

Figure 55.2 shows common radiological findings seen in inflammatory and non-inflammatory/degenerative arthritis but these changes are often seen very late in the course of the disease. The impetus is now on earlier case detection in order to prevent or delay joint destruction especially since targeted therapies are available. The imaging modality of choice in this circumstance depends on the clinical phenotype that is being suspected. Ultrasound examination of superficial joints is far more sensitive in picking up early synovial inflammation even in joints that are asymptomatic. MRI is especially useful for deeper joints, bone marrow oedema, soft tissue oedema and axial disease (Tins and Butler 2013).

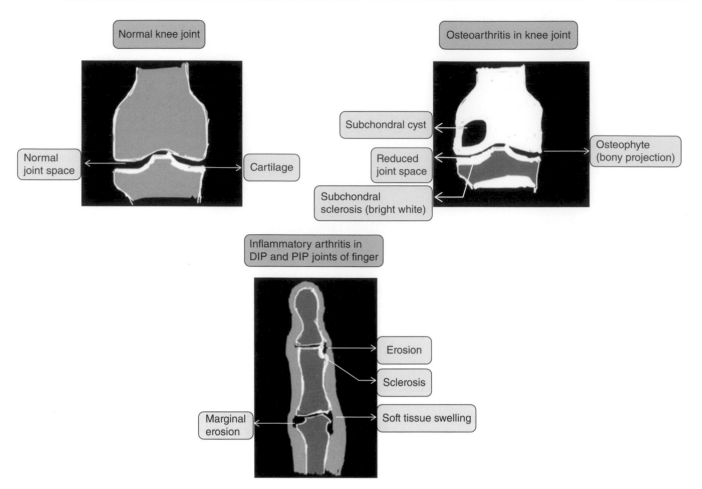

Figure 55.2 Radiologic features in osteoarthritis and inflammatory arthritis versus normal joint

55.8 SYNOVIAL FLUID ANALYSIS

Synovial fluid analysis is useful in excluding septic arthritis and hemarthrosis (bloody aspirate) from other causes of a joint effusion. Aspirating the joint to dryness also gives immediate pain relief. The primary differential rests between inflammatory arthritis and non-inflammatory arthritis. It is important to note that inflammatory arthritis includes septic arthritis, crystal arthropathies and SARDs whereas non-inflammatory arthritis includes osteoarthritis, trauma, avascular necrosis and degenerative arthritides like Charcot's disease.

The normal viscosity of synovial fluid is high, and inflammation reduces it. Synovial fluid is normally almost acellular. Inflammatory arthritis causes a WCC of up to 2000/mm^3 whilst septic arthritis causes a higher WCC of >20000/mm^3 with >95% being polymorphonuclear leucocytes. Positive microbiology from gram stain and culture cements the diagnosis of septic arthritis. Finding crystals in polarised light examination signifies a crystal arthropathy of gout (urate crystals) or pseudogout (calcium pyrophosphate crystals).

References

Lyons, R., Narain, S., Nichols, C. et al. (2005). Effective use of autoantibody tests in the diagnosis of systemic autoimmune disease. *Annals of the New York Academy of Sciences* 1050 (1): 217–228.

Newkirk, M.M. (2002). Rheumatoid factors: what do they tell us? *The Journal of Rheumatology* 29 (10): 2034–2040.

Nishimura, K., Sugiyama, D., Kogata, Y. et al. (2007). Meta-analysis: diagnostic accuracy of anti-cyclic citrullinated peptide antibody and rheumatoid factor for rheumatoid arthritis. *Annals of Internal Medicine* 146 (11): 797–808.

Tins, B.J. and Butler, R. (2013). Imaging in rheumatology: reconciling radiology and rheumatology. *Insights Into Imaging* 4 (6): 799–810.

▼

This chapter tells you how to approach muscle aches from a rheumatological perspective

▲

Muscle aches and pains = myalgia

Muscle disease = myopathy

Muscle inflammation = myositis

Example 56.1

A 69 year old woman presented with worsening generalised aches and pains over a six week period having been forced to see the doctor by her husband. PMH: nil. Medications: paracetamol.

J: SQs – *elderly woman + sub-acute myalgia. Provisional diagnoses – wide differential.*

The symptoms followed a flu-like illness with no previous history of similar symptoms. On direct questioning she reported fluctuating episodes of being unable to get up from chair or pick heavy objects. Her husband reported that she had intermittently complained of sweating. No joint symptoms, or recreational drug use. Never smoked and alcohol occasional. No new drugs, travel history, history of tuberculosis (TB) or exotic pets at home. No weight loss or other red flag symptoms. No symptoms suggestive of giant cell arteritis (GCA).

J: *Inability to rise from a chair indicates proximal muscle weakness. Could it be a proximal myopathy?*

The discriminatory factor would be objective muscle weakness since these symptoms could also be due to pain or stiffness. Identifying muscle stiffness after rest, e.g. in the mornings could point to an inflammatory disorder, e.g. polymyalgia rheumatica (PMR).

O/E: Looked well. Temperature 37.3 °C, Saturations 98% on air, RR 14, BP 140/72, Pulse 90 bpm, BMs 8 mmol l⁻¹. Cardiovascular system, RS, PA: normal. Central nervous system: No focal neurological deficits especially no evidence of proximal muscle weakness. Although she complained of pain there was no muscle tenderness or signs of synovitis. Fundoscopy: normal; temporal arteries pulsatile and non-tender.

The Hands-on Guide to Clinical Reasoning in Medicine, First Edition. Mujammil Irfan.
© 2019 John Wiley & Sons Ltd. Published 2019 by John Wiley & Sons Ltd.
Companion website: www.wiley.com/go/irfan/clinicalreasoning

Bloods: U&Es: normal. Albumin 38 g l⁻¹, ALT 60 IU l⁻¹, bilirubin 8 μmol l⁻¹, ALP 130 IU l⁻¹, CRP 200 mg l⁻¹, ESR 99 mm per hour, Hb 140 g l⁻¹, platelets 400 × 10⁹ l⁻¹, WCC 13 × 10⁹ l⁻¹, CK 150 IU l⁻¹. Autoimmune and myeloma screen pending. ECG and CXR: normal.

J: *Severity of illness – relatively well. There is no focal muscle weakness and the pattern of muscle involvement (girdle muscles) suggests PMR. The age (>50), raised ESR and CRP are in keeping with this. Although the ALT is raised, the CK is normal which implies that it is not coming from the muscles.*

Would you have requested an autoimmune screen?

Activity 56.1

(Allow few seconds!)

Autoimmune screens in these scenarios should be requested after assessing the pre-test probability of finding a SARD. This is especially since false positives are high in the elderly which may well lead the clinician down the wrong path.

Myeloma screen and USG abdomen: normal. Rheumatoid factor positive and ANA positive at 1:40. There was no history to suggest a staggered paracetamol overdose and the levels were normal (raised ALT). A rheumatology consultation was requested who suggested treatment with standard dose of prednisolone 15 mg OD for suspected PMR. They felt that the raised ALT could be a non-specific manifestation of PMR. Anti-CCP antibodies were requested (as polymyalgic RA is well described). A temperature spike of 38.3 °C was noted by the registrar who felt that a period of observation was essential prior to initiating steroids. Blood cultures were sent and an echo was requested.

Would you start the patient on prednisolone? Give reasons.

Activity 56.2

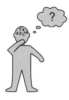

(Allow few seconds!)

The answer lies in the diagnostic certainty and the confident exclusion of mimics. Given that immunosuppressants are not a good idea in the presence of underlying untreated infections; the priority will be to exclude infections. The significantly high ESR and CRP with the temperature spikes are not typical of PMR unless there is co-existent GCA which seems unlikely here. In light of this argument the registrar's decision seems appropriate. The positive rheumatoid factor (RF) and ANA were rightly ignored as they were false positives. Moreover, a positive ANA titre at 1:40 gives a higher false positive rate than 1:160 which is the recommended cut-off.

> Three successive blood cultures, anti-CCP antibodies and the echo were negative and the patient was started on 15 mg OD of prednisolone as an in-patient. Symptoms improved dramatically within two days confirming the diagnosis of PMR and she was discharged. She remained well on follow-up two months later.

This example highlights the principles of defining the pre-test probability of disease before requesting tests. Identification of the misfits in data (high grade pyrexia) led to the cautious exclusion of underlying sepsis (especially since she was relatively well, and we had time on our side). How deep would you search for infections and at what point would you consider treatment depends on the reasonable certainty of having excluded infections since treatment is not without risks here. This is called the threshold-approach to decision making (Pauker and Kassirer 1980). Involving the patient in this decision-making process and externalising the risks helps. Further caution was exercised when she was treated as an in-patient and the therapeutic efficacy of the treatment (a characteristic of PMR) was used to confirm the diagnosis.

Example 56.2

Four weeks from onset

> A 72 year old man presents to his GP with worsening muscle aches and pains over four weeks. PMH: MI and coronary stent, HT, CKD stage 2, COPD. Medications: aspirin, clopidogrel, ramipril, bisoprolol, simvastatin, salbutamol and flixotide inhalers.

P: *SQs – elderly man + sub-acute myalgias + vascular risk factors and COPD. Provisional diagnoses – wide differential.*

> He noticed gradually worsening muscle weakness in his arms and legs and was finding it difficult to get up from a chair and pick things up. No recent change in medications, travel history or infective symptoms.

P: *Proximal muscle weakness + pain suggests PMR.*

Muscle weakness does not fit with PMR.

What other differentials can you think of assuming that he has true muscle weakness?

Activity 56.3

(Allow two minutes)

P: *All differentials of proximal myopathy, e.g. vitamin D deficiency, hypothyroidism, myasthenia gravis, muscular dystrophy, etc.*

O/E: Pulse 80 bpm, BP 140/70, Temperature 36.6 °C, RR 12 per minute. CNS: Proximal muscle weakness in hips 3/5 bilaterally and shoulders 4/5 bilaterally. Reflexes: preserved. No ocular signs or fatiguability. Plantars: down-going. Sensory examination: normal. The rest of the systemic and neurological examination: normal.

P: *severity of illness – ill. Pattern – symmetrical proximal muscle weakness with preserved reflexes = proximal myopathy. Legs are weaker than the arms.*

Eight weeks later

The GP noted that he had been on simvastatin for nearly six months since his MI. He felt that the clinical findings were in keeping with statin-induced myopathy and stopped it. He requested bloods including CK, reassured him and asked him to return in a month if symptoms were no better. Bloods: CK 450, ALT 60 and the rest normal. He returned in a month with persistent symptoms only slightly better.

P: *Should we look for other causes of proximal myopathy?*

The GP requests further bloods: FBC, ESR, U&Es, TFTs, vitamin D and liver function tests (LFTs): normal. CK 200 IU l⁻¹ and ANA positive 1:1280. CXR: normal. In view of these results he refers him to the neurologist and a rheumatologist.

What questions would you ask the patient at this stage?

Activity 56.4

(Allow three minutes)

....

....

....

....

....

Questions will have to be directed at uncovering other differentials of proximal myopathy like polymyositis, dermatomyositis, paraneoplastic myositis, etc.

Three months later

There were no skin or joint symptoms, no red flags of malignancy (to exclude dermatomyositis/CTDs). The symptoms had improved slightly but were still present. O/E: Mild proximal muscle weakness mainly in the hips of 4/5. No other focal neurological deficits. The neurologist arranged NCSs, EMG and muscle biopsy all of which showed non-specific changes but no clear evidence of inflammatory muscle disease (polymyositis, dermatomyositis, etc). The worried patient was advised to wait for the out-patient rheumatology review.

Four months later

The rheumatologist reviewed the story and an examination failed to reveal any objective muscle weakness. The symptoms were getting better and the muscle enzymes were normal. She reassured the patient that statin-induced myopathy can take up to six months to get better and the positive ANA was very likely to be drug induced (simvastatin). She followed him up in two months and his symptoms had resolved.

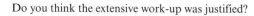

Do you think the extensive work-up was justified?

Activity 56.5

(Allow few seconds!)

Statin induced myopathy

- Ranges from simple myalgia to rhabdomyolysis.
- Can occur months after starting statin.
- CK can be normal.
- Fluvastatin and pravastatin have lesser propensity to cause myopathy.
- Drug interactions and underlying endocrine/neuromuscular disorders increase the risk of myopathy.

What this question is asking is how we make decisions to investigate further. The answer lies in a review of all the variables involved in the presentation, i.e. physician factors, patient factors and the clinical problem (Higgs et al. 2008). Physician factors such as personal emotional factors (e.g. recent complaint), local workplace context and organisational context can affect the decisions taken. For example, fear of litigation rhyming with risk-averse organisations and workplace will push the individual to over-investigate. Similarly, patient factors such as psychosocial factors and family context (e.g. anxiety about the diagnosis, sick role taken on by the patient) and the intrinsic uncertainty of the clinical problem itself will all contribute to investigation decisions.

On the whole, assuming that the clinicians were aware that statin-induced myopathy can take several months to resolve it is difficult to be critical of their actions. Indeed, failure of symptom resolution is an indication for further investigation in this context. On the other hand, we work in resource limited settings and over-investigating will only make it worse by discovering 'incidentalomas' that contribute to further unnecessary investigations, notwithstanding the expense and associated patient anxiety (Moynihan et al. 2012). It would be a personal matter of choice as to where we draw the line. Once again, shared-decision making whilst externalising our thought processes (uncertainty) with our patients will help. Knowledge of these issues is pertinent in making sound clinical decisions whilst calibrating our actions for future practice.

▼

Pre-test probability of disease influences the interpretation of test results.

Remember the threshold approach to decision making.

Be aware of overdiagnosis and the factors that lead to it.

Shared decision making with our patients is a good antidote to uncertainty.

▲

References

Higgs, J., Jones, M,A., Loftus, S., and Christensen, N. (eds), *Clinical Reasoning in the Health Professions*,.3ʳᵈ ed. Elsevier, 2008.
Moynihan, R., Doust, J., and Henry, D. (2012). Preventing overdiagnosis: how to stop harming the healthy. *BMJ (Clinical Research Ed.)* 344: e3502.
Pauker, S.G. and Kassirer, J.P. (1980). The threshold approach to clinical decision making. *The New England Journal of Medicine* 302 (20): 1109–1117.

57 Joint Pain

▼

This chapter tells you how to approach joint pain from a rheumatological perspective

▲

Example 57.1

An on-call SHO was bleeped to review a 60 year old lady with a hot, swollen, painful right wrist. She was four days into her admission with left sided community acquired pneumonia. PMH: rheumatoid arthritis, hypertension, diabetes mellitus. Medications: aspirin, bendrofluazide, perindopril, metformin, sitagliptin, leflunomide (stopped since admission), amoxycillin since admission.

P: SQs – *middle aged lady + CAP + acute monoarthritis on a background of Rheumatoid arthritis (RA) + vascular risk factors. Provisional diagnoses – flare-up of RA, septic arthritis, pseudogout, gout (bendrofluazide).*

Current smoker 40 py, alcohol 20 units per week. She had received two courses of antibiotics for her chest over the last four weeks.

O/E: Temperature 37.7 °C, Pulse 90 bpm, BP 110/70, RR 12 per minute, BMs 12 mmol l^{-1}, Saturations 94% on air. No sub-cutaneous tophi. Right wrist: overlying skin erythematous, joint swollen with effusion, tender with reduced movement. Rheumatoid hands noted. Bilateral MCP and PIP joints of the hands were slightly tender with pre-existent RA but no active synovitis. Left basal signs in keeping with CAP. Rest of the systemic examination: normal.

Bloods on admission: WCC 18 × 10^9 l^{-1}, platelets 500 × 10^9 l^{-1}, Hb 140 g l^{-1}, CRP 150 mg l^{-1}, Na$^+$ 128 mmol l^{-1}, K$^+$ 5 mmol l^{-1}, urea 16 mmol l^{-1}, creatinine 150 μmol l^{-1}; LFTs: normal, except albumin 32 g l^{-1} and Ca^{2+} 2.32 mmol l^{-1}. Previous Na$^+$ 137 mmol l^{-1}, creatinine 110 μmol l^{-1}. Sputum cultures: Streptococcus pneumoniae.

P: *severity of illness – very ill. The hyponatraemia and AKI (pre-renal) could be secondary to dehydration. I would ensure that perindopril, bendrofluazide and metformin are withheld. Could it be reactive arthritis?*

Reactive arthritis is often seen following GI and genito-urinary infections with specific micro-organisms. It is associated with spondyloarthropathies (enthesitis and extra-articular manifestations in eyes and skin) and has a predilection for weight-bearing joints of the lower limbs. This is not the picture here.

The Hands-on Guide to Clinical Reasoning in Medicine, First Edition. Mujammil Irfan.
© 2019 John Wiley & Sons Ltd. Published 2019 by John Wiley & Sons Ltd.
Companion website: www.wiley.com/go/irfan/clinicalreasoning

Identify the positive and negative clinical features in this lady that help in increasing/decreasing the likelihood of potential differentials?

Activity 57.1

(Allow three minutes)

Positive clinical features that increase the likelihood of specific diseases:

- CAP – pseudo-gout (crystal arthropathy), septic arthritis.
- Pre-existing RA – septic arthritis.

Negative clinical features that decrease the likelihood of specific diseases:

- Polyarticular inflammation with RA – flare-up of RA. However, this is unlikely since a single joint is more inflamed than the rest.
- Sub-cutaneous tophi – gout.

The SHO felt that this was a flare-up of RA since she was already known to have RA. He prescribed co-codamol given that NSAIDs were contra-indicated (AKI). He repeated the bloods and requested a rheumatology consult.

Repeat bloods: WCC $14 \times 10^9 \, l^{-1}$, Hb $120 \, g \, l^{-1}$, platelets $450 \times 10^9 \, l^{-1}$, CRP $200 \, mg \, l^{-1}$, Na^+ $134 \, mmol \, l^{-1}$, K^+ $4.5 \, mmol \, l^{-1}$, urea $10 \, mmol \, l^{-1}$, creatinine $130 \, \mu mol \, l^{-1}$, LFTs: normal, except albumin $28 \, g \, l^{-1}$; urate $0.4 \, mmol \, l^{-1}$.

P: *The normal urate rules out gout. The inflammatory markers are worsening but the AKI is better.*

Urate actually decreases with systemic inflammation. Raised urate levels help but a normal level does not exclude gout.

The rheumatologist re-visited the history and confirmed that the wrist had been painful for nearly two weeks prior to admission. The patient denied significant travel history, weight loss, eye, genito-urinary or GI symptoms (reactive arthritis). There was no history of back pain (spondyloarthropathies). The right wrist joint effusion was aspirated and sent for C&S, WCC and microscopy for gram stain and crystals. The aspirate was thin in consistency and slightly cloudy. X-ray did not show chondrocalcinosis (pseudogout).

Joint aspirate: WCC $20000/mm^3$ with 95% polymorphonuclear leucocytes, gram stain showed gram positive cocci and occasional negatively birefringent needle shaped crystals (Margaretten et al. 2007). The rheumatologist treated her for septic arthritis with vancomycin pending the sensitivity results. Bendrofluazide was stopped. Blood and synovial fluid cultures grew Streptococcus pneumoniae and the antibiotic was switched to tazocin. The patient subsequently improved and was discharged.

This example shows how faulty context formulation (a swollen wrist on a background of RA) led the SHO to diagnose a flare-up of RA. If due consideration was given to the rest of the SQs (CAP, bendrofluazide), other possibilities could have been entertained e.g.

crystal arthropathy, septic arthritis, etc. Hypothetico-deductive reasoning (if disease A is associated with finding B, the absence of finding B decreases the likelihood of disease A) as illustrated in activity 57.1 can then be used to discriminate between the hypotheses.

The key finding in this lady was that the signs and symptoms in the wrist were significantly disproportionate to those in the other joints of the hands ('monoarthritis' as stated in the SQs). This reduces the likelihood of a flare-up of RA. Pre-existing rheumatological disease increases the risk of septic arthritis and although the leflunomide was stopped it has a long half-life (up to two weeks) conferring an immunosuppressed state. Erythema of the skin overlying the affected joint raises the probability of either septic arthritis or crystal arthropathy. Lastly, crystal arthropathy can co-exist with septic arthritis and if clinical suspicion is high microscopy, culture and sensitivity (MC&S) is strongly indicated even if synovial fluid shows crystals (Zhang et al. 2006).

Example 57.2

> A 55 year old lady was referred to the Rheumatologist by the GP with a two week history of painful, swollen left wrist joint. PMH: Irritable bowel syndrome. Medications: paracetamol and codeine phosphate prn.

> J: *SQs – middle aged lady + acute monoarthritis + IBS. Provisional diagnoses – septic arthritis, reactive arthritis, crystal arthropathy, post viral arthritis* etc.

> She reported morning stiffness lasting up to an hour and was finding it difficult to work as a cleaner due to pain. There was no preceding illness or trauma. No significant travel history. No skin, eye, genito-urinary, systemic symptoms. No back pain (axial symptoms), enthesitis (pain at insertion of tendons and ligaments). She had occasional diarrhoea and constipation with her IBS but no blood or mucus per rectum. Current smoker of 40 py.

> O/E: Temperature 37.5 °C, Pulse 86 bpm, BP 130/65, RR 12. No skin rashes, nodules or tophi. No scaly skin in hidden areas (scalp, behind ears, umbilicus, natal cleft), nail-plate or nail-fold abnormalities, red eye, dactylitis (diffusely swollen 'sausage' fingers). Left wrist: signs of synovitis with swelling, tenderness and reduced range of movement but no effusion. Mild tenderness in PIP joints in the hands. Rest of the systemic examination: normal.

> J: *Revised SQs – middle aged lady + acute inflammatory oligoarthritis + IBS. Provisional diagnoses – reactive arthritis (GI symptoms with 'IBS'), peripheral spondyloarthropathy (SpA). Severity of illness – ill.*

Which rheumatological conditions are less likely owing to the absence of clinical findings described above?

Activity 57.2

(Allow three minutes)

Skin rashes, nail-fold abnormalities, systemic features – SARDs.
Skin nodules – RA, SLE, sarcoidosis.

Nail-plate abnormalities and scaly skin – psoriatic arthritis.

Lack of eye, skin, genito-urinary symptoms, axial symptoms, enthesitis, dactylitis – lessen peripheral SpA but GI symptoms seem to point to it.

> He requested some tests and prescribed naproxen for the pains. Upon follow-up in four weeks: RA, ACCP, autoimmune screen, coeliac screen U&Es, LFTs: normal; CRP 50 mg l⁻¹, ESR 60 mm per hour, WCC $12 \times 10^9 l^{-1}$, Hb 100 g l⁻¹, platelets $450 \times 10^9 l^{-1}$, MCV 84 fl, viral hepatitis serology: negative; left wrist X-ray: normal. The joint pains were slightly better on naproxen.

How would you interpret these results?

Activity 57.3

(Allow few seconds!)

J: The raised inflammatory markers (WCC, CRP, ESR and platelets) point to an inflammatory arthritis. The normocytic anaemia can represent anaemia of chronic disease with a diffuse inflammatory state. There is no laboratory evidence of a SARD.

> Given the short history and lack of clear-cut findings, the Rheumatologist diagnosed undifferentiated arthritis. She was explained that this was an interim diagnosis which could change with disease evolution. For now, she was given the reassurance of a follow-up and advised to return quicker if symptoms changed or worsened. An ultrasound scan of the hands was requested which was normal.
>
> Two months later she re-presented to the GP with fever, cough and phlegm. She was treated with antibiotics and a CXR requested. The CXR showed multiple pulmonary nodules and she was referred to the Respiratory physicians for urgent suspected cancer.

Let us pause here. Re-state the SQs and the provisional diagnoses?

Activity 57.4

(Allow two minutes)

SQs – middle aged lady + undifferentiated inflammatory arthritis + multiple pulmonary nodules + smoker + IBS. Provisional diagnoses – malignancy (with paraneoplastic arthritis), RA, SLE, sarcoidosis, granulomatosis with polyangiitis (Wegener's), subacute bacterial endocarditis, HIV with Kaposi's or TB.

The CT scan was reviewed in the multi-disciplinary meeting where it showed multiple subsolid nodules <5 mm and a follow up CT in three months was suggested. She was seen in the clinic by a respiratory registrar. There were no red flag symptoms of malignancy, features suggestive of sarcoidosis, infective endocarditis, TB or other SARDs. Given the history of undifferentiated arthritis he repeated the RF and ACCP antibodies which were positive in high titres. HIV test: negative. She was re-referred to the Rheumatologists for suspected RA with pulmonary nodules. When reviewed, the disease had evolved into a symmetric inflammatory polyarthritis in keeping with RA and the diagnosis was confirmed.

This example shows the fluid state of affairs when data is being accumulated. Variability in disease presentation and disease evolution over time constantly revise SQs. Paying attention to the SQs in flux ensures that we are consciously considering other possibilities. Specialists are increasingly working in silos where the clinical picture in its entirety can be easily relegated to the background. It is up to each one of us to exercise vigilance and ensure that the person sitting in front of us is seen in a holistic light.

▼

Ensure that the right context has been formulated using all the available SQs.

Remain vigilant to the fluid state of SQs as the disease evolves.

▲

References

Margaretten, M.E., Kohlwes, J., Moore, D. et al. (2007). Does this adult patient have septic arthritis? *Journal of the American Medical Association* 297 (13): 1478–1488.

Zhang, W., Doherty, M., Pascual, E. et al. (2006). EULAR evidence based recommendations for gout. Part I: diagnosis. Report of a task force of the standing committee for international clinical studies including therapeutics (ESCISIT). *Annals of the Rheumatic Diseases* 65 (10): 1301–1311.

58 Back Pain

▼

This chapter tells you how to approach back pain from a rheumatological perspective

▲

Example 58.1

A 72 year old man presents to A&E with a three week history of low back pain. PMH: bipolar disorder, depression, HT, COPD, end-stage renal disease (ESRD) on haemodialysis and previous alcohol excess. Medications: valproate, citalopram, losartan, alfacalcidol, erythropoietin injections, salbutamol and seretide inhalers and maintenance prednisolone 5 mg od.

J: SQs – elderly man + sub-acute back pain + psychiatry issues + ESRD on haemodialysis + history of HT, COPD, alcohol excess. Provisional diagnoses – mechanical back pain, malignancy (age), osteoporotic fracture (steroids), cord compression, spinal stenosis. I would look for red flags.

He reported gradual onset low back pain with no features suggestive of cord compression or spinal stenosis. No history of trauma, malignancy or weight loss. The pain was worse at night and co-codamol helped. Previous history of mechanical back pains in his 50s.

O/E: Pulse 86 bpm, BP 140/70, Temperature 37.3 °C, RR 14 per minute, BMs 10 mmol l^{-1}, Saturations 96% on air. Diffuse tenderness over lumbar spine, no focal neurological deficits; straight leg raising test: normal; rest of the systemic examination: normal. Lumbar spine X-ray: normal. Bloods: Hb 110 g l^{-1}, platelets 200 × 10^9 l^{-1}, WCC 10 × 10^9 l^{-1}, CRP 40 mg l^{-1}, Na$^+$ 134 mmol l^{-1}, K$^+$ 4.5 mmol l^{-1}, urea 10 mmol l^{-1}, creatinine 150 μmol l^{-1}, LFTs: normal, except albumin 30 g l^{-1}, globulin 40 g l^{-1}, Corrected Ca^{2+} 2.3 mmol l^{-1}.

J: There are no sinister features.

The A&E doctor suggested continuing co-codamol and advised to return if symptoms did not settle. He returned in one week with worsening back pain. The clinical findings were similar. The nurses commented that he was able to walk around the department and suggested that it might be drug-seeking behaviour given the psychiatric and alcohol history. He was discharged on ibuprofen for pain relief and advised to return if concerned.

J: A second admission raises concerns especially since the pain is not settling. I wonder if there is an underlying cause.

The Hands-on Guide to Clinical Reasoning in Medicine, First Edition. Mujammil Irfan.
© 2019 John Wiley & Sons Ltd. Published 2019 by John Wiley & Sons Ltd.
Companion website: www.wiley.com/go/irfan/clinicalreasoning

He re-presented three days later with intractable pain localised to L1 and was admitted. A repeat lumbar spine x-ray showed collapsed L1. CXR: normal. Bloods: Hb 100 g l⁻¹, MCV 82 fl, platelets 150 × 10⁹ l⁻¹, WCC 12 × 10⁹ l⁻¹, CRP 60 mg l⁻¹, Na⁺ 135 mmol l⁻¹, K⁺ 5 mmol l⁻¹, urea 12 mmol l⁻¹, creatinine 170 μmol l⁻¹; LFTs: normal, except albumin 26 g l⁻¹, globulin 40 g l⁻¹, corrected Ca^{2+} 2.2 mmol l⁻¹, PO_4^- 1.8 mmol l⁻¹, ALP 130 IU l⁻¹; serum electrophoresis: normal. He was treated for an osteoporotic fracture given the history of chronic steroid use, and prescribed oramorph for pain relief.

Can you think of any other causes for the collapsed L1 in this context?

Activity 58.1

(Allow two minutes)

....

....

....

....

....

J: *the myeloma screen is negative, and the bone profile does not suggest metastases. Can the CRP be raised due to the fracture?*

Not really and certainly not to this extent. Given the age of the patient, malignancy continues to be on the differential. Other causes include bacterial osteomyelitis including TB.

On day three of admission he spiked a temperature of 38 °C and blood cultures were sent. A urine dipstick showed protein 2+, blood 2+, leucocytes and nitrites positive and was sent for culture. He was treated for a presumed UTI.

J: *If he did not have urinary tract symptoms, shouldn't we be looking for another source?*

Quite right!

The blood cultures grew *Staphylococcus aureus*. The back pain prompted a spinal MRI which showed findings consistent with vertebral body osteomyelitis of L1 and an echo was normal. In retrospect, it came to light that he had had several courses of high dose steroids for exacerbations of COPD over the last two months which in combination with the haemodialysis line inserted recently resulted in discitis/osteomyelitis. He was treated with appropriate antibiotics for osteomyelitis and the haemodialysis line was removed, cultured and replaced at a different site. He was also continued on bisphosphonate prophylaxis.

Unpacking principle: Failure to elicit daily steroid use >5 mg and a recent haemodialysis line insertion misled the clinicians. Red flags of back pain here were age >50, pain not relieved by rest, immunosuppression and risk of osteoporosis (steroids) (Chou 2014). Seeking seemingly excessive pain relief is a yellow flag. These factors should have alerted the clinician to seek out further information. Why did this not happen? One possibility is 'attribution' error which labelled the patient's recurrent attendances as drug seeking behaviour (negative stereotype – past psychiatric issues and alcohol dependence). A recent diagnosis of mechanical back pain also kept its momentum (diagnosis momentum) through subsequent admissions.

The lack of a robust inflammatory response in the bloods was also contributory. The elderly are often unable to mount an effective inflammatory response and the steroids don't help. We must exercise extra caution when a patient is on steroids as inflammatory conditions like sepsis, peritonitis from perforation, etc. can present atypically. A fortuitous blood culture result led the team to the right diagnosis in this case which may not always happen.

Example 58.2

> A 35 year old man was seen by the GP registrar for a six week history of joint pains in the hands. PMH: 10 year history of mechanical back pain, asthma. Medications: symbicort and salbutamol inhalers.

> P: *SQs – young man + sub-acute joint pains + mechanical back pain + asthma. Provisional diagnoses – rheumatological disease but needs refinement whether single, oligo or polyarticular disease.*

> The small joints of his hands were intermittently painful and swollen. Recently the left wrist had become tender causing difficulty with his work as a computer analyst. On direct questioning he admitted to morning stiffness in the joints. There were no preceding skin, eye, genito-urinary or gastro-intestinal symptoms. No travel history.
>
> O/E: Temperature 36.5 °C, Pulse 82 bpm, BP 130/70. Hands: bilaterally symmetrical MCP, PIP joint swelling and synovial tenderness. No joint effusions, nail-fold infarcts, tophi or calcinosis. He surmised that this represented RA and requested anti-CCP. On the following visit, the CCP was positive and he was referred to rheumatology.

What differentials can you think of in this context?

Activity 58.2

....
....
....
....
....

(Allow three minutes)

> P: *This is polyarticular disease. I can only think of RA and probably CTDs.*
>
> Differentials include RA, spondyloarthropathies (SpA) including reactive arthritis, crystal arthropathies, e.g. chronic gout, CTD related arthropathies.

> He was seen by the rheumatologist who elicited a 10 year history of 'mechanical' back pain, which when probed further suggested an inflammatory aetiology, i.e. worse at rest (e.g. night) and better with movement. He confirmed symmetric polyarthropathy in the hands and continued to examine the feet. Dactylitis of the right third and fourth toes with enthesitis of right Achilles tendon was found which the patient had put down to a sprain (Brockbank et al. 2005). He also had evidence of psoriatic plaques in the natal cleft (hidden areas of psoriasis). A diagnosis of psoriatic arthropathy was made and treatment initiated.

Why did the GP registrar miss the diagnosis but not the rheumatologist?

Activity 58.3

(Allow few seconds!)

Knowledge deficits can certainly account for the different outcomes but assuming that they were similar we can try to work out the reasons from a clinical reasoning perspective.

Representativeness error: It is possible that the symmetrical polyarthropathy of the hands invoked the prototype of RA since this was its typical presentation. This led to the knee-jerk response of requesting the RF. Rule-based/deterministic/categorical reasoning tells us that a standard response (blood tests for RF and autoimmune screen) is elicited upon encountering a familiar scenario (symmetric polyarthropathy). The prevalence of CCP positivity in psoriatic arthritis varies between 6% and 16% which is interestingly associated with an aggressive and erosive polyarticular disease (Bogliolo et al. 2005). The positive result misled the GP registrar into falsely confirming RA. Remember that test results should be interpreted in conjunction with the pre-test probability of disease and RA was less likely here owing to the presence of axial disease.

Unpacking principle: The previous example illustrated this in history taking whilst this example shows it in action in clinical examination. The rheumatologist kept an open mind despite the label of RA on the referral letter. This avoided premature closure leading to a thorough history (back pain) and clinical examination (foot examination). It is wise to remember that there are no short-cuts in eliciting history and physical signs, but this can only happen when our mind is open to different possibilities. Activity 58.2 illustrates how representativeness error can be countered in daily practice.

▼

A thorough history and clinical examination can unravel other diagnoses but this can only happen if we keep our mind open to different possibilities.

Always produce a list of differential diagnoses as a matter of routine practice. This will counter most cognitive errors including representativeness error.

Steroids can mask inflammation and cause atypical disease presentations.

Never forget examination of feet in musculoskeletal assessment.

▲

References

Bogliolo, L., Alpini, C., Caporali, R. et al. (2005). Antibodies to cyclic citrullinated peptides in psoriatic arthritis. *The Journal of Rheumatology* 32 (3): 511–515.

Brockbank, J.E., Stein, M., Schentag, C.T., and Gladman, D.D. (2005). Dactylitis in psoriatic arthritis: a marker for disease severity? *Annals of the Rheumatic Diseases* 64 (2): 188–190.

Chou, R. (2014). In the clinic. Low back pain. *Annals of Internal Medicine* 160 (11): ITC6–ITC1.

59 Multi-System Disease

▼
This chapter tells you how to approach multi-system disease from a rheumatological perspective
▲

Always exclude malignancy and infection in multi-system disease before considering autoimmune conditions.

Example 59.1

> A 65 year old woman presented to the medical admissions unit with a three week history of increasing malaise, lethargy and loss of appetite. The GP had treated her with clarithromycin for acute bronchitis a week ago with no impact on symptoms. PMH: hypertension and diabetes mellitus for which she took atenolol and metformin.

> J: *SQs – Middle aged woman + subacute non-specific systemic symptoms + vascular risk factors. Provisional diagnoses – Infection, non-resolving pneumonia if it was one.*

> Poor diabetes control is another possibility.

> ET had declined from half a mile to 100 yards on the flat secondary to tiredness. She denied any localising infective symptoms. On direct questioning she admitted to occasional night sweats with fever. No relevant travel history or exposure to tuberculosis. The diabetes was well controlled.

> J: *Tiredness seems to be significant. The night sweats make me think of sepsis or haematological malignancies.*

> O/E: Elevated BMI. Pulse 86 bpm, RR 14 per minute, BP 140/70, Temperature 37.5 °C, Saturations 94% on air and BMs 12 mmol l^{-1}. Systemic examination: normal; no lymphadenopathy.
>
> CXR and ECG: normal. Hb 100 g l^{-1}, MCV 88 fl, WCC 14 × 10^9 l^{-1}, platelets 500 × 10^9 l^{-1}, CRP 60 mg l^{-1}, ALT 60 IU l^{-1}, ALP 350 IU l^{-1} and albumin 32 g l^{-1}. Blood film: thrombocytosis; clotting: normal; U&Es: normal. Urine dipstick: positive for leucocytes, blood 1+ and protein 1 +.

> J: *Severity of illness – relatively well. Working diagnosis – UTI.*

> Note that there are no urinary symptoms. The lowish albumin, elevated platelets and normocytic anaemia seem to point towards a chronic inflammatory condition. The mild LFT dysfunction could be due to clarithromycin or acute cholangitis.

The Hands-on Guide to Clinical Reasoning in Medicine, First Edition. Mujammil Irfan.
© 2019 John Wiley & Sons Ltd. Published 2019 by John Wiley & Sons Ltd.
Companion website: www.wiley.com/go/irfan/clinicalreasoning

She was empirically treated with trimethoprim for a UTI. Urine cultures were however negative. USG abdomen: fatty infiltration and normal common bile duct. The liver dysfunction was put down to the recent antibiotics.

J: *There is no evidence of cholangitis.*

The LFTs settled, but after an initial improvement, the inflammatory markers increased again by day 5. She started to spike temperatures (>38 °C) intermittently. A repeat CXR showed some subtle infiltrates in the left base and she was switched to intravenous piperacillin/tazobactam for a presumed hospital acquired pneumonia (HAP). Urine and blood cultures were sent. A single blood culture bottle grew coagulase negative *Staphylococcus aureus* which was ignored as a common skin contaminant. Urine culture: negative.

I would ensure that the skin (cellulitis), joints (septic arthritis) and central nervous system (meningo-encephalitis) are examined for localising signs of sepsis.

Inflammatory markers grumbled along with CRP 40 mg l⁻¹, WCC 11 × 10⁹ l⁻¹ and intermittent temperature spikes. Clinically she continued to feel ill. There were no new clinical findings. On day 10 she developed purplish discolouration of the tips of the right index and ring fingers. ECG: sinus tachycardia. Urine dipstick: positive for blood 2+ and protein 2+. U&Es: normal electrolytes, urea 12 mmol l⁻¹ and creatinine 150 μmol l⁻¹. Surgical consultation ruled out major arterial thrombosis. An autoimmune screen was requested.

J: *Could it be drug-induced?*

Good point! Piperacillin/tazobactam can occasionally cause drug fever and acute interstitial nephritis but it would not explain the purplish discolouration of the fingers.

She continued to deteriorate despite antibiotics and developed severe hypotension and tachycardia. Following a brief admission to ITU she succumbed to the illness. At post-mortem she was found to have aortic valve marantic endocarditis (Non-bacterial thrombotic endocarditis-NBTE). The autoimmune screen was negative.

Where do you think things went wrong?

Activity 59.1

(Allow three minutes)

....
....
....
....
....
....
....

One could argue that the final diagnosis was academic, but it just as well could have been something treatable hence it is worth evaluating what went wrong.

Failure to trigger hypotheses: It appears that the right hypothesis was never triggered (infective endocarditis or its clones). Critics would even point out that her physicians exhibited 'search satisficing' where soft signs like positive urine dipstick were labelled UTI or subtle basal changes were labelled HAP since they were convenient and alternative possibilities were never explored. However, in the heat of events unfolding we can all imagine succumbing to the errors that her physicians fell for. How can we avoid this?

Often it is the context or working space that we define that helps in generating the right hypotheses. Framing the right context helps in triggering the right hypotheses. Utilising differential diagnoses is another way of considering other diagnostic possibilities.

Framing the context or working space: A prolonged hospital admission often obscures the evolving circumstances. Re-visiting the SQs and chunking them into medical phrases would help. This scenario is a fairly common occurrence in hospital settings where it seems to be morphing into fever of unknown origin (FUO). Three broad categories make up the vast majority of FUOs – infections, malignancies and CTDs.

The purplish discolouration in combination with the AKI triggered the single hypothesis of CTDs when other differentials should have also been considered. Infective endocarditis exhibits immune phenomena including glomerulonephritis, Osler's nodes and Roth spots mimicking an autoimmune condition. The purplish discolouration of the fingers in this case was due to micro emboli from the valvular endocarditis resulting in a localised immune-mediated vasculitis. These represent minor criteria in modified Duke's criteria. In our readings we should endeavour to identify the constellation of clinical findings that should trigger specific hypothesis. For example, sub-acute constitutional symptoms + AKI + digital micro emboli = infective endocarditis, atrial myxoma, CTDs. Of note, NBTE requires a high index of suspicion especially since it does not cause the classic clinical findings of murmurs, etc.

Example 59.2

A 70 year old woman presented with new onset confusion over one week. PMH: HT, IHD, CKD stage 2, arthritis. Medications: aspirin, lisinopril, diltiazem, atorvastatin, bendrofluazide, hypromellose eye drops, glandosane spray and co-codamol.

P: *SQs – elderly woman + acute confusion + vascular risk factors. Provisional diagnoses – infection (CNS or extra-cranial), CVA, encephalopathy (metabolic, hypertensive or infective).*

There were no localising infective symptoms. O/E: Pulse 90 bpm, BP 146/90, Saturations 95% on air, Temperature 38.3 °C, BMs 12 mmol l^{-1}, RR 16 per minute. No signs of cellulitis, septic arthritis, spinal tenderness (discitis), meningeal irritation. Mental status changes with inability to recall all three words and an abnormal clock drawing test (CDT) but no altered conscious level. Rest of the systemic examination: normal. Confusion assessment method (CAM) screen: positive for delirium.

ECG, CXR and urine dipstick: normal. Bloods: Hb 98 g l^{-1}, MCV 85 fl, platelets 150 × 10^9 l^{-1}, WCC 12 × 10^9 l^{-1}, CRP 30 mg l^{-1}; U&Es, bone profile and LFTs: normal.

P: *The cause of the delirium is not clear from the data so far. Would a primary CNS infection cause this presentation?*

Yes, encephalitis can certainly present as acute confusion. Normocytic anaemia with mild CRP rise could also indicate a sub-acute inflammatory process once infection is excluded.

A CT head and LP were performed to exclude meningo-encephalitis. CT head: small vessel disease, LP: normal. She was initially started on empiric ceftriaxone and acyclovir both of which were stopped, and she was switched to co-amoxiclav. Her family reported that she had become increasingly forgetful over the last month with a reduced appetite and half stone weight loss.

Re-state the SQs and re-frame the context?

Activity 59.2

(Allow two minutes)

....
....
....
....
....
....
....

P: *SQs – elderly woman + delirium + red flag symptoms (weight loss). Provisional diagnosis – malignancy.*

Day 5: CT thorax, abdomen and pelvis: normal. The temperature spikes continued. Re-examination failed to reveal any new findings. Repeat bloods: Hb 96 g l⁻¹, MCV 82 fl, platelets 120 × 10⁹ l⁻¹, WCC 10 × 10⁹ l⁻¹, CRP 30 mg l⁻¹, ESR 80 mm per hour; rest of bloods: normal, except albumin 28 g l⁻¹. Three sets of blood cultures: negative. Myeloma screen: negative.

On day 7 she complained of acute right sided pleuritic chest pain. A computerised tomography pulmonary angiogram did not reveal any PE. An SHO looking after the patient wondered if she could have SLE requested an autoimmune screen. The antinuclear antibody (ANA) (1:320) and RF were positive. The consultant humoured her and checked the presentation against the criteria for SLE. Since she did not meet >4 criteria (arthritis, serositis – pleuritic chest pain, positive ANA) the diagnosis was abandoned. He wondered if she could instead have Giant Cell Arteritis given the raised ESR, normocytic anaemia and constitutional symptoms but the lack of headache made this less likely.

P: *I thought we should not be using classification criteria for diagnosis.*

They shouldn't be but clinicians tend to. A rheumatology opinion would be useful in such cases.

The co-amoxiclav was stopped on day 8 but she remained confused. On day 10 she had a self-terminating seizure. There were no metabolic abnormalities that could explain the seizure. A neurology consultation was requested with an MRI head. The MRI showed diffuse cerebral oedema and periventricular hyperintensities. The neurologist raised the possibility of cerebral lupus and a rheumatology review confirmed the same. Prednisolone was started which slowly improved the cognitive dysfunction over the next few months.

This example shows how guidelines/decision-support aids and scoring systems have the potential to be misused. Classification criteria in Rheumatology have been designed to be used on a population-wide basis for research purposes. They were not designed to be used at an individual level for diagnosis. Moreover, all patients with SLE do not progress in the same manner and therefore do not always satisfy the criteria especially in the early course of their disease. Indeed late-onset SLE in the elderly has been shown to have a variable presentation (as in this case) when compared to those whose disease manifests earlier resulting in a delay in diagnosis (Lazaro 2007; Arnaud et al. 2012). On the other hand, the CAM tool was used appropriately to screen for delirium when symptoms were presumed to be acute.

The phenomenon of 'zebra retreat' can also be seen very clearly in this example. The heuristic of 'if you hear hoof-beats think of horses not zebras' has been so deeply ingrained in clinicians that a rare diagnosis is rarely entertained. The prohibitive cost of specialised tests coupled with self-doubt and a fear of being ridiculed by peers makes clinicians backtrack on their clinical hunch. This has been eloquently termed the 'zebra retreat' where sometimes there truly is a zebra in the herd of horses and it takes courage to stand firm in one's convictions (Croskerry 2002).

In hindsight, the presence of sicca symptoms (artificial tears and saliva in medication list) with multi-system features (constitutional, musculoskeletal, haematological, neurological dysfunction, serositis and positive immunological tests) point to the possibility of late-onset SLE.

▼

Framing the right context helps in triggering the right hypotheses.

The elderly often tend to have atypical presentations.

Never hesitate to make esoteric diagnoses if the situation demands but always have an eye on the base-rate (disease prevalence) to guide you.

Recognise the limitations of clinical guidelines and scoring systems and ensure that your patient meets the characteristics of the test population from which the guidelines were formulated.
▲

References

Arnaud, L., Mathian, A., Boddaert, J., and Amoura, Z. (2012). Late-onset systemic lupus Erythematosus. *Drugs & Aging* 29 (3): 181–189.

Croskerry, P. (2002). Achieving quality in clinical decision making: cognitive strategies and detection of bias. *Academic Emergency Medicine: Official Journal of the Society for Academic Emergency Medicine* 9 (11): 1184–1204.

Lazaro, D. (2007). Elderly-onset systemic lupus erythematosus: prevalence, clinical course and treatment. *Drugs & Aging* 24 (9): 701–715.

▼

This section gives you an overview of common clinical conditions from a clinical reasoning perspective

▲

This section is for those of you who need a refresher of the common clinical conditions that will be encountered on your placements. There is little to be gained by reproducing what can be easily obtained from any standard textbook of medicine, so I shall attempt to highlight practical real-world issues that will help in reaching a diagnosis, deciding on appropriate investigations and picking the right treatment.

Each of the clinical conditions is discussed under the headings of diagnosis, investigations and treatment, where relevant. The information has been provided in phrases to economise on space and crystallise the important points in a nutshell. By extension, it is by no means exhaustive or detailed, yet it will focus your attention to the salient features that is often missing from textbooks.

Where indicated, likelihood ratios of relevant clinical findings have been provided in brackets under the diagnostic headings. These can be used in conjunction with the pre-test probability to arrive at a post-test probability-thereby increasing or decreasing the likelihood of the diagnosis in question. This will be one way of ensuring that you individualise the interpretation of clinical findings in the patient in front of you and deliver truly personalised care.

The Hands-on Guide to Clinical Reasoning in Medicine, First Edition. Mujammil Irfan.
© 2019 John Wiley & Sons Ltd. Published 2019 by John Wiley & Sons Ltd.
Companion website: www.wiley.com/go/irfan/clinicalreasoning

▼

This section gives you an overview of common clinical conditions in Respiratory medicine

▲

61.1 ASTHMA

Often an out-patient diagnosis and occasionally a diagnosis on emergency admission.

Diagnosis
- Characterised by reversible airways obstruction (laboratory based).
- Historical features that make this diagnosis more likely: Episodic SOB/cough, diurnal variation in symptoms, well between exacerbations (normal ET/ADLs), personal (childhood) or family history of asthma/atopy, steroid responsiveness (although this is subjective).
- Smoking can confound/worsen asthma/cause co-existent COPD.

Investigations
- Spirometry is obstructive.
- Bronchodilator reversibility test – FEV_1 increases by >12%.
- If spirometry is normal, do mannitol challenge test to look for bronchial hyper-responsiveness and a drop in FEV_1.

Treatment
- Inhaled corticosteroids mainstay of therapy.
- Follow British Thoracic Society asthma guidelines.

61.2 COPD

Prevalence ~12% (Adeloye et al. 2015)

Often an out-patient diagnosis and occasionally a diagnosis on emergency admission.

Diagnosis
- Symptom of breathlessness which worsens over time.
- Positive LRs: smoker >40 py (12), auscultatory wheezing (4.4), maximum laryngeal height ≤4 cm (4.2), forced expiratory time ≥9 seconds (6.7) (Straus et al. 2000; Garcia-Pachon 2002).

Investigations
- COPD is an obstructive airways disease that progressively worsens over time. Remember that parenchymal emphysema alone (one of the phenotypes) may not show obstruction but is diagnosed with a low gas transfer factor on PFTs.
- FEV_1 does not always correlate with symptoms.
- Owing to all of the above, the diagnosis and classification has limitations.

Treatment
- Steroids and bronchodilators relieve symptoms but do not affect mortality. The economically efficient model which affects long-term outcomes on a population-wide basis is smoking cessation > vaccinations > pulmonary rehabilitation > inhaled pharmacotherapies. The most evidence based intervention that affects mortality is smoking cessation and long-term oxygen therapy (the last when indicated).

The big difference between asthma and COPD is that the former when treated has a normal life-expectancy.

The Hands-on Guide to Clinical Reasoning in Medicine, First Edition. Mujammil Irfan.
© 2019 John Wiley & Sons Ltd. Published 2019 by John Wiley & Sons Ltd.
Companion website: www.wiley.com/go/irfan/clinicalreasoning

61.3 PNEUMONIA

Diagnosis

- A combination of pulmonary infective symptoms with an inflammatory response on blood tests, positive sputum microbiology and a radiographic evidence of consolidation (gold standard) → working diagnosis of pneumonia.
- Above, minus radiographic consolidation = acute bronchitis or infective exacerbation of underlying chronic airways disease (asthma/COPD).
- Remember that clinical judgement (severity of illness) should supplement implementation of scoring systems like CURB65 and local microbiology guidelines.
- Simultaneously, remember that adherence to these helps in preventing long-term bacterial resistance patterns and emergence of opportunistic pathogens like clostridium.
- The likelihood ratios for various clinical findings in pneumonia are discussed in Chapter 1.

Investigations

- CXR as above.
- Microbiological evidence (sputum or blood) of infective organism.
- The last is not essential for diagnosis, but is especially helpful in the setting of chronic lung disease to identify colonisation and narrowing the spectrum of antibiotic therapy.

Treatment

- Working diagnosis of pneumonia should be accompanied by an exposition of its context, e.g. community acquired pneumonia, hospital acquired pneumonia, aspiration pneumonia, opportunistic infection, ventilator associated pneumonia. This ensures that the right empiric antibiotic therapy is given based on the likely pathogen before microbiological evidence can narrow the spectrum of antibiotic therapy.

61.4 PULMONARY EMBOLISM (PE)

Diagnosis

- Symptomatology correlates with pathology, i.e. acute pleuritic chest pain → peripheral emboli (closer to the pleura), whereas acute breathlessness → central emboli (nowhere near pleura but cause obstruction in main pulmonary arteries and lack of blood flow in pulmonary circulation causes hypoxia and SOB).
- Always assess pre-test probability prior to requesting tests either by Gestalt or scoring systems like Wells score.
- The prevalence of PE with their LRs in the three categories stratified by Wells simplified score are: low 1.3 (LR 0.13), 16 (LR 1.9), and 41 (LR 5.9) respectively (Wells et al. 2001).
- Positive LR of D-dimer is 1.7.
- Negative LR of D-dimer is 0 for both low and moderate pre-test probability of PE on Well's score. It therefore effectively excludes the diagnosis of a PE (Perrier et al. 2004).

Investigations

- ABG – hypoxia, increased A-a gradient, hypocapnia.
- ECG- sinus tachycardia, $S_IQ_{III}T_{III}$.
- Recognise the limitations of d-dimer and Wells score.
- The suggested investigation of an acute PE is a CTPA (central PE) and chronic thrombo-embolic pulmonary hypertension (CTEPH) is V/Q scan (more sensitive and discriminates proximal large vessel disease from peripheral small vessel disease). However, the choice of test depends on several factors, including the institutional preference and expertise.
- The results of imaging must be interpreted with the pre-test probability of a PE.
- Echo is useful to assess right heart dysfunction in massive PE.
- Troponin helps with risk stratification.

Treatment

- If the diagnosis is suspected, treatment should be initiated if the risk/benefit ratio is favourable.
- Choices include LMWH, warfarin with LMWH cover until INR therapeutic or newer oral anticoagulants (NOACs).
- Patient preference and views should contribute to the choice of therapy.
- LMWH preferred in patients with malignancy.
- Thrombolysis in massive PE and selected cases of submassive PE again based on risk/benefit ratio.
- Pulmonary embolism severity index (PESI) gives prognostic information on mortality (look it up on the internet/apps).

61.5 PLEURAL EFFUSION

Diagnosis
- Often sub-acute history of breathlessness.
- Look for aetiology during clinical assessment, e.g. red flag symptoms with pleural effusion → malignant effusion, infective symptoms with effusion → parapneumonic effusion or empyema.
- Bilateral effusions are usually due to a 'failure' (liver, heart, renal, gastrointestinal – protein-losing enteropathy).
- caveat: heart failure can also cause unilateral effusion.
- Exudates are often due to pleural inflammation or lymphatic blockage.
- Transudates are often due to interstitial pulmonary edema due to increased hydrostatic pressure.
- Dullness to percussion (LR 8.7) increases the likelihood of pleural effusion whilst reduced tactile vocal fremitus (LR 0.21) reduces the likelihood (Wong et al. 2009).

Investigations
- Ultrasound-guided pleural aspiration and classification using Light's criteria.
- Diagnosing a transudate or an exudate narrows the differentials.
- Exudative effusion – medical thoracoscopy has the diagnostic advantage of pleural biopsies under direct vision (therefore higher yield) and therapeutic advantage of draining the fluid and talc poudrage to prevent recurrence all in one sitting.

Treatment
- Treat the cause.
- Symptomatic treatment includes therapeutic thoracentesis.
- Malignant effusions can be treated symptomatically with thoracentesis and pleurodesis to prevent recurrence.
- Indwelling pleural catheters can be used as palliative treatment for malignant effusions.

61.6 PNEUMOTHORAX

Diagnosis
- Acute breathlessness or pleuritic chest pain
- Primary spontaneous pneumothorax implies no underlying chronic lung disease and secondary pneumothorax implies otherwise, e.g. asthma.
- Smoking increases the risk of pneumothorax.
- Tension pneumothorax is identified by its accompanying haemodynamic instability (low BP and tachycardia).

Investigations
- CXR – remember that a pneumothorax is distinguished from a bulla by the convex lung margin.
- BTS guidelines base their therapeutic decisions on the size of the pneumothorax on a CXR but it is wise to recall that the true volume of a pneumothorax cannot be estimated on a two dimensional film.
- Look at the opposite lung to identify an undiagnosed pre-existing lung disease.

Treatment
- Follow BTS guidelines.
- Prevention of recurrence can be medical (talc pleurodesis) or surgical (pleurectomy).
- Smoking cessation.
- Can fly one week after lung re-expansion or two weeks after traumatic pneumothorax resolution.
- Can never go deep sea diving unless a definitive pleural procedure has been done to prevent recurrence.

61.7 INTERSTITIAL LUNG DISEASE (ILD)

Diagnosis
- The diagnosis is often a combination of clinical-radiological-pathological findings with disease behaviour over time influencing the final diagnosis.
- Often a sub-acute presentation with breathlessness and cough but can occasionally present for the first time as an acute exacerbation.
- Idiopathic pulmonary fibrosis is the most common ILD.
- ILDs in the setting of CTD, sarcoidosis and drug induced ILDs are particular sub-groups that should be on the radar of a general physician.

- Smoking can worsen or in some cases cause ILD, e.g. Respiratory bronchiolitis-associated interstitial lung disease (RBILD).
- Pulmonary hypertension is a common complication of chronic ILDs.

Investigations
- PFTs showing restriction with a low gas transfer factor are a common finding in ILD.
- High resolution computed tomography shows reticulo-nodular, reticular, or cystic lung disease.
- Lung biopsy (surgical or transbronchial cryobiopsy) in some instances.
- Echo can confirm pulmonary hypertension.

Treatment
- Specific treatments aimed at controlling disease progression is where we are at present, e.g. pirfenidone in Idiopathic Pulmonary Fibrosis.
- General principles of therapy include treating the underlying disease (CTDs), smoking cessation (RBILD), withdrawing causative drugs, treating cor pulmonale, supplementary oxygen when indicated, pulmonary rehabilitation and vaccinations to prevent respiratory tract infections.

61.8 LUNG CANCER

Diagnosis
- Smoking is the single most common risk factor.
- Often a late presentation but can also present as an incidental finding on CT scans, e.g. solitary pulmonary nodule.
- Symptoms can be myriad or none but commonly include systemic features like weight loss with respiratory complaints like cough or haemoptysis.
- Think of the symptoms on an anatomical model from inside out, e.g. lymphadenopathy → pulmonary mass effects, e.g. breathlessness, cough, haemoptysis → pleural effusion → rib pain from metastases → cord compression from thoracic metastases → distant metastases mass effects or paraneoplastic syndromes.
- Broadly classified into small cell carcinoma or non-small cell carcinoma (NSCLC) the latter being more common.

Investigations
- Tissue diagnosis, e.g. bronchoscopy is paramount since treatment is fairly toxic or involves major surgery.
- Staging of disease is primarily done to identify patients who would benefit from curative surgery and to provide prognostic information.
- PFTs are useful to assess patients physiologically before subjecting them to treatment, e.g. surgery or haemo-radiotherapy.

Treatment
- Small cell carcinoma is extremely chemosensitive but relapses very quickly giving it a very poor prognosis.
- NSCLC on the other hand is more indolent but carries a relatively better prognosis in general especially if surgically resected.
- Chemo-radiotherapy is often aimed at slowing disease progression although newer stereotactic radiotherapy procedures and targeted molecular drugs have been quite successful in some instances.
- Smoking cessation improves therapeutic outcomes.

References

Adeloye, D., Chua, S., Lee, C. et al. (2015). Global and regional estimates of COPD prevalence: systematic review and meta-analysis. *Journal of Global Health* 5 (2): 20415.

Garcia-Pachon, E. (2002). Paradoxical movement of the lateral rib margin (Hoover sign) for detecting obstructive airway disease. *Chest* 122 (2): 651–655.

Perrier, A., Roy, P.M., Aujesky, D. et al. (2004). Diagnosing pulmonary embolism in outpatients with clinical assessment, D-dimer measurement, venous ultrasound, and helical computed tomography: a multicenter management study. *The American Journal of Medicine* 116 (5): 291–299.

Straus, S.E., McAlister, F.A., Sackett, D.L. et al. (2000). The accuracy of patient history, wheezing, and laryngeal measurements in diagnosing obstructive airway disease. CARE-COAD1 Group. Clinical Assessment of the Reliability of the Examination-Chronic Obstructive Airways Disease. *JAMA* 283 (14): 1853–1857.

Wells, P.S., Anderson, D.R., Rodger, M. et al. (2001). Excluding pulmonary embolism at the bedside without diagnostic imaging: management of patients with suspected pulmonary embolism presenting to the emergency department by using a simple clinical model and d-dimer. *Annals of Internal Medicine* 135 (2): 98–107.

Wong, C.L., Holroyd-Leduc, J., Straus, S.E. et al. (2009). Does this patient have a pleural effusion? *Journal of the American Medical Association* 301 (3): 309.

▼
This section gives you an overview of common clinical conditions in Cardiology
▲

62.1 ATRIAL FIBRILLATION

Diagnosis

- Often an incidental finding (asymptomatic) or can present with symptoms of breathlessness and heart failure.
- Loss of the 'atrial kick' contribution to cardiac output unmasks heart failure and the rapid rate shortens the time for ventricular filling (diastole) leading to symptoms.
- The sluggish blood flow in the atrium and atrial appendage causes thrombus formation with potential for systemic embolism, e.g. stroke.
- Examination uncovers associated heart failure and in some instances the cause for AF, e.g. Hyperthyroidism, valvular heart disease, or sepsis.

Investigations

- ECG to confirm the rate and irregular rhythm.
- Echo to assess structural heart disease – LA diameter (influences success rate of cardioversion), co-existent LV dysfunction (increased mortality, thromboembolic risk, and influences therapeutic choices), underlying valvular lesions.
- TFTs.

Treatment

- Always treat underlying cause if found.
- Two important decisions – rate or rhythm control strategy and decisions on anticoagulation.
- No difference in mortality or morbidity between the two strategies but rhythm control strategy is often tried first for symptom relief and potentially less cardiac structural remodelling in new onset AF especially if no underlying cause found.
- LV dysfunction + AF digoxin, overt heart failure + AF – beta blockers ± digoxin for symptom relief, preserved LV function + AF – β blocker or calcium channel blocker.
- Anticoagulation decisions are based on CHA_2DS_2 – Vasc risk score balanced against bleeding risk score, e.g. HASBLED (Lip et al. 2010; Pisters et al. 2010).
- These scoring systems have limitations since the risk factors are not equivalent to the event rate, they have a range and do not have equal weighting.
- In general, higher embolic risk patients receive the greatest benefit from anticoagulation (absolute risk reduction) which often offsets the bleeding risk.
- No difference in therapeutic efficacy between warfarin or NOACs.

62.2 HEART FAILURE (HF)

From an epidemiological stand-point, the most prevalent diseases in the population are IHD and DM with vascular risk factors like hypertension, smoking, obesity, and hypercholesterolemia. So, you wouldn't be wrong to guess that the cause of heart failure in your patient is IHD but remember that the aetiology can be either functional (e.g. IHD, HT), structural (e.g. valvular heart disease), or metabolic (e.g. sepsis).

Three practical clinical categories of left heart failure:

- Low ejection fraction (EF) with elevated end-diastolic filling pressures – (systolic dysfunction).

The Hands-on Guide to Clinical Reasoning in Medicine, First Edition. Mujammil Irfan.
© 2019 John Wiley & Sons Ltd. Published 2019 by John Wiley & Sons Ltd.
Companion website: www.wiley.com/go/irfan/clinicalreasoning

- Normal EF with elevated filling pressures – (diastolic dysfunction, provided other causes like restrictive structural heart disease, intermittent ischemia, and high output cardiac failure are excluded). Remember that diastolic dysfunction can exist without producing HF with preserved EF, e.g. normal ageing process.
- Low EF with normal filling pressures, can be asymptomatic (e.g. post MI which should still be treated since it improves prognosis).

Diagnosis

- HF is a clinical diagnosis with no technological gold standard.
- It occurs when the heart is:
  - Not contracting very well – systolic dysfunction, HF with reduced EF $\leq 40\%$ (HF_rEF), or
  - Not relaxing very well – diastolic dysfunction, a risk factor for HF with preserved EF $\geq 50\%$ (HF_pEF).
- Mortality is lower in diastolic than systolic HF.
- Clinical features that increase the post-test probability of HF in someone presenting with breathlessness in the emergency department are (all have LRs > 2): overall clinical impression, history of HF, orthopnoea, paroxysmal nocturnal dyspnoea (PND), S3, pulmonary rales, ankle oedema, elevated JVP, ECG evidence of AF, and radiographic pulmonary venous congestion or interstitial oedema (Wang et al. 2005).
- $BNP < 100\,pg\,ml^{-1}$ (0.09) reduces the likelihood of HF the most especially in the presence of airway disease.

Investigations

- ECG – look for sinus tachycardia, anterior Q waves, and AF which increase the probability of HF.
- CXR – look for pulmonary venous congestion and interstitial oedema.
- Limitations of echo – EF does not predict symptom severity or diagnose HF, it merely confirms clinical suspicions, same as elsewhere in medicine.

Treatment

- Treat the cause.
- Lifestyle changes for IHD, vascular risk factors, e.g. smoking cessation, weight reduction, etc.
- Drug therapy – to reduce morbidity/mortality.
- β blockers (carvedilol, bisoprolol, or metoprolol SR), ACEi or ARB, aldosterone antagonists, diuretics, and digoxin, the last two do not have mortality benefit.
- Treat AF if present.
- Cardiac resynchronization therapy, e.g. PPM/ICD insertion.
- Cardiac transplantation in appropriate context.
- Cardiac rehabilitation and in end-stage HF, palliation.
- Treat underlying cause in HF_pEF, e.g. hypertension.
- Treat elevated filling pressures in HF_pEF with cautious diuretics as over diuresis can drop filling pressures in an already small, stiff LV which will drop cardiac output and BP.

62.3 ACUTE CORONARY SYNDROME (ACS)

ACS implies suspected myocardial ischemia. The diagnosis utilises all three elements of clinical assessment, ECG and cardiac biomarkers. It covers a broad range of syndromes starting with unstable angina (UA), Non-ST elevation MI (NSTEMI), and ST elevation MI (STEMI). The first two are indistinguishable at presentation and a troponin rise in NSTEMI distinguishes it from UA. However, they both signify high risk. STEMI is a class apart since it demands prompt coronary intervention.

Diagnosis

- In patients presenting with undifferentiated chest pain to the emergency department with a non diagnostic ECG, the clinical features that carry the highest LRs for ACS include: pain radiating to both arms (4.1), radiation to right arm (3.8), vomiting (3.5), ex-smoker (2.5) (Goodacre et al. 2003). HEART score of 7–10 has the highest LR of 13 for diagnosing ACS (Fanaroff et al. 2015).
- Characteristics of chest pain that decrease the likelihood of ACS are the 3 Ps – pleuritic, positional, or reproducible on palpation (Swap and Nagurney 2005).
- Remember that left bundle branch block (LBBB) is also a criterion for reperfusion therapy in STEMI and chest pain is not essential for the diagnosis of MI.

Investigations
- A normal ECG quite reliably rules out an MI but does not discriminate those who might still need close observation since 7% of these can still have an MI (Goodacre et al. 2003)
- Serial ECGs are needed to evaluate ACS
- Do not exclude ACS on the basis of a normal ECG whilst the patient is having chest pain (Chase et al. 2006)
- Serial troponin T or I levels help in ruling in or ruling out ACS and risk stratification but remember they can be normal in UA which is a clinical diagnosis
- Cardiac troponin, especially troponin I is very specific to myocardium therefore it always indicates myocardial damage, however the mechanism of damage may not always be coronary thrombosis
- Causes of false positive troponin elevations broadly arise from myocardial damage from:
  - Supply-balance mismatch, e.g. tachyarrhythmias.
  - Direct myocardial damage due to myocarditis or toxicity, e.g. drugs.
  - Indeterminate cause, e.g. sepsis related myocardial permeability and increased stress on the myocardium promoting leakage of troponins into the circulation.

Troponins can remain elevated up to one to two weeks after an MI.

Treatment
- Primary PCI for STEMI or fibrinolysis if former unavailable.
- Drug therapy for STEMI similar to NSTEMI with regimens based on the interventional strategy chosen.
- Risk-stratify using TIMI or GRACE score in patients with NSTEMI.
- Rule of thumb – early invasive strategy if moderate/high risk score.
- High pre-test probability of ACS → start therapy whilst waiting for troponin results, i.e. oxygen if hypoxic, morphine if in pain, nitroglycerine if in pain, or hypertensive, dual-antiplatelet therapy (aspirin + clopidogrel), anticoagulation therapy, IV/PO beta blocker, e.g. metoprolol if on-going chest pain, tachycardia or hypertension, and no contra-indication within 24 hours, high-dose statin. Remember to stop the anticoagulation therapy in accordance with the treatment strategy used –
  - Invasive strategy: stopped at end of PCI or
  - Conservatively managed: continued for duration of hospitalisation up to eight days.

62.4 INFECTIVE ENDOCARDITIS (IE)

Diagnosis
- Remember to ascertain the pre-test probability of IE and then apply the modified Duke criteria to diagnose IE using your clinical judgement.
- These criteria were developed for left sided native valve IE and therefore have lower sensitivity for IE in other settings.
- Resolution of clinical signs and symptoms ≤4 days after institution of antibiotics makes IE less likely.
- Remember to include IE in the differential for autoimmune conditions.

Investigations
- Contrary to the popular myth, blood cultures do not have to coincide with temperature spikes (Riedel et al. 2008).
- IE and other conditions like infected intravascular devices are associated with continuous bacteraemia unlike the intermittent bacteraemia seen in conditions like pneumonia or UTI.
- Two blood culture sets can be taken sequentially from two different sites at the same time and another set taken at an interval of four to six hours.
- Optimal volume of blood in each bottle is 10 ml (Weinstein 1996).
- At least four blood culture sets are needed if the pre-test probability of a common contaminant is high.
- A trans-oesophageal echo (TEE) is more sensitive than a trans-thoracic echo (TTE) which is especially useful in the setting of prosthetic valves or if the pre-test probability of IE is high despite a negative TTE.
- Follow-up blood cultures are needed to document clearing of bacteraemia after successful antibiotic therapy.

Treatment

- Standard duration of bactericidal antibiotics for IE is six weeks but varies with context.
- Empiric therapy can be started if pre-test probability is high following blood cultures.
- Conditions that increase the probability of IE are history of IE, prosthetic valves, repaired congenital heart disease, or valve regurgitation in a transplanted heart – all indications for antibiotic prophylaxis prior to instrumentation involving mucosal disruption especially in the setting of an ongoing infection.

62.5 HYPERTENSION

Commonly screened in primary practice and rarely picked up in secondary care. Difficult to control hypertension and possible secondary hypertension referred to secondary care for further investigations.

Diagnosis

- The prevalence of hypertension in the developed world is 25%.
- Diagnosed non-invasively on multiple readings as per national guidelines (NICE in UK).
- Once diagnosed, calculate 10 year cardiovascular risk and look for target-organ damage, i.e. renal (urine protein:creatinine ratio), examine fundi for hypertensive retinopathy and an ECG to look for left ventricular hypertrophy (LVH) in particular.

Investigations

- Treatment resistant hypertension and suspected secondary hypertension will have to be investigated in more detail to ascertain the aetiology (e.g. endocrine, renal causes).
- Assessing for the presence of other vascular risk factors (diabetes mellitus, hyperlipidaemia) is important to reduce the overall cardiovascular risk.

Treatment

- Lifestyle advice (healthy diet, exercise, weight loss, smoking cessation) is the cornerstone of therapy even in patients on antihypertensives.
- Treatment reduces risk of developing cardiovascular disease (coronary artery disease and cerebrovascular disease).
- National guidelines recommend treatment based on the BP reading.
- Treatment should be started immediately if they have already demonstrated evidence of end-organ damage (MI, stroke, etc.) or have accelerated hypertension.
- Risk reduction with treatment is in proportion to the estimated risk of developing cardiovascular disease, i.e. the greatest benefit is seen in the highest risk individuals (Sundström and Neal 2015).
- Therefore, treatment trends are now moving towards a risk based strategy rather than the actual BP reading, e.g. calculate the absolute risk reduction for the patient in front of you, explain the benefits of antihypertensive therapy in them and start therapy if benefits outweigh risks (Wallis et al. 2002).

62.6 AORTIC STENOSIS (AS) USED AS A PROTOTYPE OF VALVULAR HEART DISEASE

Think of it in patients presenting with exertional chest pain, breathlessness, and syncope. These three symptoms are in fact markers of severe AS indicating the need for valve replacement.

Diagnosis

- Clinical features that increase the likelihood of AS (LR > 2): exertional syncope, slow rising carotid pulse, late peaking in intensity of murmur, soft S2, presence of S4, reduced pulse pressure (Etchells et al. 1997).

Investigations

- Diagnosis confirmed by echocardiogram and cardiac catheterization.

Treatment

- Surgical candidates – valve replacement is indicated in symptomatic patients ideally before LVEF is reduced.
- Valve replacement can be combined with other cardiac surgical procedures if indicated, e.g. CABG.
- Non-surgical candidates, i.e. intermediate to high surgical risk – consider Transcatheter aortic valve implantation (TAVI) or medical management ± palliation.

References

Chase, M., Brown, A.M., Robey, J.L. et al. (2006). Prognostic value of symptoms during a normal or nonspecific electrocardiogram in emergency department patients with potential acute coronary syndrome. *Academic Emergency Medicine: Official Journal of the Society for Academic Emergency Medicine* 13 (10): 1034–1039.

Etchells, E., Bell, C., and Robb, K. (1997). Does this patient have an abnormal systolic murmur? *JAMA* 277 (7): 564–571.

Fanaroff, A.C., Rymer, J.A., Goldstein, S.A. et al. (2015). Does this patient with chest pain have acute coronary syndrome? *JAMA* 314 (18): 1955.

Goodacre, S.W., Angelini, K., Arnold, J. et al. (2003). Clinical predictors of acute coronary syndromes in patients with undifferentiated chest pain. *QJM: Monthly Journal of the Association of Physicians* 96 (12): 893–898.

Lip, G.Y.H., Nieuwlaat, R., Pisters, R. et al. (2010). Refining clinical risk stratification for predicting stroke and thromboembolism in atrial fibrillation using a novel risk factor-based approach: the euro heart survey on atrial fibrillation. *Chest* 137 (2): 263–272.

Pisters, R., Lane, D.A., Nieuwlaat, R. et al. (2010). A novel user-friendly score (HAS-BLED) to assess 1-year risk of major bleeding in patients with atrial fibrillation. *Chest* 138 (5): 1093–1100.

Riedel, S., Bourbeau, P., Swartz, B. et al. (2008). Timing of specimen collection for blood cultures from febrile patients with bacteremia. *Journal of Clinical Microbiology* 46 (4): 1381–1385.

Sundström, J. and Neal, B. (2015). Replacing the hypertension control paradigm with a strategy of cardiovascular risk reduction. *European Heart Journal – Quality of Care and Clinical Outcomes* 1 (1): 17–22.

Swap, C.J. and Nagurney, J.T. (2005). Value and limitations of chest pain history in the evaluation of patients with suspected acute coronary syndromes. *JAMA* 294 (20): 2623.

Wallis, E.J., Ramsay, L.E., and Jackson, P.R. (2002). Cardiovascular and coronary risk estimation in hypertension management. *Heart (British Cardiac Society)* 88 (3): 306–312.

Wang, C.S., FitzGerald, J.M., Schulzer, M. et al. (2005). Does this Dyspneic patient in the emergency department have congestive heart failure? *Journal of the American Medical Association* 294 (15): 1944.

Weinstein, M.P. (1996). Current blood culture methods and systems: clinical concepts, technology, and interpretation of results. *Clinical Infectious Diseases: An Official Publication of the Infectious Diseases Society of America* 23 (1): 40–46.

63 Nephrology

▼

This section gives you an overview of common clinical conditions in Nephrology

▲

Intrinsic renal disease can be glomerular, tubular, interstitial, or vascular in keeping with the components of a kidney.

Figure 63.1 shows how the various glomerulonephritides can be conceptualised using the urinary findings of proteinuria and haematuria. At one end of the spectrum is the nephrotic syndrome with only proteinuria and no haematuria. The other end has nephritic syndrome with predominant haematuria and some proteinuria. As we move from the nephrotic to the nephritic end we see that proteinuria gradually diminishes but persists whilst haematuria gradually increases. At various points on this spectrum lie the different glomerulonephritides which are composed of varying proportions of proteinuria and haematuria. Two conditions namely SLE and IgA nephropathy span across the spectrum since they can present anywhere along this line.

Clinical classification and histological patterns help narrow down the aetiology of glomerulonephritis. However, it is to be appreciated that nephritic and nephrotic syndromes can overlap and co-exist, and it is only renal biopsy that can clearly identify the cause, E.g. post-streptococcal GN can initially present as nephritic

The spectrum of glomerular diseases

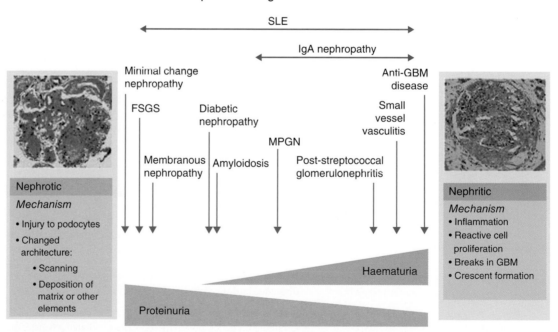

Figure 63.1 Source: Turner, N. 2017. *Glomerulonephritis explained - Educational resources for renal medicine* [Online]. Available at: http://www.edrep.org/pages/resources/glomerulonephritis.php [Accessed: 30 November 2017]. Reproduced with permission of Professor Neil Turner.

Table 63.1 Discriminatory features between nephritic and nephrotic syndrome

	Nephritic syndrome	Nephrotic syndrome
Clinical features	Predominant haematuria Hypertension	Predominant proteinuria Oedema Hypertension Hyperlipidaemia Protein leakage resulting in various manifestations like infections by capsulated organisms, venous and arterial thrombosis, hypothyroidism, etc.
Urinalysis	*Active urinary sediment* Dysmorphic red cells, red cell casts, and *variable* proteinuria.	*Bland urinary sediment* Heavy proteinuria
Serum creatinine eGFR	High Low	Often normal Often normal
Pathological features	*Proliferative GN* Mesangial cell injury. Glomerular filtration barrier injury leading to active urinary sediment (see above). Glomerular parietal epithelial cell injury causing crescent formation. Indirect podocyte injury due to inflammation in the vicinity causing variable proteinuria. Intense inflammatory infiltration.	*Non-proliferative GN* Podocyte injury leading to proteinuria alone. Matrix deposition. Little inflammatory component since podocytes are separated from the circulation by the Glomerular Basement Membrane (GBM).

syndrome and in the late stages with nephrotic syndrome. Histological patterns have their own shortcomings in that they are 'descriptive' and each pattern can have several causes, e.g. membranous glomerulonephritis can be due to SLE, chronic hepatitis B infection, malignancy, or drugs. Table 63.1 shows the principal differences between nephritic and nephrotic syndrome.

63.1 ACUTE AND CHRONIC RENAL FAILURE: SEE CHAPTERS 19 AND 20

63.2 URINARY TRACT INFECTION (UTI)

The prevalence of asymptomatic bacteriuria in a woman of reproductive age is 5%. The pre-test probability of a UTI rises to 50% if this person presents with one or more urinary symptoms (Bent et al. 2002). Cystitis presents with dysuria, frequency, urgency, suprapubic pain, and haematuria. Pyelonephritis presents with fever, chills, costovertebral angle tenderness ± symptoms of cystitis.

Diagnosis
- When an underlying condition (e.g. diabetes mellitus) increases the chances of treatment failure it is called a complicated UTI.
- Uncomplicated UTI can be treated with simple short course antibiotic regimens and therefore establishing its presence changes management.
- Four symptoms that increase the likelihood of a UTI include dysuria, frequency, haematuria, and back pain.
- Four symptoms that decrease the likelihood include vaginal symptoms of irritation and discharge and the absence of dysuria and frequency.

Investigations
- Combined dipstick positivity to nitrite and leucocyte esterase has a LR of 4.2 but a negative test does not rule out UTI (Hurlbut and Littenberg 1991).
- If the dipstick is negative but symptoms suggest UTI, the post-test probability remains high at 20%, which means a urine culture will have to be sent to exclude UTI.

Treatment
- Uncomplicated UTI can be treated empirically with short course regimens in accordance with local microbiology guidelines.
- Asymptomatic bacteriuria should only be treated in the context of pregnancy or planned urinary tract instrumentation.

63.3 HYPOVOLEMIA

Diagnosis
- Volume status assessment is an integral part of clinical assessment in nephrology.
- LRs of clinical findings that increase the likelihood of hypovolemia not due to blood loss: urine specific gravity >1.020 (11) in healthy, young adults; capillary refill time >2 seconds in adult men, >3 seconds in adult women, and >4 seconds in elderly (6.9); pulse increment from supine to standing >30 bpm (1.7) (Schriger and Baraff 1988; Bartok et al. 2004).
- Increased likelihood of hypovolemia due to blood loss: postural pulse increment >30 bpm and postural dizziness preventing them from standing.

63.4 NEPHROLITHIASIS

Diagnosis
- Calcium oxalate or calcium phosphate is the most common urinary tract stone.
- Typical pain and haematuria are the most discriminating features for nephrolithiasis, but the absence of haematuria does not exclude it.
- Remember to exclude a long list of differentials in the vicinity, e.g. ectopic pregnancy, appendicitis – think of the anatomical structures in this location.
- Stones can be complicated by infections and obstruction which can be the presenting symptoms.

Investigations
- Definitive test – non-contrasted CT.
- Pregnant patients – USG scan.

Treatment
- Conservative management for stones <10 mm with NSAIDs or opioids for analgesia and hydration.
- Urology referral if conservative management fails or there are stone related complications.
- Preventive therapy depends on composition of stone.

References

Bartok, C., Schoeller, D.A., Sullivan, J.C. et al. (2004). Hydration testing in collegiate wrestlers undergoing hypertonic dehydration. *Medicine and Science in Sports and Exercise* 36 (3): 510–517.

Bent, S., Nallamothu, B.K., Simel, D.L. et al. (2002). Does this woman have an acute uncomplicated urinary tract infection? *JAMA* 287 (20): 2701–2710.

Hurlbut, T.A. and Littenberg, B. (1991). The diagnostic accuracy of rapid dipstick tests to predict urinary tract infection. *American Journal of Clinical Pathology* 96 (5): 582–588.

Schriger, D.L. and Baraff, L. (1988). Defining normal capillary refill: variation with age, sex, and temperature. *Annals of Emergency Medicine* 17 (9): 932–935.

Turner, N. 2017. Glomerulonephritis explained - Educational resources for renal medicine [Online]. Available at: http://www.edrep.org/pages/resources/glomerulonephritis.php [Accessed: 30 November 2017].

▼

This section gives you an overview of common clinical conditions in Neurology

▲

64.1 STROKE

Prevalence of stroke in patients presenting with relevant neurological findings is 10%.

Diagnosis
- Stroke is a clinical diagnosis.
- Three signs increase the likelihood of stroke: facial paresis (14), arm drift (4.2), and abnormal speech (5.2) (Goldstein and Simel 2005).
- Remember to clinically localise the lesion in the cortex or sub-cortical region based on the presence or absence of cortical signs like graphaesthesia, speech problems, etc.
- Try to decipher the aetiology of stroke by looking for carotid bruits (athero-embolic risk), AF (cardio-embolic risk), DVT (paradoxical embolism from venous circulation through Patent Foramen Ovale to arterial circulation).
- NIHSS score predicts prognosis and gives severity of neurological deficit.

Investigations
- Non-contrasted CT head is essential in excluding haemorrhagic stroke prior to thrombolysis for an ischaemic stroke.
- Absence of confirmatory signs of an ischaemic stroke on CT does not preclude thrombolysis in individuals with a high post-test probability of stroke, i.e. a high clinical suspicion of stroke.
- Supplementary tests to assess vascular risk factors (hypertension, hyperlipidaemia, diabetes mellitus, smoking), tests to delineate aetiology of stroke like ECG, echo, carotid dopplers bearing in mind the absolute benefits of pursuing this approach, e.g. eligibility for carotid endarterectomy.

Treatment
- Thrombolysis in eligible individuals with ischaemic stroke.
- Clopidogrel for secondary prevention.
- Combined aspirin and clopidogrel can be used in the presence of recent acute coronary events.
- Warfarin or NOACs for cardio-embolic stroke from AF.
- Continue with antihypertensive therapy if already on it prior to stroke.
- Treat accompanying hyperglycaemia, fever, dehydration.
- Do not treat hypertension in acute stroke unless needed prior to thrombolysis or evidence of target-organ damage.
- Follow National Institute of Clinical Excellence guidelines for stroke management.
- Carotid endarterectomy in eligible candidates.

64.2 TRANSIENT ISCHAEMIC ATTACK (TIA)

Diagnosis
- Prevalence as in stroke.
- ABCD[2] score helps in risk stratification.
- It was designed to be used in primary care settings.
- The revised definition of TIA where the presence of brain infarction on imaging regardless of the duration of symptoms portends a higher risk of further strokes.
- This in combination with studies that showed poor predictive power of ABCD[2] especially in hospital settings means that this score has limitations (Stead et al. 2011; Amarenco et al. 2012).

A – Age > 60 = 1
B – BP ≥ 140/90 = 1
C – Clinical features (unilateral hemiparesis = 2, speech disturbance = 1, other = 0)
D² – Duration (≥60 min = 2, 10–59 = 1, and < 10 min = 0), Diabetes mellitus = 1

Investigations
- Directed at uncovering mechanism of TIA.
- ECG (AF), cardiac examination (cardio-embolic source), carotid dopplers (large artery anterior circulation TIA), identify vascular risk factors.
- CT head or MRI (more sensitive).

Treatment
- Vascular risk factor reduction
- Specific treatment directed at aetiology – AF (anticoagulation), carotid artery stenosis (endarterectomy), etc.

64.3 MENINGITIS

Diagnosis
- Absence of all three features of fever, neck stiffness, and altered mental status reduces the likelihood of bacterial meningitis (Attia et al. 1999).
- Individual signs of meningeal irritation like Kernig's, Brudzinski's and neck stiffness lack sensitivity but have good specificity.
- Therefore their absence does not exclude meningitis.
- Age >60, immunocompromised state, seizure within one week of presentation, previous CNS disease and focal neurological deficits predict abnormality on CT head, indicate the need for CT head prior to LP (Hasbun et al. 2001). This should however not delay antibiotic therapy.

Investigations
- CT head as discussed in the preceding section prior to LP.
- LP to confirm microbiological evidence of bacterial meningitis which is the gold standard.

Treatment
- Delayed antibiotic therapy increases mortality in bacterial meningitis.
- Hypotension, altered mental status, and seizures at presentation predict high mortality (Aronin et al. 1998).
- Dexamethasone improves neurological outcomes in community acquired pneumococcal meningitis and should be given before or together with the first dose of antibiotic in suspected bacterial meningitis.

64.4 ENCEPHALITIS

Diagnosis
- Altered mental status, seizures, and focal neurological deficits.
- Immunocompromised state widens the differential for aetiology.
- Think of non-infectious causes as well, e.g. tumours, paraneoplastic syndromes, cerebral vasculitis, Acute Disseminated Encephalomyelitis, etc. which may be amenable to therapy.
- Seizures and diffuse cerebral oedema predict poor prognosis.

Investigations
- CT/MRI showing temporal lobe involvement points to HSV encephalitis.
- LP: CSF showing increased red cells in the right context points to HSV encephalitis.
- CSF should be sent for viral PCRs – HSV, enteroviruses.

Treatment
- Early acyclovir therapy improves mortality and morbidity
- Patients with low pre-test probability of encephalitis (normal mental state, normal CT, and CSF WCC < 5 cells mm^{-2}) who have a negative HSV PCR on CSF can have their acyclovir discontinued (Tyler 2004).

64.5 EPILEPSY

Figure 64.1 shows a concept map for seizures (Fisher et al. 2017). It illustrates how epilepsy forms only a part of the overall schema of seizures. Seizures can occur due to structural, infective, immune, genetic, or metabolic causes. The definition of epilepsy as per the International League against Epilepsy framework is also shown (Fisher et al. 2014).

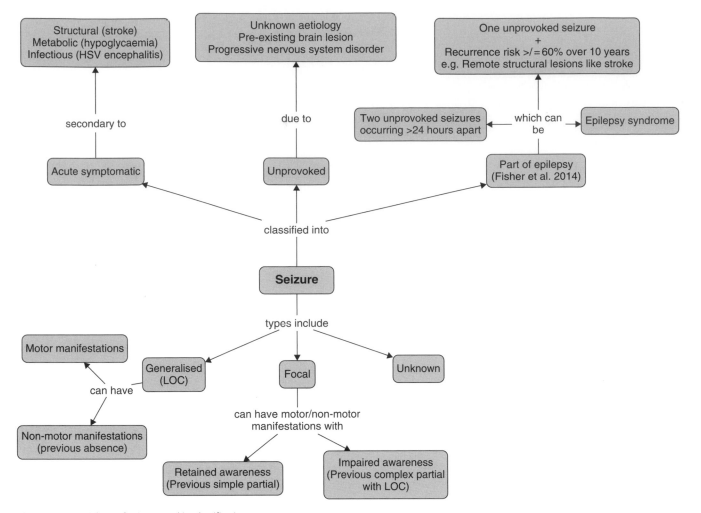

Figure 64.1 Aetiology of seizures and its classification

Broadly speaking, seizures are classified into generalised and focal with a second layer of motor or non-motor manifestations. Focal seizures then have a third layer of impaired or retained awareness.

If the seizure activity starts only in one part of the brain it is called focal. The site of the brain involved determines the symptoms of what we call 'aura'. If the seizure is not accompanied by loss of consciousness (LOC) they are called focal seizures with retained awareness. However, if the seizure activity then spreads to involve the rest of the brain resulting in LOC or sometimes just loss of awareness of the surroundings we call it a focal seizure with impaired awareness. This is usually associated with repetitive behaviours or 'automatisms' like grimacing, lip smacking or occasionally walking or running too.

If the seizure activity starts in all parts of the brain simultaneously they are called generalised seizures which can be of several types ranging from muscle stiffening (tonic), rhythmic muscle jerking (clonic), both (tonic–clonic), sudden loss of tone in muscles (atonic), brief muscle contractions (myoclonic), and finally staring into space with no loss of muscle tone (absence).

Diagnosis
- Epilepsy is a difficult diagnosis to make.
- Up to 25% of patients with 'epilepsy' have a diagnosis of psychogenic non-epileptic seizures (Szaflarski et al. 2000).
- Seizures can occur in the setting of syncope (hypoxia), sleep disordered breathing, etc.
- History is the most vital part of clinical assessment with witness accounts helping make the diagnosis.

- Tongue biting has a high specificity for epilepsy compared to urinary incontinence.
- First seizure assessment needs to bear in mind the various precipitants including medical disorders as treating the underlying aetiology can 'cure' the seizure.
- Do not forget to explain the advice from Driver and Vehicle Licensing Agency to individuals who drive.

Investigations

- There is not much role for measuring serum prolactin in routine evaluation of seizures but can be used to differentiate it from pseudo seizures depending upon the type of seizure (raised in up to half of patients with generalised tonic clonic seizures (GTCS) and focal seizures with impaired awareness).
- Video EEG monitoring has a role to play in the diagnosis of epilepsy.
- Neuroimaging has a role in provoked seizure assessment to ascertain structural brain lesions like stroke.
- LP, inter-ictal EEG and ECG are indicated in relevant contexts.

Treatment

- Treat the cause in provoked seizures ± anti-epileptic therapy.
- Anti-epileptic therapy is initiated based on several factors including the risk of recurrent seizures, permanence of underlying neurological conditions, e.g. scar from old stroke, side effect profile, patient preferences, and co-morbidities.
- Anti-epileptics can be deferred after a single unprovoked seizure depending on individual risk profile, benefits, and patient preferences.
- Broad spectrum anti-epileptics like lamotrigine, valproate, clobazam, topiramate, and levetiracetam can be used in both generalised or focal seizures.
- Narrow spectrum anti-epileptics like carbamazepine, phenytoin, and gabapentin are used in focal seizures including those evolving into generalised seizures.

64.6 HEADACHE

Diagnosis

P – Pulsating
O – Duration of 4–72 hours
U – Unilateral
N – Nausea
Ding – Disabling

- The POUNDing mnemonic helps in classifying headaches into migraine (higher prevalence in general population) or non-migraine headaches.
- Score of 4 (LR 24), 3 (LR 3.5), ≤2 (LR 0.41).
- Clinical findings which increase the likelihood of finding an abnormality on imaging with LRs in brackets: cluster-type headache (11), abnormal findings on neurological examination (5.3), undefined headache (non-migraine, cluster, or tension type) (3.8), headache with aura (3.2), aggravated by exertion, or valsalva (2.3), headache with vomiting (1.8).
- Normal neurological examination (0.71), not aggravated by valsalva (0.7), not associated with vomiting (0.46) and defined type headache (cluster, migraine, or tension) (0.66) reduced the likelihood of an abnormal brain scan (Detsky et al. 2006).
- Prevalence of significant intra-cranial pathology in chronic headache – 1% and in thunder-clap headache – 43%.
- Use clinical judgement in all other scenarios.

References

Amarenco, P., Labreuche, J., and Lavallée, P.C. (2012). Patients with transient ischemic attack with ABCD2 <4 can have similar 90-day stroke risk as patients with transient ischemic attack with ABCD2 ≥4. *Stroke* 43 (3): 863–865.

Aronin, S.I., Peduzzi, P., and Quagliarello, V.J. (1998). Community-acquired bacterial meningitis: risk stratification for adverse clinical outcome and effect of antibiotic timing. *Annals of Internal Medicine* 129 (11): 862–869.

Attia, J., Hatala, R., Cook, D.J., and Wong, J.G. (1999). The rational clinical examination. Does this adult patient have acute meningitis? *Journal of the American Medical Association* 282 (2): 175–181.

Detsky, M.E., McDonald, D.R., Baerlocher, M.O. et al. (2006). Does this patient with headache have a migraine or need neuroimaging? *Journal of the American Medical Association* 296 (10): 1274.

Fisher, R.S., Acevedo, C., Arzimanoglou, A. et al. (2014). ILAE official report: a practical clinical definition of epilepsy. *Epilepsia* 55 (4): 475–482.

Fisher, R.S., Cross, J.H., D'Souza, C. et al. (2017). Instruction manual for the ILAE 2017 operational classification of seizure types. *Epilepsia* 58 (4): 531–542.

Goldstein, L.B. and Simel, D.L. (2005). Is this patient having a stroke? *JAMA* 293 (19): 2391–2402.

Hasbun, R., Abrahams, J., Jekel, J. et al. (2001). Computed tomography of the head before lumbar puncture in adults with suspected meningitis. *New England Journal of Medicine* 345 (24): 1727–1733.

Stead, L.G., Suravaram, S., Bellolio, M.F. et al. (2011). An assessment of the incremental value of the ABCD2 score in the emergency department evaluation of transient ischemic attack. *Annals of Emergency Medicine* 57 (1): 46–51.

Szaflarski, J.P., Ficker, D.M., Cahill, W.T. et al. (2000). Four-year incidence of psychogenic nonepileptic seizures in adults in Hamilton county, OH. *Neurology* 55 (10): 1561–1563.

Tyler, K.L. (2004). Herpes simplex virus infections of the central nervous system: encephalitis and meningitis, including Mollaret's. *Herpes: The Journal of the IHMF* 11 (Suppl 2): 57A–64A.

65 Gastroenterology

▼

This section gives you an overview of common clinical conditions in Gastroenterology

▲

65.1 CIRRHOSIS

Diagnosis

- Early diagnosis of cirrhosis can facilitate intervention which can improve the prognosis.
- Clinical features with the highest likelihood ratios (LRs) predicting cirrhosis are: ascites (7.2), platelets count <160 (6.3), spider angiomata (6.3), and the Bonacini cirrhosis discriminant score > 7 (9.4).
- Platelet count >160 (0.29) and absence of hepatomegaly (0.37) reduces the likelihood of cirrhosis (Udell et al. 2012).
- The Bonacini score consists of platelet count, ALT/AST ratio, and INR (Bonacini et al. 1997).
- The highest LRs for ascites are: increased abdominal girth (4.1), weight gain (3.2), ankle swelling (2.8), fluid wave (5.3), and shifting dullness (2.1).
- The absence of ankle oedema makes ascites very unlikely (LR- 0.1) (Chongtham et al. 1998; Williams and Simel 1992).
- Alcohol is by far the most common cause of cirrhosis in the developed world.
- Screening questionnaires vary with what we are trying to detect and our patient population.
- Prevalence of alcohol excess in primary care is up to 18%.
- CAGE is useful to detect alcohol abuse and dependence (Aertgeerts et al. 2004).
- TWEAK and T-ACE are useful to screen women (Bradley et al. 1998).
- AUDIT-C is useful to detect problem drinking which is not the same as abuse or dependence (Fiellin et al. 2000).
- Remember screening tests do not make the diagnosis. A positive screening test should be followed by in-depth history to diagnose the problem.

Investigations

- Tests to ascertain the aetiology of cirrhosis should be guided by the initial evaluation of the patient including history, physical examination and baseline investigations.
- Liver biopsy is not essential in all cases but can be useful in scenarios where the aetiology is in doubt and will alter management, e.g. transplantation.
- Imaging studies often include ultrasonography as first line.
- Results as always must be interpreted in the clinical context.
- MRI with its higher sensitivity is especially useful in diagnosing haemochromatosis and complications of cirrhosis.

Treatment

- Directed at the cause.
- Most common cause in the western world being alcohol excess, abstinence greatly improves the prognosis.
- Complications of cirrhosis should be managed as per national guidelines, e.g. British Gastroenterology Society/NICE guidelines.
- Liver transplantation in appropriate contexts.
- MELD-Na score offers a prognostic model which is also being used to prioritize patients awaiting liver transplantation (Kim et al. 2008).

The Hands-on Guide to Clinical Reasoning in Medicine, First Edition. Mujammil Irfan.
© 2019 John Wiley & Sons Ltd. Published 2019 by John Wiley & Sons Ltd.
Companion website: www.wiley.com/go/irfan/clinicalreasoning

65.2 UPPER GI BLEED

Diagnosis

- Clinical features that increase the likelihood of an upper GI bleed include: history of black stool or melena (5.1–5.9), melenic stool on PR examination (25), ratio of urea to creatinine >30 (7.5), and blood on nasogastric lavage (9.6).
- Blood clots in stool reduce the likelihood of UGIB (0.05).
- Features that increase the likelihood of severe UGIB requiring urgent intervention include: blood on nasogastric lavage (3.1), tachycardia >100 bpm (4.9), and Hb < 80 g l⁻¹ (4.5–6.2).
- Blatchford score of 0 reliably identifies patients who do need urgent intervention (Srygley et al. 2012).

Investigations and treatment

- See clinical example 51.1 and follow national guidelines.

General points to consider in the management of UGIB in patients with liver disease:

- Treat concomitant uremia, sepsis, and vitamin K deficiency.
- Plasma volume expansion can worsen portal pressures and potentiate variceal bleeding. Hence blood products like cryoprecipitate are preferred to fresh frozen plasma (FFP).
- Short of global tests of haemostasis like thromboelastography it is worth looking at platelet count and fibrinogen levels and correcting them as necessary.
- Consider desmopressin (vasopressin) or platelet transfusions for low platelets prior to procedures as per guidelines.
- Clinical evidence of Accelerated Intravascular Coagulation and Fibrinolysis (AICF) – oozing from skin puncture sites, low fibrinogen levels, high D-dimer levels point to hyperfibrinolysis which can be treated with antifibrinolytics. The liver produces all clotting factors except factor VIII (endothelium), and XIII A-subunit (bone marrow). Therefore normal factor VIII levels in AICF can be used to distinguish it from disseminated intravascular coagulation (DIC).

65.3 INFLAMMATORY BOWEL DISEASE (IBD)

Diagnosis

- Think of this diagnosis in patients who present with diarrhea and blood per rectum.
- Patients may also have systemic symptoms of fever, fatigue, weight loss which can bring in several differentials especially infective diarrhea.
- Extra-intestinal manifestations (joint, skin, eye, DVT, arterial thrombosis, pulmonary complications) can give a clue with regards to the possibility of IBD.
- Features that increase the likelihood of a severe exacerbation of colitis include: loose bloody stools >6 per day temperature ≥ 37.5 °C, pulse ≥9- bpm, Hb < 105 g l⁻¹, erythrocyte sedimentation rate (ESR) > 30 mm per hour.
- Other markers of severity are low albumin and high platelet count.
- Complications include toxic megacolon (colon diameter > 6 cm or caecal diameter > 9 cm + systemic toxicity).
- Features suggestive of Crohn's disease – perianal disease, absence of rectal inflammation, presence of ileitis, focal inflammation with granulomas on endoscopy.

Investigations

- Stool for MC&S and Clostridium difficile, colonoscopy when indicated (not in severe colitis).
- AXR to exclude colonic dilatation in patients with severe colitis.

Treatment

- Multidisciplinary management including colorectal surgeon and dietician for patients with severe exacerbation of colitis.
- IV corticosteroids, IV fluids, stool chart.
- Failure to respond – Gastroenterology referral if not already done.
- Surgery when fails to respond to maximal medical therapy or develops life-threatening complication like bowel perforation.
- Follow British Gastroenterology and NICE guidelines (Mowat et al. 2011).

65.4 PEPTIC ULCER DISEASE (PUD)

Diagnosis
- Suspected in patients with dyspepsia ± drugs like NSAID use.
- Largely asymptomatic but if symptomatic, features include epigastric pain, food-provoked, or empty stomach epigastric discomfort, nausea.
- Always think of other anatomical structures in close proximity of epigastric pain, e.g. inferior wall MI.
- Complications: bleeding, perforation, fistula, gastric outlet obstruction.

Investigations
- Barium studies, contrasted CT scans, can be done but upper GI endoscopy has the highest sensitivity + provides tissue for histology.
- *Helicobacter pylori* tests should be done in all patients found to have peptic ulcers.
- In presence of active UGIB, *H. pylori* breath tests can be done but not stool antigen tests.
- In endoscopically diagnosed peptic ulcers, biopsy urease test can be done concurrently.
- *H. pylori* eradication should be confirmed four weeks after treatment.

Treatment
- *H. pylori* eradication therapy + PPI.
- Maintenance PPI therapy in recurrent PUD.

References

Aertgeerts, B., Buntinx, F., and Kester, A. (2004). The value of the CAGE in screening for alcohol abuse and alcohol dependence in general clinical populations: a diagnostic meta-analysis. *Journal of Clinical Epidemiology* 57 (1): 30–39.

Bonacini, M., Hadi, G., Govindarajan, S., and Lindsay, K.L. (1997). Utility of a discriminant score for diagnosing advanced fibrosis or cirrhosis in patients with chronic hepatitis C virus infection. *The American Journal of Gastroenterology* 92 (8): 1302–1304.

Bradley, K.A., Boyd-Wickizer, J., Powell, S.H., and Burman, M.L. (1998). Alcohol screening questionnaires in women: a critical review. *Journal of the American Medical Association* 280 (2): 166–171.

Chongtham, D.S., Singh, M.M., Kalantri, S.P. et al. (1998). Accuracy of clinical manoeuvres in detection of minimal ascites. *Indian Journal of Medical Sciences* 52 (11): 514–520.

Fiellin, D.A., Reid, M.C., and O'Connor, P.G. (2000). Screening for alcohol problems in primary care: a systematic review. *Archives of Internal Medicine* 160 (13): 1977–1989.

Kim, W.R., Biggins, S.W., Kremers, W.,.K. et al. (2008). Hyponatremia and Mortality among Patients on the Liver-Transplant Waiting List. *New England Journal of Medicine* 359 (10): 1018–1026.

Mowat, C., Cole, A., Windsor, A. et al. (2011). Guidelines for the management of inflammatory bowel disease in adults. *Gut* 60 (5): 571–607.

Srygley, F.D., Gerardo, C.J., Tran, T., and Fisher, D.A. (2012). Does this patient have a severe upper gastrointestinal bleed? *JAMA* 307 (10): 1072–1079.

Udell, J.A., Wang, C.S., Tinmouth, J. et al. (2012). Does This Patient With Liver Disease Have Cirrhosis? *Journal of the American Medical Association* 307 (8): 832–842.

Williams, J.W. and Simel, D.L. (1992). The rational clinical examination. Does this patient have ascites? How to divine fluid in the abdomen. *Journal of the American Medical Association* 267 (19): 2645–2648.

66 Geriatric Medicine

▼

This section gives you an overview of common clinical conditions in Geriatric Medicine

▲

66.1 DEMENTIA

Diagnosis
- Reference standard in most studies is DSM-IV.
- Prevalence in people aged >65 is 6–16% with a rising prevalence with increasing age.
- Several screening tools exist, and the tool selected in your clinical practice should bear in mind the population being screened (e.g. education level, primary language), the purpose of screening, the cognitive domains being tested, and ease of use.
- Highly sensitive tests are useful to detect early cognitive impairment whilst highly specific tests are useful to confirm the diagnosis of dementia.
- Remember that co-existent depression can invalidate dementia screening tools since they will be falsely positive.
- Median positive LR for mini mental state examination (MMSE) is 9.5 and it varies with the cut-off point used.
- Informant reported memory problems has a LR of 6.5 (Holsinger et al. 2007).
- The mini-cog is not limited by the subject's education or language and has a LR of 6.5 and MoCA (Montreal Cognitive Assessment) has a comparable diagnostic performance with MMSE for detecting mild cognitive impairment (LR 4.7) (Tsoi et al. 2015).
- Positive screening tests should be confirmed with more detailed tests to diagnose dementia.
- Above all, the history should be congruent with the results of neurocognitive tests.

Investigations
- Vitamin B12, TFTs.
- CT head when diagnosis is in doubt, rapid decline in cognition, focal signs and pragmatically when findings would reassure patients, and their relatives, however the last may be contentious.

Treatment
- Alzheimer's – cholinesterase inhibitors for mild to moderate dementia, symptomatic treatment of behavioural disturbances.
- Vascular dementia – risk factor modification and treatment.
- Avoid alcohol excess.
- Multi-disciplinary management – nutritional support, physiotherapy, occupational therapy.
- Managing polypharmacy, falls risk, psychosocial support, and end-of life care.

66.2 PARKINSON'S DISEASE

Diagnosis
- Prevalence 1–2%.
- Unfortunately, no technological reference standard exists so studies have used autopsy or serial neurological assessment.
- Symptoms with significant positive LRs: difficulty in rising from chair (1.9–5.2), difficulty in turning in bed (13), difficulty opening jar (6.1).
- Signs: rigidity with bradykinesia (4.5), rigidity (2.8), glabella tap (4.5).
- Absence of rigidity and bradykinesia has a negative LR of 0.12 (Rao et al. 2003).

The Hands-on Guide to Clinical Reasoning in Medicine, First Edition. Mujammil Irfan.
© 2019 John Wiley & Sons Ltd. Published 2019 by John Wiley & Sons Ltd.
Companion website: www.wiley.com/go/irfan/clinicalreasoning

Investigations
- No imaging studies are diagnostic of Parkinson's.
- DaTscan has a role in differentiating idiopathic or Parkinson's plus syndromes from drug induced Parkinson's or essential tremor, however its sensitivity/specificity are reportedly similar to a clinical diagnosis by an experienced clinician.

Treatment
- Levodopa is the mainstay of therapy.
- Treatment is individualised.
- Lowest possible dose with least side effects and most efficacy should be selected.
- Options include levodopa + peripheral dopa decarboxylase inhibitor, dopamine agonists (pramipexole, rotigotine, apomorphine), monoamine oxidase B inhibitors, and catechol-o-methyl transferase inhibitors.

66.3 DELIRIUM: SEE CHAPTERS 40 AND 44

66.3.1 Osteoporosis

Diagnosis
- Prior probability depends on age and ethnicity.
- Fracture risk assessment tool (FRAX) predicts 10 years probability of fracture for an untreated patient (Sheffield.ac.uk 2017).
- Risk categories generated are used for diagnosis rather than intervention.
- Therapy should be individualised using the FRAX risk score, individual risk factors, patient preferences, and cost effectiveness.
- Dose dependent risk of osteoporosis in patients on prednisolone.
- Relative risk of hip fracture at prednisolone dose <2.5 mg (0.99), 2.5–7.5 mg (1.77), and >7.5 mg (2.27).
- Risk returns to baseline rapidly upon cessation of prednisolone (Van Staa et al. 2000).

66.4 DEPRESSION

Diagnosis
- Lifetime prevalence varies from 3% in Japan to 16.9% in U.S. (Andrade et al. 2003).
- Prevalence in older adults – 2% in primary care and 30% in hospital (Beekman et al. 1999; Koenig et al. 1997).
- Screening tools are equally effective in picking up depression and the ideal tool varies with the population being screened, time available, and intention of screening.
- The median positive LR for all tools is 3.3 and median negative LR is 0.12 (Williams et al. 2002).
- The PHQ-9 is brief, has modules for other psychiatric illnesses and is useful to assess treatment response with a positive LR of 7.3 (Kroenke et al. 2001).
- Like elsewhere, screening tests do not make the diagnosis but will have to be followed up by detailed assessment ± treatment if positive.

References

Andrade, L., Caraveo-Anduaga, J.J., Berglund, P. et al. (2003). The epidemiology of major depressive episodes: results from the International Consortium of Psychiatric Epidemiology (ICPE) Surveys. *International Journal of Methods in Psychiatric Research* 12 (1): 3–21.

Beekman, A.T., Copeland, J.R., and Prince, M.J. (1999). Review of community prevalence of depression in later life. *The British Journal of Psychiatry: The Journal of Mental Science* 174: 307–311.

Holsinger, T., Deveau, J., Boustani, M. et al. (2007). Does this patient have dementia? *Journal of the American Medical Association* 297 (21): 2391.

Koenig, H.G., George, L.K., Peterson, B.L. et al. (1997). Depression in medically ill hospitalized older adults: prevalence, characteristics, and course of symptoms according to six diagnostic schemes. *The American Journal of Psychiatry* 154 (10): 1376–1383.

Kroenke, K., Spitzer, R.L., Williams, J.B. et al. (2001). The PHQ-9: validity of a brief depression severity measure. *Journal of General Internal Medicine* 16 (9): 606–613.

Rao, G., Fisch, L., Srinivasan, S. et al. (2003). Does this patient have Parkinson disease? *Journal of the American Medical Association* 289 (3): 347–353.

Sheffield.ac.uk. 2017. WHO Fracture Risk Assessment Tool (FRAX). [online] Available at: www.sheffield.ac.uk/FRAX [Accessed 26 Nov. 2017].

Van Staa, T.P., Leufkens, H.G., Abenhaim, L. et al. (2000). Use of oral corticosteroids and risk of fractures. *Journal of Bone and Mineral Research: The Official Journal of the American Society for Bone and Mineral Research* 15 (6): 993–1000.

Tsoi, K.K., Chan, J.Y., Hirai, H.W. et al. (2015). Cognitive tests to detect dementia. *Journal of the American Medical Association: Internal Medicine* 175 (9): 1450.

Williams, J.W., Noël, P.H., Cordes, J.A. et al. (2002). Is this patient clinically depressed? *Journal of the American Medical Association* 287 (9): 1160–1170.

▼

This section gives you an overview of common clinical conditions in Endocrinology

▲

Most common clinical conditions in endocrinology have been discussed in detail in Chapters 26–28. Hence, I shall limit myself to a couple of conditions that I thought will be useful from a practical point of view.

67.1 DIABETES MELLITUS (DM)

67.1.1 Newly Diagnosed Diabetes Mellitus

Prevalence in the western world~8%.

Diagnosis
- Traditional phenotypes: Type 1 DM – younger, low body mass index (BMI), osmotic symptoms, diabetic ketoacidosis (DKA); Type 2 DM – older, higher BMI, insulin resistance, hyperosmolar hyperglycaemic non-ketotic state (HHS).
- Facts: Increasing world-wide prevalence of obesity means Type 1 diabetics can be obese, DKA can also occur in Type 2; Type 1 can also occur in older age.
- Solution: ≥2 of – acute symptoms, age <50 years, BMI <25 kg m^{-2} and personal or family history of autoimmune disease have a likelihood ratio (LR) of 3.1 to predict positive autoantibodies in keeping with Type 1 DM – by extension these factors should make you think of insulin therapy at presentation (Fourlanos et al. 2006).

Investigations
- See Chapter 28.

Treatment
- Type 1 DM individuals have absolute insulin deficiency.
- Therefore, start insulin at 0.2–0.4 units kg^{-1}; 40–50% of this dose should be given as long-acting insulin and the remainder split pre-meals as regular or rapid acting insulin.
- Type 2 DM – relative insulin deficiency ± insulin resistance.
- Lifestyle modification, risk factor reduction.
- Decision to start pharmaceutical therapy and target HbA$_1$C is individualised within reason.
- Follow NICE guidance with regards to choice of drugs.
- Regardless of the classification type of DM, individuals who have weight loss and exhibit increased ketogenesis, i.e. present with DKA should be treated with insulin initially and continued in type 1 DM.

67.2 DIABETIC EMERGENCIES

Diagnosis
- DKA as the name suggests is characterised by ketoacidosis i.e. not ketonuria but ketonemia (≥3 mmol l^{-1}) + elevated anion gap (>10) metabolic acidosis (pH < 7. 3).
- HHS is non-ketoacidotic but characterised by hyperglycaemia (> 33.3 mmol l^{-1}) and hypersomolality.
- DKA can be hyperglycaemic (>11 mmol l^{-1} – standard treatment) or euglycemic (treated with additional intravenous dextrose).
- Look for precipitants, e.g. infection, cocaine abuse, MI, pancreatitis, missed insulin, etc.

The Hands-on Guide to Clinical Reasoning in Medicine, First Edition. Mujammil Irfan.
© 2019 John Wiley & Sons Ltd. Published 2019 by John Wiley & Sons Ltd.
Companion website: www.wiley.com/go/irfan/clinicalreasoning

Investigations
- Venous blood gas, electrolytes, serum ketones (beta-hydroxybutyrate).
- CXR, urine dipstick, ECG.
- DKA is accompanied by a non-specific rise in serum amylase and lipase.
- Therefore, co-existent pancreatitis will have to be diagnosed by clinical examination and imaging.

Treatment
- Follow National and local guidelines.
- Mainstay of therapy is intravenous fluids (isotonic saline), potassium replacement and weight based fixed rate intravenous insulin, in that order.
- Treat precipitating factors.
- If known diabetic on insulin – subcutaneous long acting insulin should be continued.
- Multi-disciplinary management with diabetes team, specialist nurse, dietician, community nurse support, GP, etc.

67.3 DIABETIC LARGE FIBRE NEUROPATHY

- Prevalence~23–79%.

Diagnosis
- Pattern: distal symmetric sensory or mixed polyneuropathy.
- Loss of joint position, vibration and ankle reflexes are the earliest manifestation.
- Absence of vibration sensation with a 128 Hz tuning fork has a LR of 16–35 and pressure sensation with a 5.07 Semmes Weinstein monofilament has a LR of 11–16 (Kanji et al. 2010).
- Normal sensation effectively excludes large fibre peripheral neuropathy, but on-going symptoms can point to small fibre neuropathy.
- Loss of pain sensation, vascular insufficiency, and autonomic dysfunction contribute to diabetic foot ulcers.
- Neuropathic pain is distinguished from peripheral vascular disease by its location (feet more than calves), worsening with rest and improving on mobilising and character of the pain (burning).

Investigations
- Atypical presentation warrants electro-diagnostic studies.

Treatment
- Ensure good glycaemic control, regular foot surveillance, and patient education.
- Drugs like antidepressants (amitryptiline, duloxetine), anticonvulsants (gabapentin), or topical therapies (capsaicin) can be used for painful diabetic neuropathy.
- Note that most painful neuropathy resolves spontaneously over time.

67.4 HYPOTHYROIDISM

Diagnosis
- Community prevalence 0.1–2%.
- Clinical features with significant positive LRs in brackets: coarse skin (3.2), dry skin (2.1), periorbital puffiness obscuring curve of malar bone (15), hypothyroid speech (2.8), delayed relaxation time of ankle reflex (12.8), bradycardia <60 bpm (3.88) (Zulewski et al. 1997; Indra et al. 2004).

67.5 HYPERTHYROIDISM

Diagnosis
- Prevalence 1.3% which rises to 4–5% in older women.
- Clinical features with significant positive LRs in brackets: tachycardia >100 bpm (2.5), apathy (10.3), weight loss (5) (Trivalle et al. 1996).

References
Fourlanos, S., Perry, C., Stein, M.S. et al. (2006). A clinical screening tool identifies autoimmune diabetes in adults. *Diabetes Care* 29 (5): 970–975.
Indra, R., Patil, S.S., Joshi, R. et al. (2004). Accuracy of physical examination in the diagnosis of hypothyroidism: a cross-sectional, double-blind study. *Journal of Postgraduate Medicine* 50 (1): 7–10.
Kanji, J.N., Anglin, R.E., Hunt, D.L. et al. (2010). Does this patient with diabetes have large-fiber peripheral neuropathy? *Journal of the American Medical Association* 303 (15): 1526.
Trivalle, C., Doucet, J., Chassagne, P. et al. (1996). Differences in the signs and symptoms of hyperthyroidism in older and younger patients. *Journal of the American Geriatrics Society* 44 (1): 50–53.
Zulewski, H., Müller, B., Exer, P. et al. (1997). Estimation of tissue hypothyroidism by a new clinical score: evaluation of patients with various grades of hypothyroidism and controls. *The Journal of Clinical Endocrinology & Metabolism* 82 (3): 771–776.

68 Rheumatology

▼

This section gives you an overview of common clinical conditions in Rheumatology

▲

Most common clinical conditions in rheumatology have been discussed in detail in Chapters 53–55.

68.1 TEMPORAL ARTERITIS/GIANT CELL ARTERITIS (GCA)

Diagnosis
- Prevalence ~0.2%. Increases with increasing age (>50 years) and varies with ethnicity (higher in Scandinavians).
- Think of it in patients presenting with fever of unknown origin.
- Combination of clinical features are more predictive of GCA than individual findings.
- Positive LRs: Jaw claudication (6.9), diplopia (3.7, scalp tenderness (3.1), jaw claudication + reduced vision (44) (Younge et al. 2004).
- Negative LRs: ESR <50 (0.44) (Mohamed and Bates 2002).
- Younge et al. (2004) have also produced a multivariate model which can be used to calculate the probability in patients aged >50 years.

Investigations
- ESR is more helpful in ruling out the disease than ruling in but remember that ESR can be easily out-weighed by the presence of other clinical findings.
- Temporal artery biopsy – skip lesions are a problem; biopsy can still be done up to 7–10 days after starting glucocorticoid therapy.

Treatment
- Glucocorticoids are the mainstay of therapy ± steroid sparing drugs.

68.2 GOUT

Diagnosis
- Prevalence ~2% in adult men and postmenopausal women.
- Gout score >8 has a probability of 82.5% for diagnosing gout in someone who presents with an acute monoarthritis (Janssens et al. 2010).
- This model was developed to diagnose gout in a primary care population without the need for joint aspiration.
- An intermediate risk category on this score necessitates joint aspiration to exclude the diagnosis.

Investigations
- Joint aspiration for synovial fluid analysis shows urate crystals which can clinch the diagnosis in the majority both in acute attacks and in-between attacks.

Treatment
- Acute attack treated with NSAIDs, glucocorticoids, or colchicine.
- Prophylaxis is with allopurinol (xanthine oxidase inhibitor) or uricosuric drugs + colchicine to prevent acute attacks during the initiation of prophylactic drugs.

References

Janssens, H.J.E.M., Fransen, J., van de Lisdonk, E.H. et al. (2010). A diagnostic rule for acute gouty arthritis in primary care without joint fluid analysis. *Archives of Internal Medicine* 170 (13): 1120–1126.

Mohamed, M.S. and Bates, T. (2002). Predictive clinical and laboratory factors in the diagnosis of temporal arteritis. *Annals of the Royal College of Surgeons of England* 84 (1): 7–9.

Younge, B.R., Cook, B.E. Jr., Bartley, G.B. et al. (2004). Initiation of glucocorticoid therapy: before or after temporal artery biopsy? *Mayo Clinic Proceedings* 79 (4): 483–491.

Index

Page numbers in italics refer to figures and those in bold refer to tables

The Hands-on Guide to Clinical Reasoning in Medicine, First Edition. Mujammil Irfan.
© 2019 John Wiley & Sons Ltd. Published 2019 by John Wiley & Sons Ltd.
Companion website: www.wiley.com/go/irfan/clinicalreasoning